Yoga for Children

Step-By-Step

Yamini Muthanna

Disclaimer

- This book is not intended to be a substitute for the medical advice of physicians. The reader should regularly consult a physician in matters relating to his/her health and particularly with respect to any symptoms that may require diagnosis or medical attention.
- This book is not advising you against any physiotherapy, sport or training or exercises. Like all exercises or forms of physical training, the yoga poses mentioned here may have some inherent risks. Readers are advised to take full responsibility for their safety. Before practising the exercises described in this book, be sure that you are trained by a professional. Do not take risks beyond your scope of experience, aptitude, training and comfort level.
- Although the author and the publisher have made every effort to ensure that the information in this book is accurate, the author and publisher disclaim any liability to any party or any loss, damage or disruption caused by errors or omissions, whether such errors or omissions result from negligence, accident or any other cause.
- The asanas listed in this book are culled from the author's personal experience and from teaching students for over three decades.
- This book is a yoga practice manual. It does not belong to any particular school of yoga.

First Published in 2022 by

Om Books International

Corporate & Editorial Office
A-12, Sector 64, Noida 201 301
Uttar Pradesh, India
Phone: +91 120 477 4100
Email: editorial@ombooks.com
Website: www.ombooksinternational.com

Sales Office
107, Ansari Road, Darya Ganj
New Delhi 110 002, India
Phone: +91 11 4000 9000
Email: sales@ombooks.com

Photographer: Prashanth K. Nagaraja, Mysore

ISBN: 978-93-94547-01-8

Printed in India

10 9 8 7 6 5 4 3 2 1

For all you beautiful kids out there...

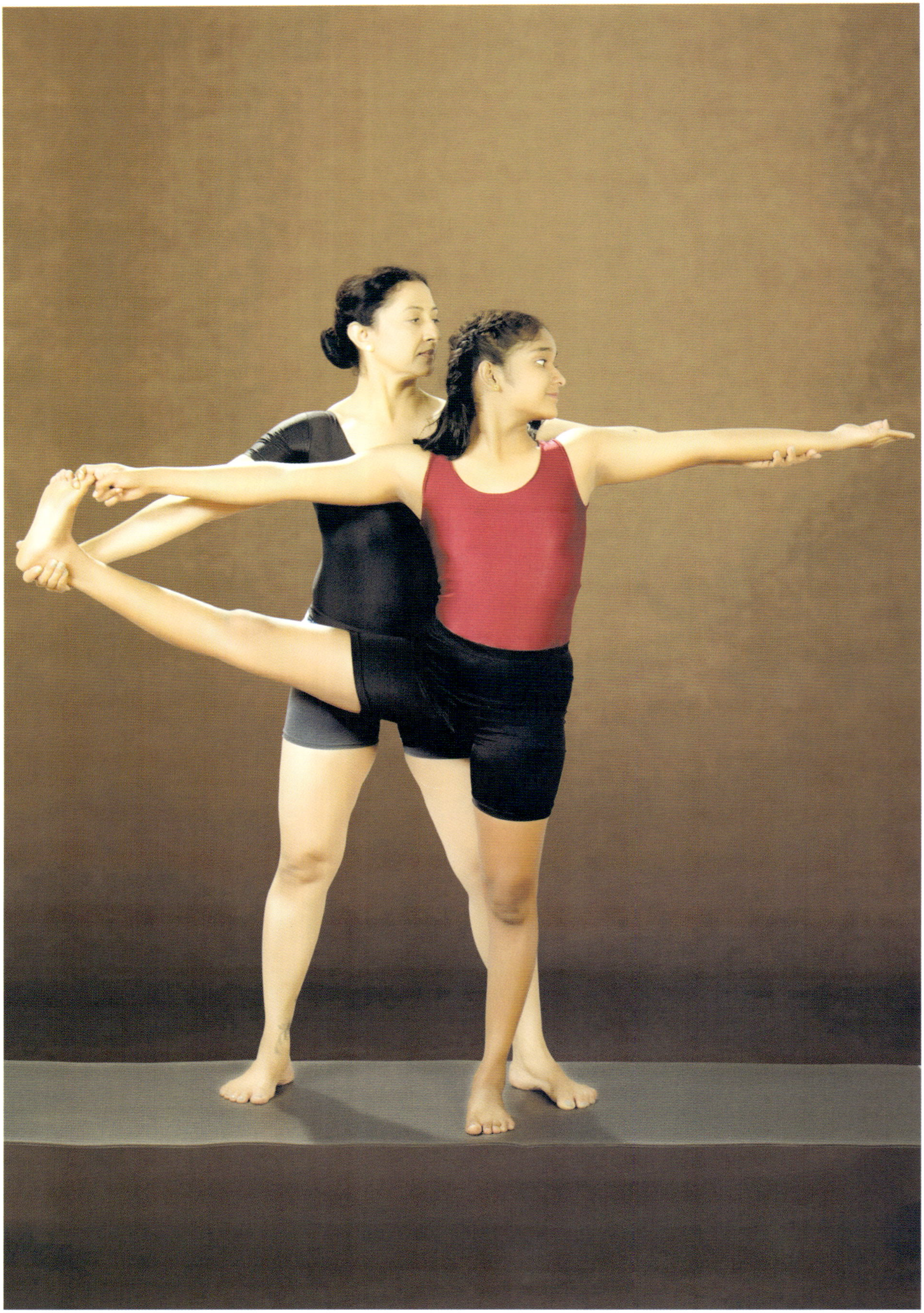

CONTENTS

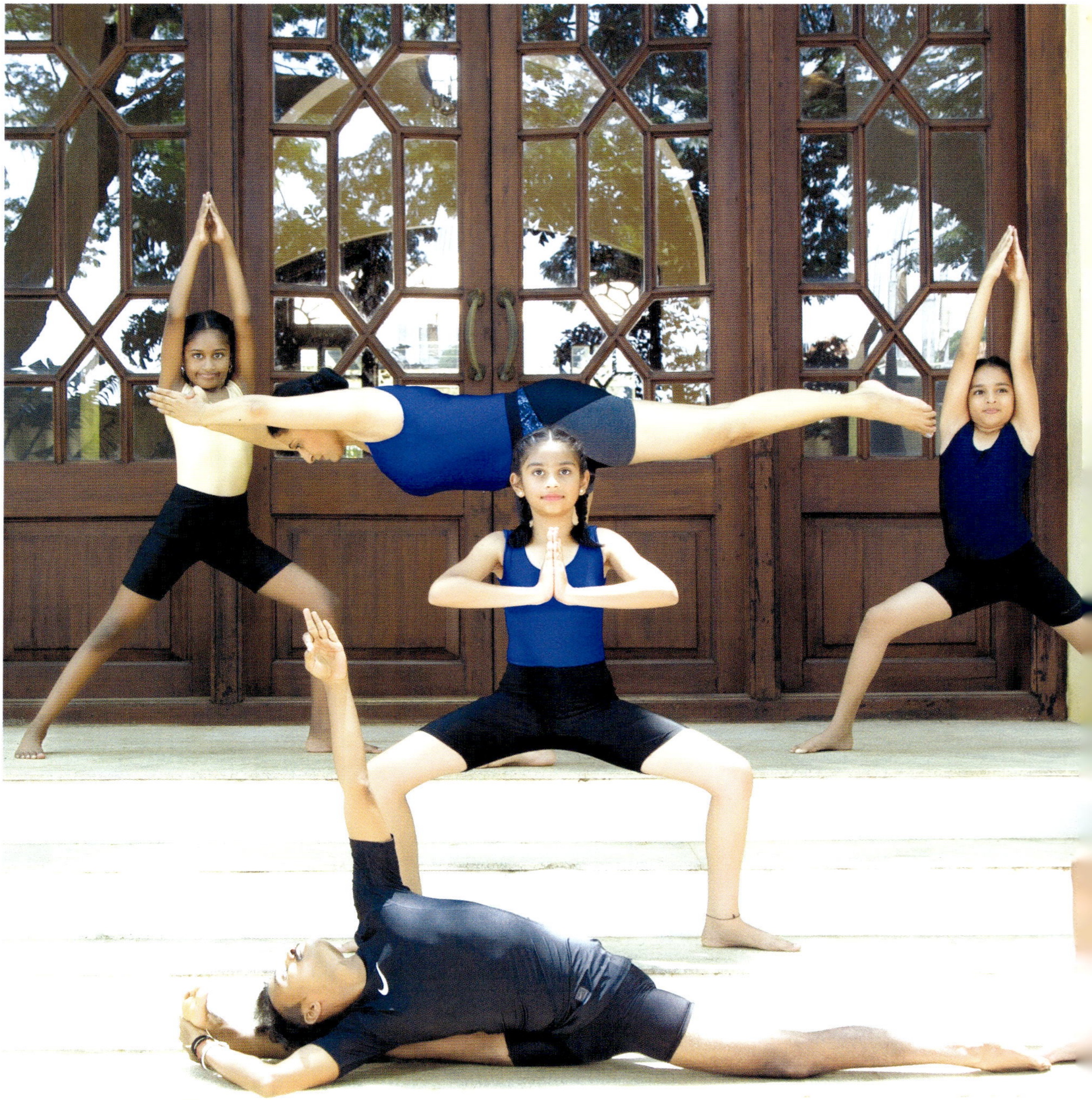

INTRODUCTION

A Note from the Acharya to Parents

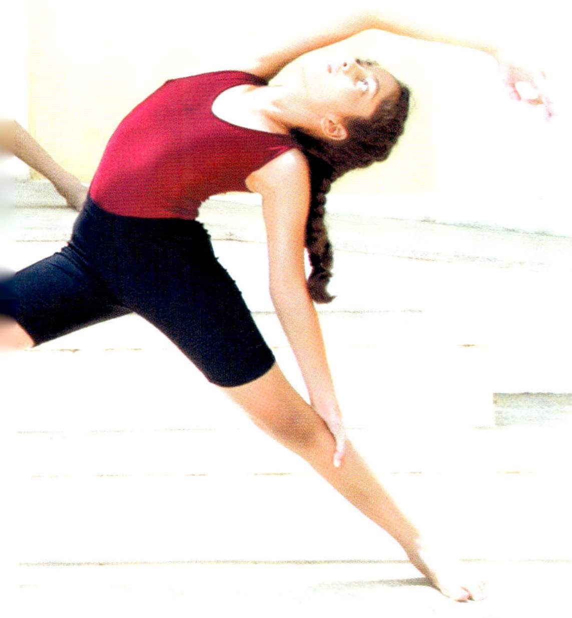

My humble suggestion to all parents is that you participate in this reading and learning experience with your kids. Yoga provides a wealth of knowledge, which increases with age and it will accompany the practitioners in various stages of their growth.

As a teacher of Indian classical dance and traditional Hatha Yoga, I take great pleasure in interacting with kids. I get to observe them away from the pressures of school and the comfort of their home, while they are learning something so new and vivid. Each child has a different response. Some are caught in a dilemma and hover between their own instincts, their parents' interest and the teacher's guidance. Eventually, I get to watch their minds expand. It is amazing to see them self-express through modes of external communication as they interact with art. This is the best part of my job! I get to help them express their emotions and manage them artistically.

Children from all over the world and with different aptitudes come to my *shaala* (school) to learn yoga or classical Indian dance. There are varied reasons for children to join. Some are very keen and curious, some gifted and some are eager to learn. Most of the time, parents want to keep their children occupied as they believe that the performing arts is a good form of physical exercise and helps in achieving excellence. Fair enough.

Integrating yoga into a child's lifestyle is a great idea. Yoga like all art forms is not aptitude oriented. Not all kids are inclined or interested to learn an art form, but yoga can be interesting as they get to explore their body and mind, challenge it and change it if they wish to. It's totally their call. You will agree

The book covers a five-point yoga programme:

1 Social Aspect relates to social behaviour. A few points have been selected from the texts of the *Yoga Sutra.* I have adapted some of these to suit modern times to help children understand them better.

2 Emotional Aspect relates to feelings and a positive attitude.

3 Physical Aspect relates to the physical dimensions of the body and covers the practice of kriyas, asanas and Pranayama.

4 Intellectual Aspect relates to mental abilities. The chapter on asanas, Pranayama and kriyas covers this aspect of development.

with me that all kids need an outlet to cope with the pressures of the modern-day education system and lifestyle. There has been a lot of research showing that children today face a lot of stress. When stressed, the child starts to express this overwhelming feeling physically, which eventually results in a specific behaviour which could become a part of his/her personality. The kind of stress varies from child to child depending on their age and the environment they are in.

We as adults may brush off some things as unimportant, which can cause even more stress in the child. Parents and teachers should recognise this stress and address it immediately. The most important thing is to help them cope with the way they are feeling, and make them understand and address the issue without dismissing it as exaggerated or unnecessary. Choosing to practise yoga is a good way to calm these sensations and bring harmony to the mind and help him/her understand the nature of his/her journey.

This book features yoga poses along with step-by-step guidance and detailed instructions for you to help and guide your child. The sequencing patterns are categorised addressing some of the issues children may have to cope with in their growing years. I have addressed them as per my personal experience and based on my observations while interacting with children. There could be any number of factors influencing a child's stress levels. The best way is to stay alert. If you observe any peculiar behaviour in the child, a counsellor's or doctor's opinion would go a long way in helping you understand it. However, to initiate the child into the practice of yoga using this book, it is important that a parent guides the child as it can be overwhelming for the child to see so much information in the book. Let children choose a routine that appeals to them. And parents can then start a discussion with the child and make him/her understand the reason for their intuitive choice. Often the child's intuition is spot on.

To give an example: imagine your child has an exam coming up in a few days. Your child's nervousness may lead him/her to naturally choose a sequence that helps with this anxious and nervous energy. The parent can point this out to the child, start a discussion and make the child aware of his/her feelings. This exercise can also be used as a tool to determine your child's frame of mind and delve deeper into the root cause of problems the child is not ready to reveal. In fact, the asanas listed here can be performed along with the child to encourage him/her to pursue a practice. Eventually the child will be able to use the book as a guide for his/her daily practice without your help. The chosen asanas are challenging and form a well-balanced set of sequences, and they are to be practised consistently to achieve best results. By encouraging the child to understand this book, it can become a helpful guide to them during his/her growing years.

5 Spiritual Aspect relates to the development of a simple spiritual understanding. Children grow every day, physically, mentally and emotionally. Physical growth is obvious while emotional growth is difficult to notice unless it is monitored closely. The indication of emotions can be recognised by behaviour. Happiness, sadness, disappointment, anticipation, satisfaction, anxiety, love and anger are all general emotions dealt with by each kid in a different way. This is what defines a child's personality.

It is important to initiate the child into the practice with proper care and knowledge because eventually the child might want to practise on his/her own. I have come across children at the beginner level completely rooted and disciplined in their practice. They do not need reminders anymore. They enjoy yoga immensely and the fruits of their discipline can be noticed in all walks of their life. You will meet some of these little practitioners in this book.

The sequences introduced here are traditional, simple and easy to remember. The book also introduces some basic principles which are from the *Yoga Sutra* (see Chapter 1). It is very important for children to remember that yoga is not a physical exercise, but a discipline that will help them enjoy life better as they grow up. There are specific codes of conduct that need to be followed while initiating a practice of yoga asanas so that the child can reap the maximum benefit.

Pictures and illustrations of yoga poses have been incorporated in this book. Each asana has a guidance table and an illustrated demonstration. This will help you instruct the child to construct an asana and follow a sequence. Cautions and benefits are also explained for each asana.

It is ideal for a child to initiate the practice with proper instructions under the guidance of a trained yoga practitioner or Guru for better alignment and construction of the asanas. Technique and corrections of asanas are best done by a teacher or a parent who is already a practitioner of yoga. This book cannot replace a Guru's training.

The sequencing pattern and asanas are suitable for children from the ages of 8–18. They could practise the asanas like a dedicated yoga practice with Surya Namaskar and asana routine as per traditional sequencing order or practise them along with their sports activities or other physical training routines.

The objective of this book is to share the knowledge of yogic practices that can benefit children. It is structured to help inculcate healthy habits, values and a sense of discipline in them.

Each generation of children face a set of tough challenges. The biggest ill-effects of stress-induced conditions on today's children are blood pressure, headaches, breathing problems, etc which is common these days. Stress causes malfunctioning of the organs of the body. At a physiological level, it can lead to hormonal dysfunction, change in heart rate, resulting in psychological problems like lack of concentration, memory loss, lethargy, anger, fear, etc.

Since yoga is a step-by-step holistic routine that trains the mind to manage stress, it is good to introduce children to this discipline as early as possible. Yoga asanas combined with Pranayama is the solution to many avoidable mental and health issues. Regular practise will empower children to cope with the adverse effects of stress very efficiently.

A Note from the Acharya to Children

"It's better to build strong children than to repair grown-ups."–Anonymous

Namaste and a big hello from me to all you kids out there!

I already know that you have a million things to do in the day. Your schedules are packed–school work, homework, extra-curricular activities, tuitions... But you are doing a fantastic job! This book is meant to give you more power and more energy.

If you've picked up this book, that means you want to

> Let me introduce myself first. I am a mother of two grown-up children. I am also a teacher who runs a yoga and Classical Indian dance school. I get to meet and teach over a hundred students every day. Over 30 years, I have seen how yoga has benefitted kids like you and adults like your parents as well! This book is for all of you to learn the art of yoga.

learn something about yoga. So, what is yoga?

Crazy stretches, right?

Wrong. Yoga is not just weird poses or stretches to exercise the body. It is an interesting art with evolved techniques to get the benefit of good health throughout your life. It teaches you how to have a better life.

Before you come to any conclusions, you have to try yoga asanas first. Once you make yoga a part of your daily routine, you will begin to see many changes in your body and mind which will make a big difference in your life ahead.

I want to share this secret with you. At one point of time, I did not think that kids like you needed to practise yoga. I felt that you should go outdoors and play. But times have changed. The roads are congested and there are hardly any playgrounds around. But if there is one near your house, you must go out and play at least for an hour. If you do not have a playground near your house or if your school homework does not permit you to go out, then yoga is a perfect choice for you.

It is the responsibility of elders in the community to make sure that you grow up in the best circumstances. As teachers, it is our job to equip you, a potential warrior, for this battlefield called 'life', with the proper tools. Yoga is valuable knowledge and has the power to remove imbalances and keep your mind and body strong and healthy. This book is a perfect guide to help you slowly and steadily absorb the practice of yoga and master some valuable techniques to enhance your future.

When you embark on your practice, many questions will arise in your mind. How does this asana help me stay healthy? Which part of the body does it affect? How should I frame my body before, during and after the asana? How does yoga improve concentration?

This book might answer most of those questions. It's not enough to do the asanas alone; you need to understand the underlying philosophy eventually. You can read Patanjali's *Yoga Sutra* when you are older. For now, I have simplified some of the important aspects for you so that you can benefit from the distilled version of the teachings. The pictures

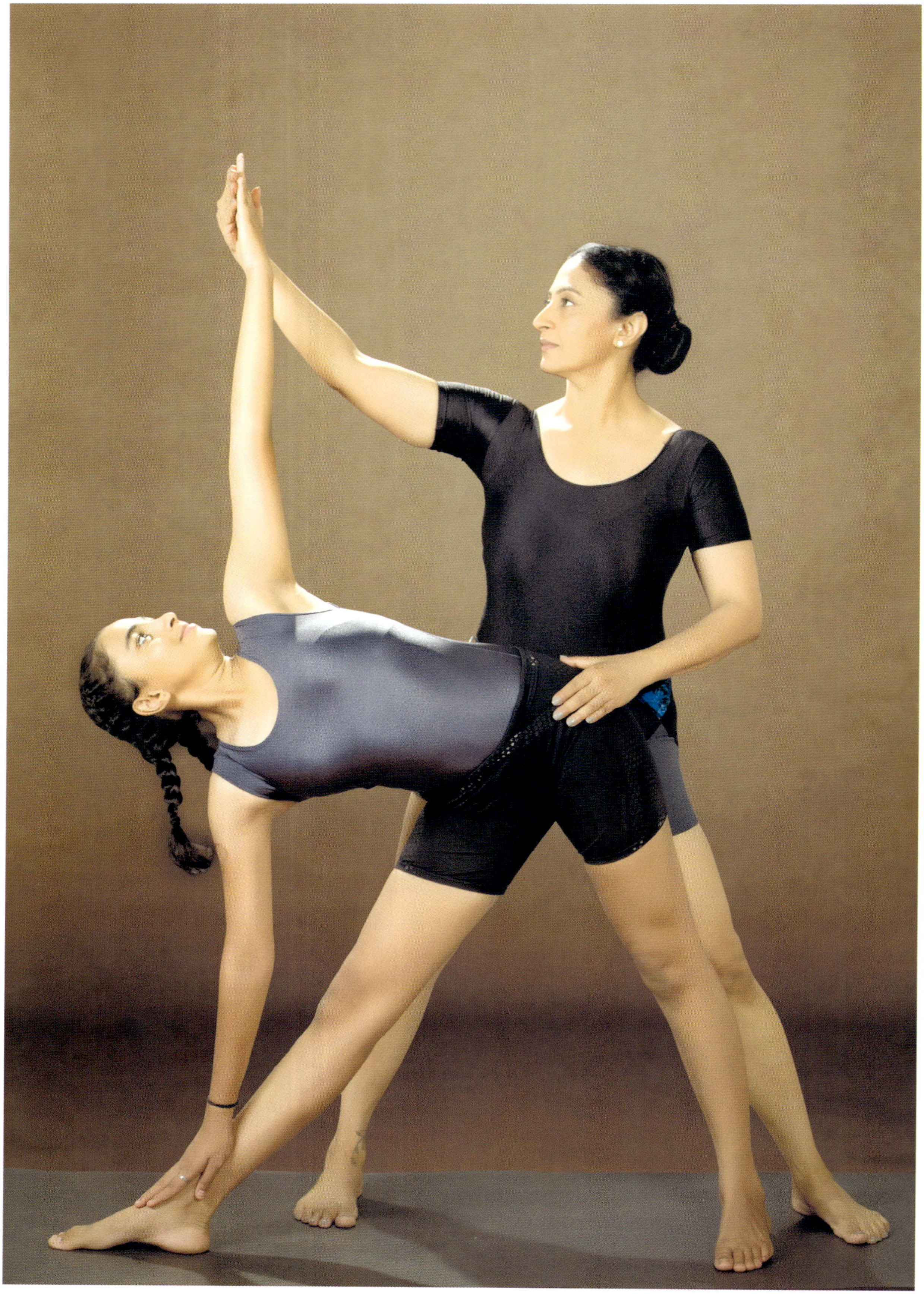

in the book feature young yogis and yoginis who will inspire you to keep working on your practice and emulate the Warrior Kids.

If you have doubts, you can ask your parents or any adult in your family to help you to read this book. But please make a note of the instructions. You can ask them to join in when you practise yoga asanas. In fact, you can teach them too! That will be fun! All of you can become stronger, healthier and happier together.

This book also explains in simple terms the philosophy of yoga as explained in the original text called the *Yoga Sutra*, which was written 3,000 years ago. Yoga though ancient is timeless in terms of knowledge and values.

I really enjoyed working on this book. I am sure that you, my dear children, are on your way to becoming true warriors like the wonderful Warrior Kids featured in these pages.

—**Acharya Yamini Muthanna**

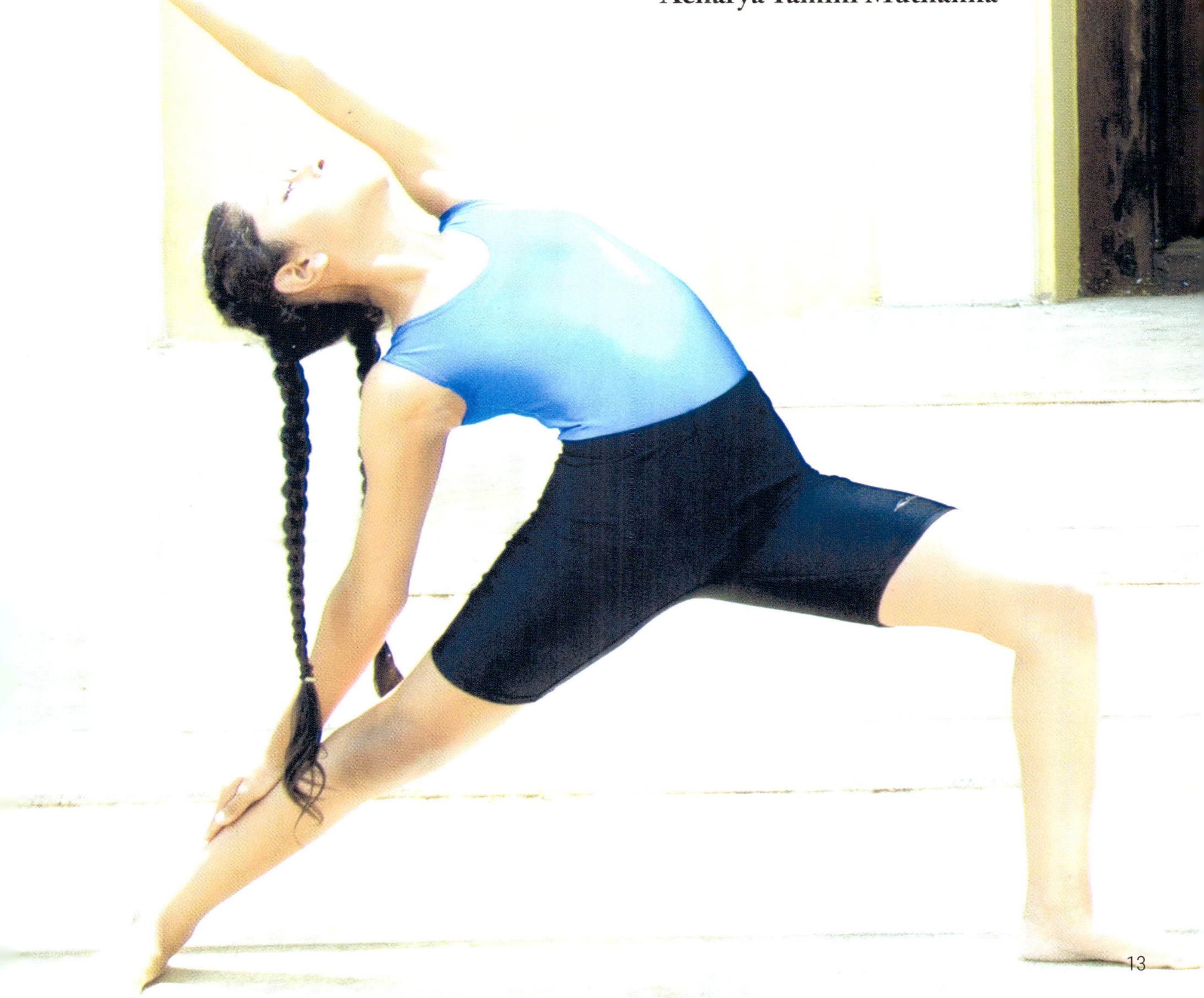

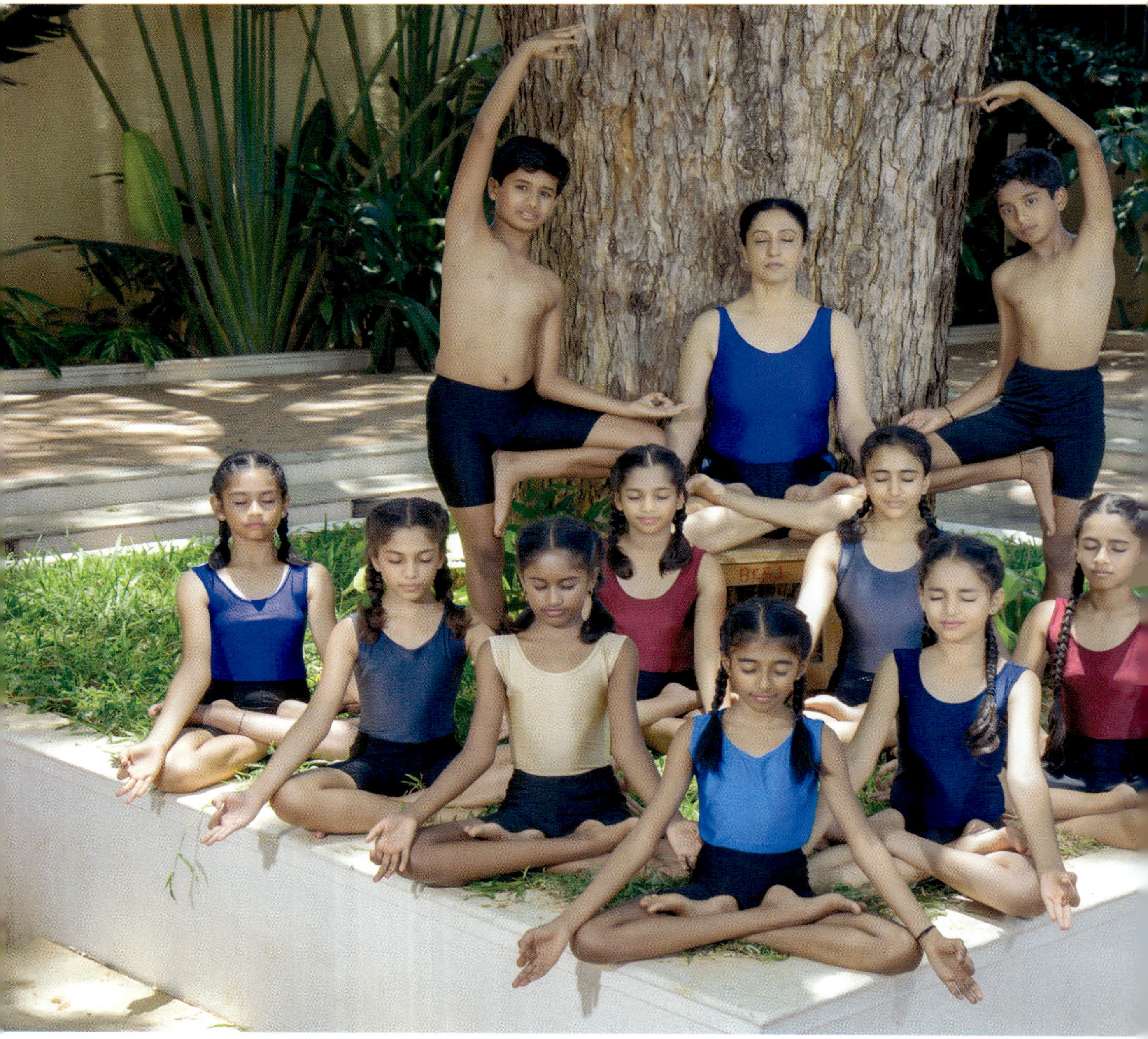

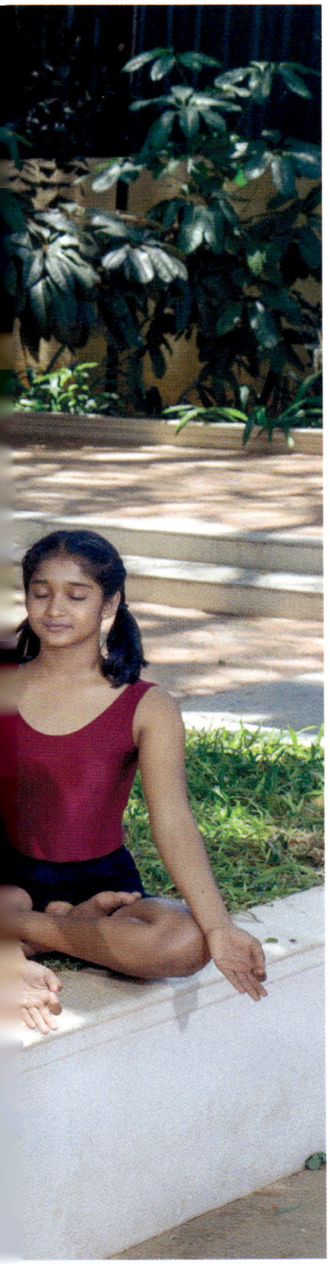

Meet the YOGA WARRIORS

The kids featured here are real-life Yoga Champions. They practise in the beautiful city of Mysore in Karnataka, India. Mysore is said to be the yoga Capital of the world as people from all over come here to practise yoga. I have heard that people from Hollywood also come here to learn the art of yoga from various Gurus. The children who are presented in this book practise yoga under their master, Rudresh Yogi. You will meet him too. They practise every day and their parents are pleased with their progress.

HAMSINI. S

Ten-year-old Hamsini. S has been practising yoga for a year. Her parents, Reethu and Shivkumar HB are thrilled with her progress and are encouraging her to continue her practice. They initiated Hamsini to practise yoga to strengthen her memory and improve her general wellbeing. Now, Hamsini is a champion of yoga and doing very well in her studies as well as sports. Her teachers and parents are very proud of her.

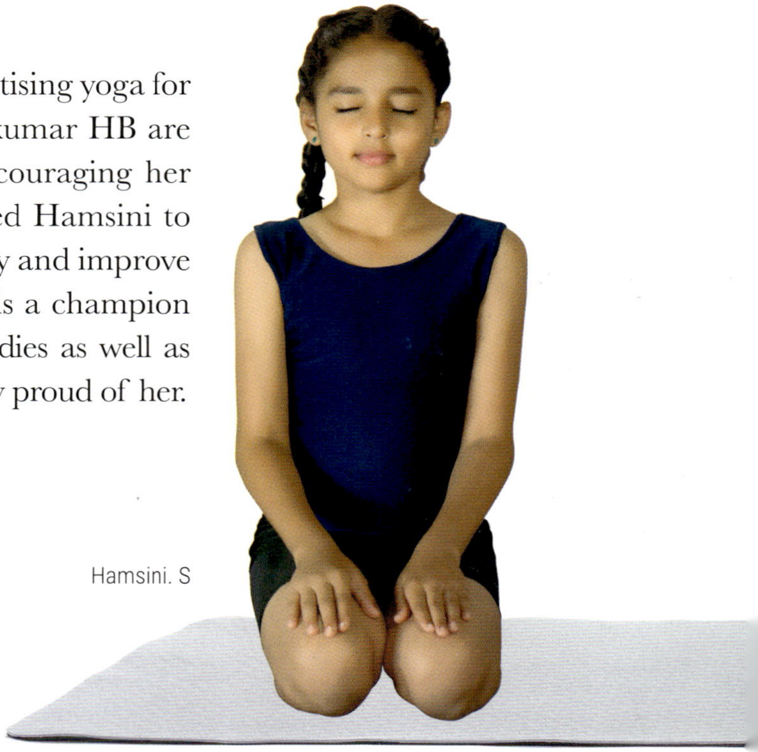

Hamsini. S

ASHWARYA. K AND ANUSHA. K

Meet the 13-year-old twins Ashwarya. K and Anusha. K They have been practising yoga for five years. They say that they have benefitted immensely since they started practising yoga. Their concentration has improved in everything, be it sports or academics. They feel strong and flexible and have made their school and parents very happy. Their parents, KS. Kumar and Lakshmi Kumar, are proud of their girls. They say that they themselves practise yoga and therefore know its benefits. They see that their girls are growing to be strong, confident and very focused. They enjoy watching them practise yoga and perfect the asanas together.

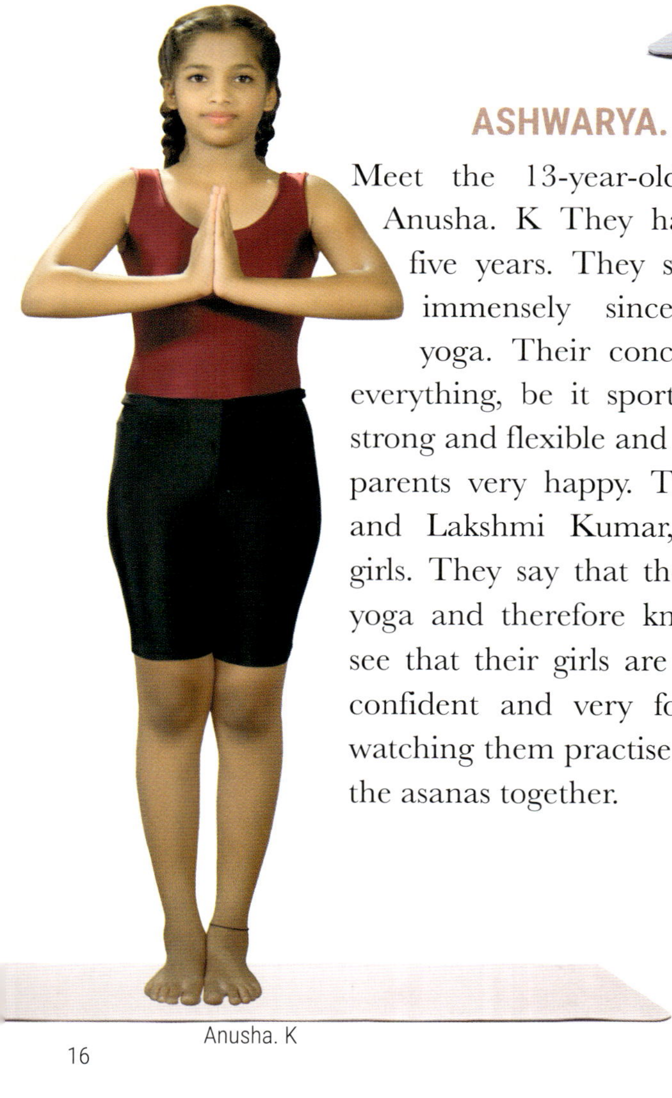

Anusha. K

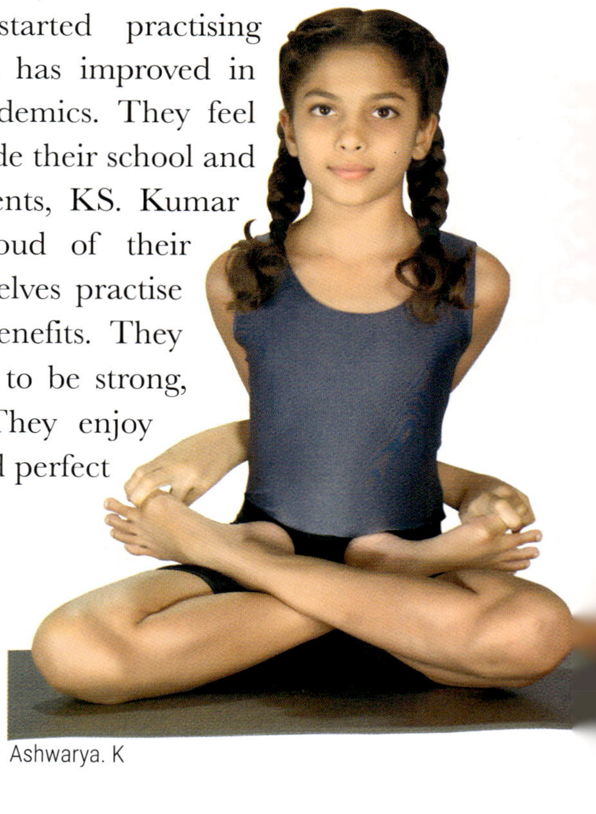

Ashwarya. K

PRATEEKSHA. GS

Eleven-year-old Prateeksha. GS has been practising yoga for three years. Her parents, Suresh. G.S and Dr. Pratibha. JP, wanted their child to study Yoga as they believed that breathing exercises or Pranayama created a sense of calmness in her. Yoga postures also helped her create a sense of balance and foster confidence and creativity. The asanas are the best way to stay healthy and be connected to the body.

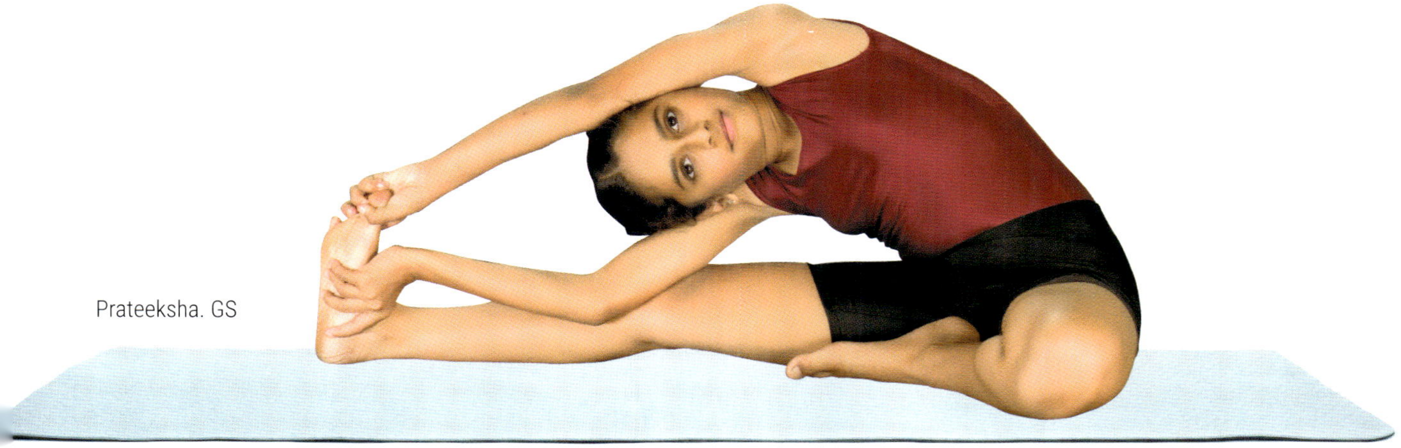

Prateeksha. GS

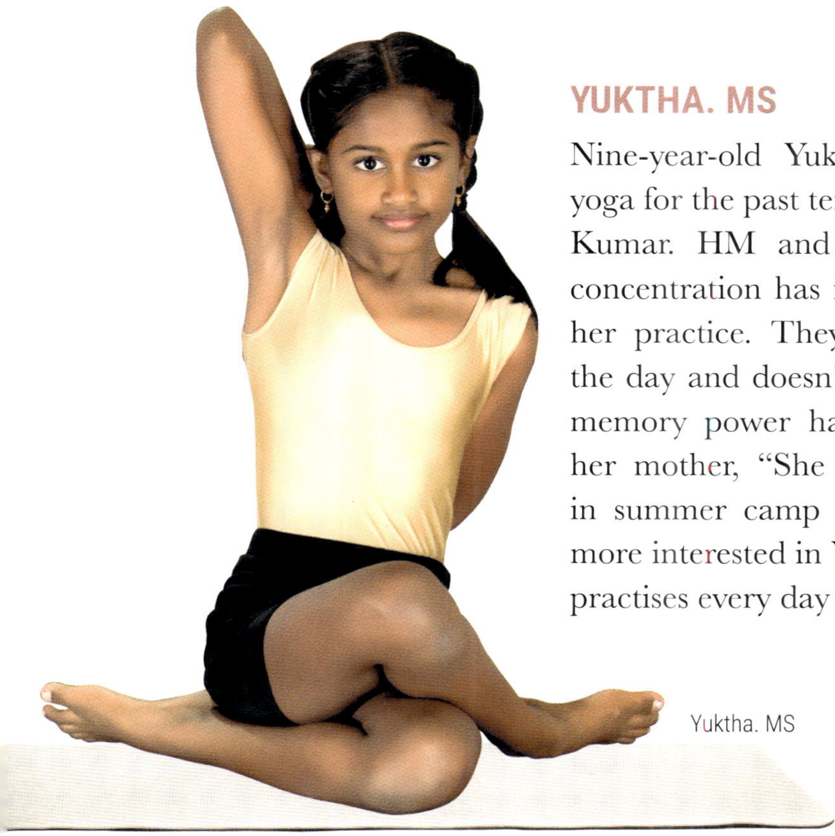

Yuktha. MS

YUKTHA. MS

Nine-year-old Yuktha. MS has been practising yoga for the past ten months. Her parents, Shantha Kumar. HM and Roopa. KJ, believe that her concentration has improved ever since she started her practice. They say she is active throughout the day and doesn't tire at all. Her immunity and memory power have increased remarkably. Says her mother, "She used to attend Patanjali Yoga in summer camp every year. There she became more interested in Yoga and meditation." Now, she practises every day and is a Yoga Champion.

SIYYA POOVIAH. K

Twelve-year-old Siyya Pooviah. K has been practising yoga for six years. Her parents, KA. Pooviah and Dr. N. Babitha Thimmaiah, were fully aware of the benefits of yoga. They say that yoga has boosted the self-esteem of their child and instilled confidence in their daughter. They say that their daughter's fondness for yoga is inspired by her yoga teacher. They also add, "Yoga enables my child to learn self-control and thereby also enhances her focus and awareness and enables her to calm the mind. It's a great way to facilitate strategic 'playtime."

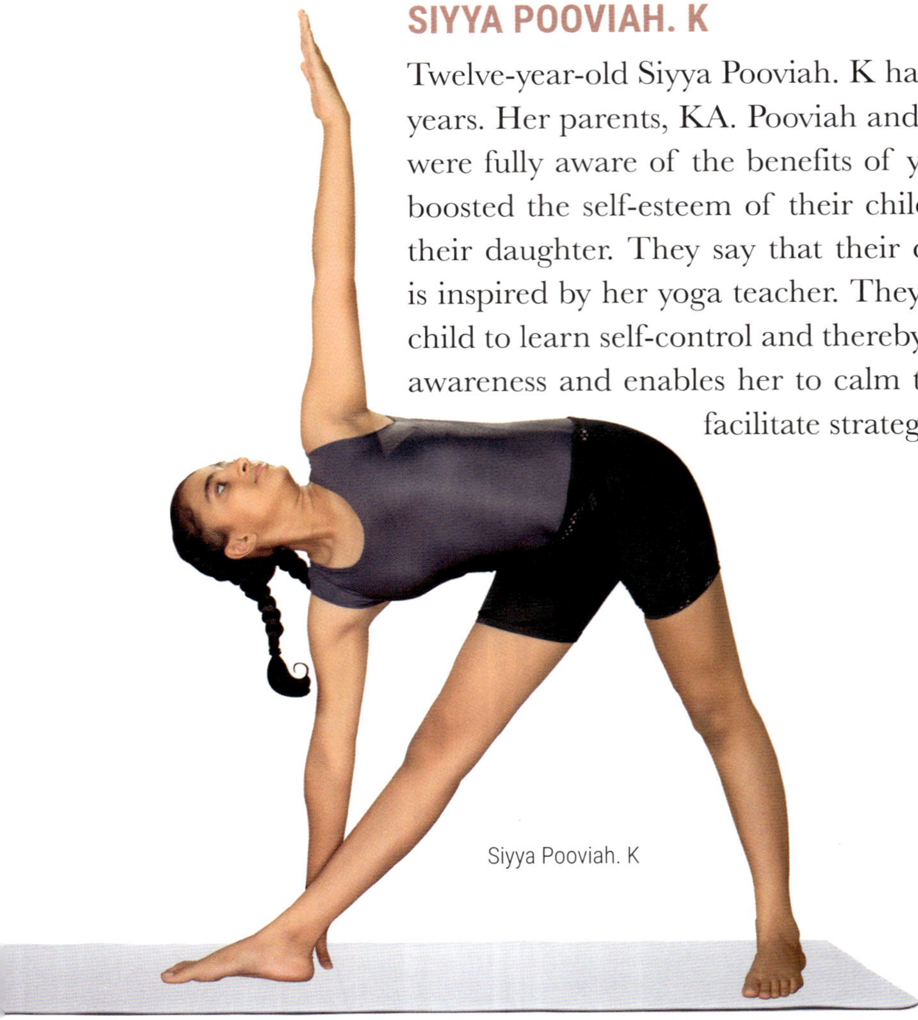

Siyya Pooviah. K

RISHITHA MANOHAR

Twelve-year-old Rishitha Manohar says that she feels very good while practising yoga and it has become a part of her life. She feels that it is good for her health and thanks her parents for initiating her into the practice. Her parents, Manohar and Manjula, are extremely happy with her progress and bless her with support and encouragement.

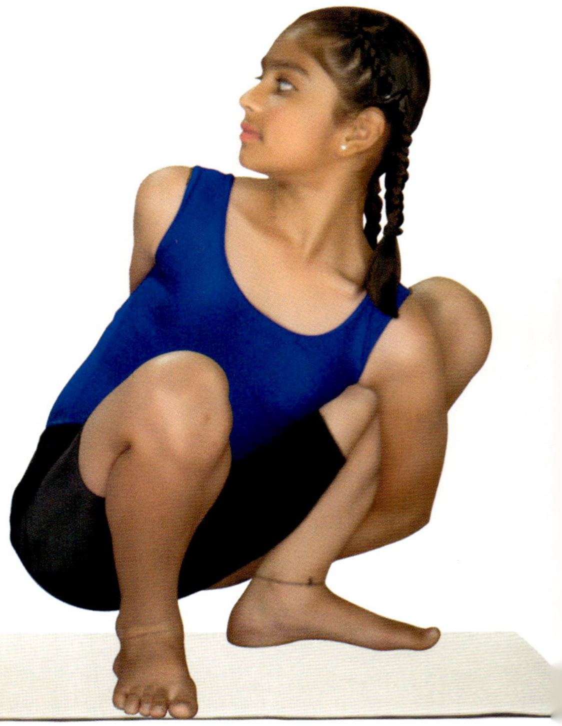

Rishitha Manohar

KUSHI K. SURESH

Thirteen-year-old Kushi K. Suresh was initiated to practise yoga as she had some health problems and delay in growth. Kushi has done very well ever since and can perform complicated asanas with ease now. She is a yoga champion. Her confidence and self-esteem have improved. Her parents are very happy. Kushi has become very disciplined and she is happy now according to her parents, Suresh. KR and Suma. NT.

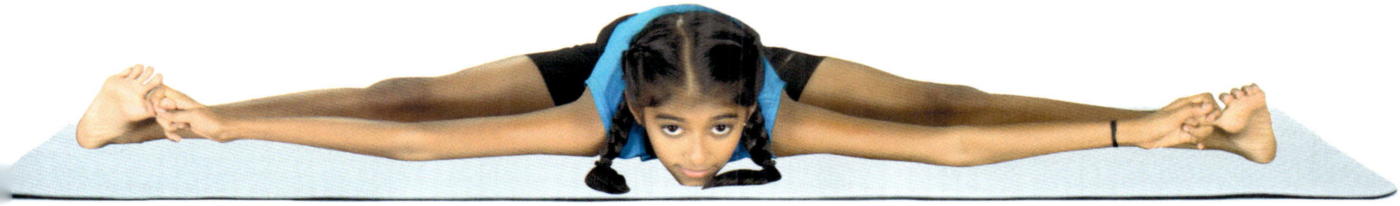

Kushi K. Suresh

KP. PRIYADARSHAN

Twelve-year-old KP. Priyadarshan has been learning yoga for many years now. He says that he enjoys the healthy feeling he gets with the practice of yoga. He feels stronger and has more focus now. He practises daily to feel good. He also says that if he doesn't practice yoga he feels lazy. His parents, Prasanna Kumar and Deepa, are very proud of their son. They say that he is always full of energy and he works hard to achieve his goals. They are happy that he is so disciplined at such a young age and has won many accolades after he began to practise yoga. He won the Prathiba Puraskar Award for 2019 for excellence at the junior level.

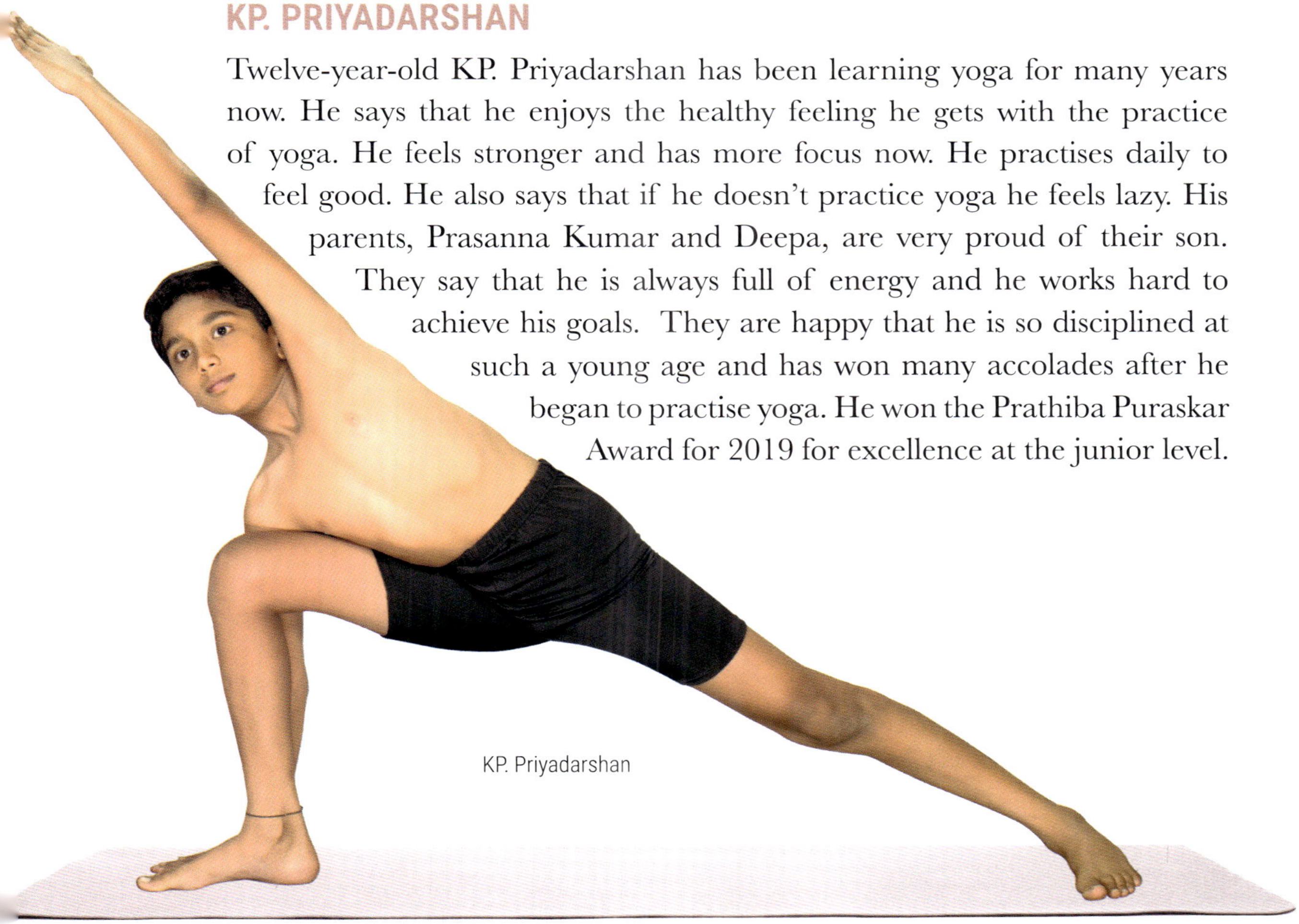

KP. Priyadarshan

AMULYA NARAYAN

Thirteen-year-old Amulya Narayan has been practising yoga for five years. Her concentration has improved in studies and co-curricular activities. "My physical strength, stamina and flexibility have increased a lot too," she says. Her father, Narayan. BK, wanted her to undergo total development at the physical as well as the mental level. "Yoga is an education. It is the best way to achieve excellence and see tangible results," says Narayan.

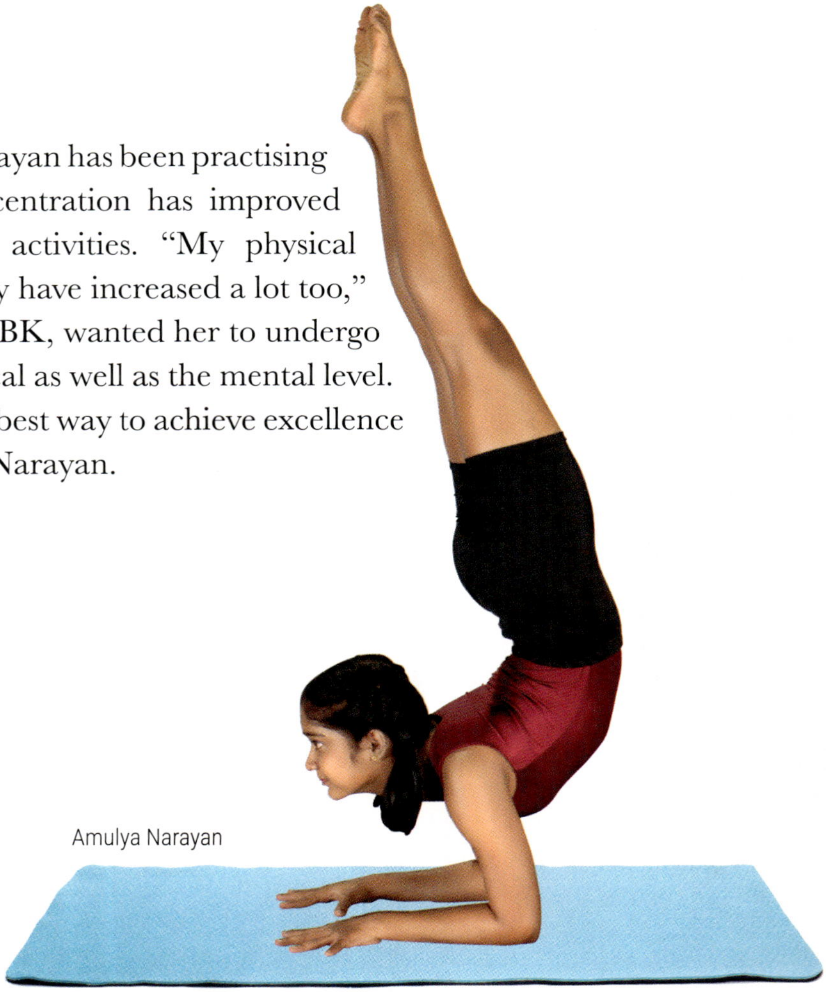

Amulya Narayan

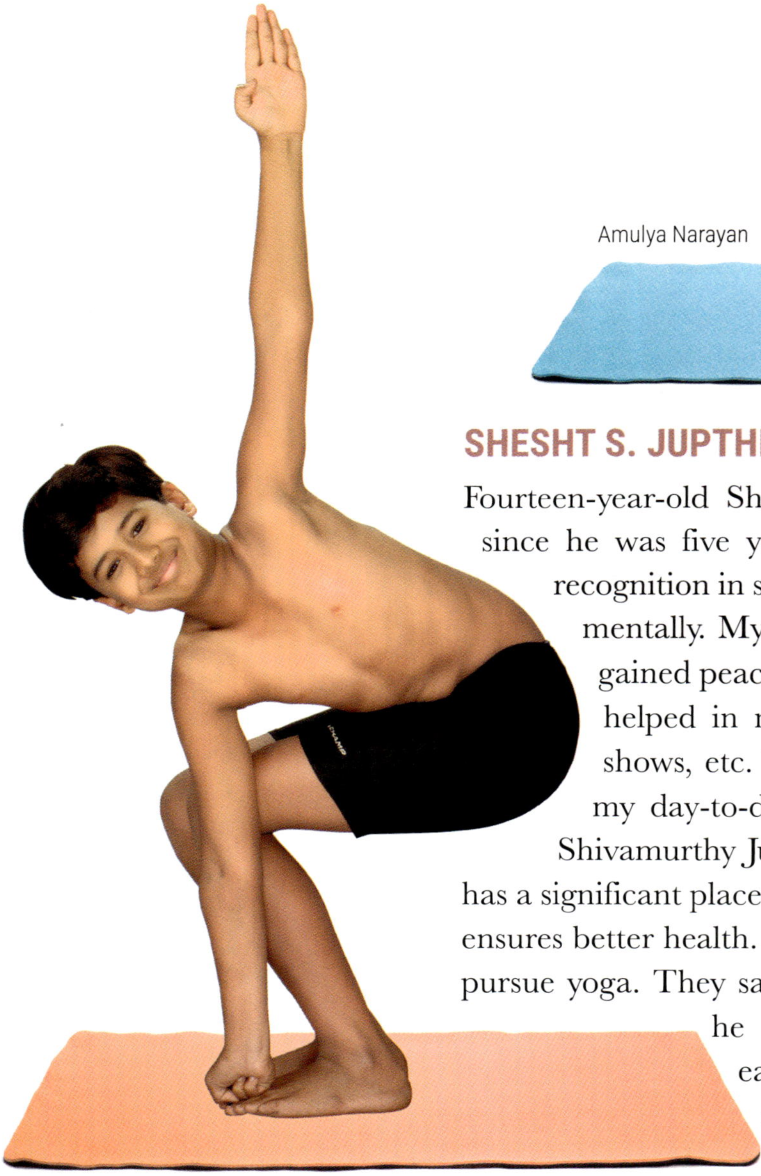

Shesht S. Jupthimath

SHESHT S. JUPTHIMATH

Fourteen-year-old Shesht S. Jupthimath has been practising since he was five years old. He says, "Yoga has given me recognition in society. It has benefitted me physically and mentally. My concentration has improved and I have gained peace of mind. Practising different asanas has helped in my performance in films, dramas, stage shows, etc. Yoga has also helped me to be active in my day-to-day life." Shesht's parents, Kalpana and Shivamurthy Juptimath, have always believed that yoga has a significant place in Indian culture and that asana practice ensures better health. This is why they encouraged their son to pursue yoga. They say, "We noticed a glow on his face when he practised. As he continues practising each and every asana, his self-confidence improves and he is motivated to practise further. He is an extremely disciplined boy. We are very proud of him."

MASTER RUDRESH (YOGA TEACHER)

Master Rudresh. CL is from a town called Kaduru. He trains champions of yoga and the kids who are featured in this book. He has been teaching yoga for many years. Master Rudresh studied Industrial and Production Engineering at the National Institute of Engineering, Mysore. He felt that his yoga skills would benefit society more and decided to take up teaching it instead of pursuing a career in Engineering. His grandfather was a practitioner of yoga and encouraged him to study it. Master Rudresh started learning yoga at the age of 10. He studied with various gurus and practises continuously.

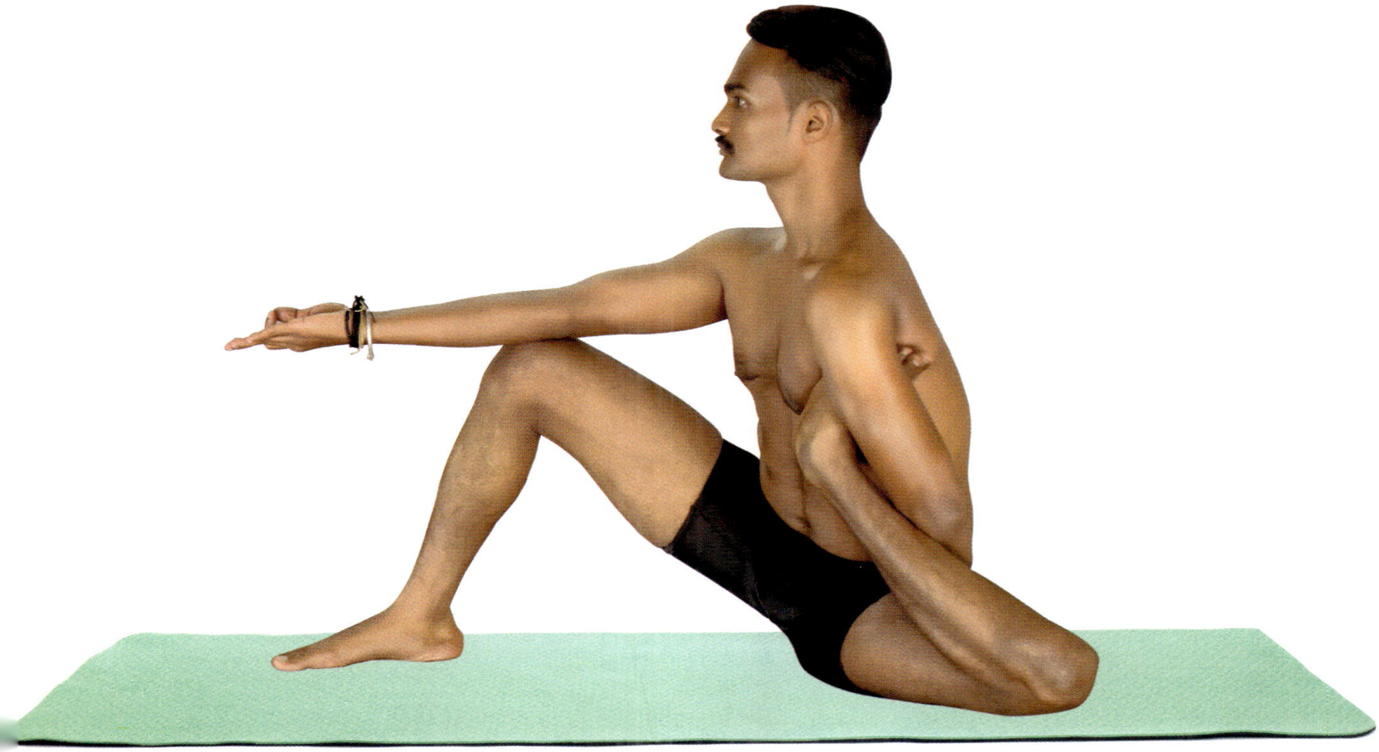

Master Rudresh (Yoga Teacher)

Rudresh has won many gold and silver medals in State and Central-level yogasana competitions. He is an eight-time winner of the State Champion of Champion title. He was the 2009 State Men's Champion of Champion conducted by the Karnataka State Amateur Yoga Association. He was also the recipient of the National Bronze Medal in the 14–17 age group category conducted by the Yoga Federation of India.

Master Rudresh worked as a freelance yoga teacher in China in 2016. He now works as a yoga teacher at Samhitha Yogashala Mysore and as a freelance children's yoga teacher. He is a Yoga Instructor at Sri Narayanananda Universal Yoga Ashrama, Hinkal, Mysore.

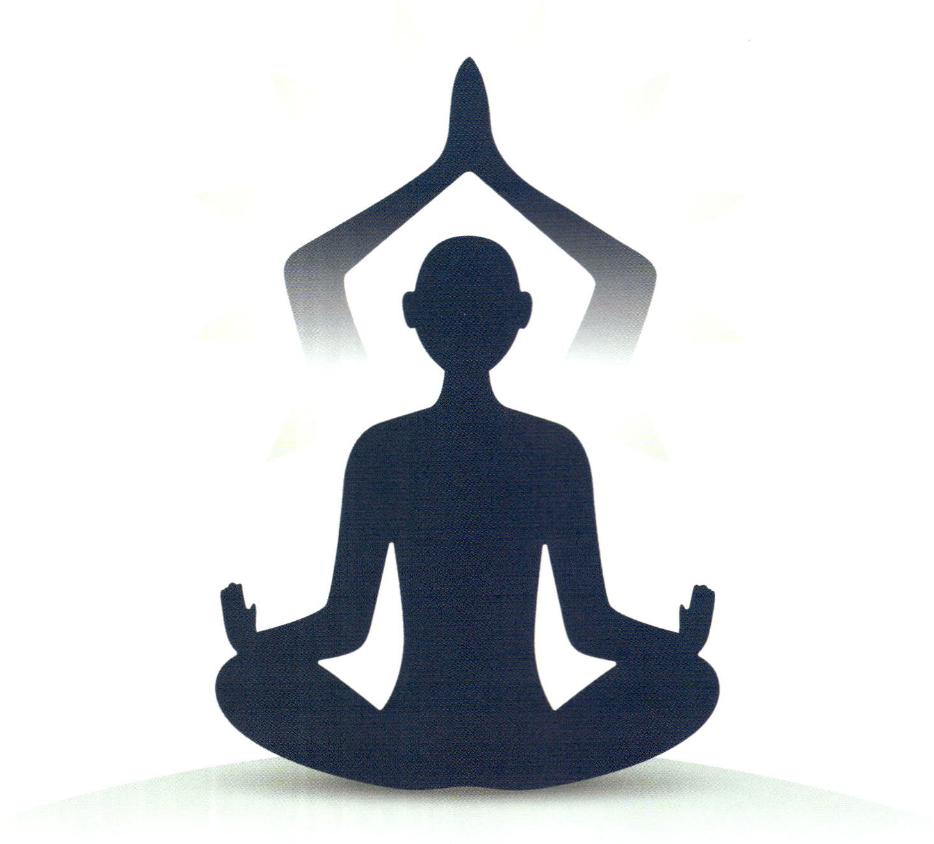

SECTION A

YOGA AND PHILOSOPHY

Chapter 1

Yoga is not just physical exercise. It is knowledge that helps you to lead a life of contentment and peace. Life can get very complicated at times. The goal of the *Yoga Sutra* is to show the path of knowledge to let us overcome the complexities in life. Sage Patanjali studied in great detail the main cause of these complexities and documented some solutions in the form of sutras. Sutras (threads of great knowledge) are short verses or one-liners of knowledge (knowledge bombs), but when expanded they can become an ocean of knowledge, which you will find relevant at all stages of your life. The information in the *Yoga Sutra* is timeless and precious. It is for everyone who wants to live a happy life.

Sage Patanjali has a wonderful theory. He explains that all of us have problems. Both kids and adults have problems, but they are different issues. Problems exist and most of them originate in our minds! Sage Patanjali proves that the solution also lies within us. The solution he suggests in the sutras are not to make the problems magically go away, but to understand them and change the way to perceive them. Genius, isn't it? This means that the way we look at a certain issue can influence the way we respond to the issue. The sutras teach you to meet challenges with a smile. Nothing is impossible in life if you have the right perspective.

So, the practice of yoga helps create an overall positivity that can eventually lead to excellence. By training the mind and body not to be affected by painful circumstances, the text of the sutras attempts to create a sense of freedom from what causes suffering in the mind. Sage Patanjali mentions in the text that by training the mind to deal with disturbances, we can overcome pain and suffering. If the mind is not disturbed, then there will be freedom from the pain and suffering associated with all our problems.

Sutra I.33 (Parental guidance required to explain this sutra)

| | Maitrikarunamuditopeksanam

Sukhadukhapunyavisayanam

Bhavanatascittaprasadanam | |

(When we look around we see different kinds of people, some happy some less happy. Some are doing good for the society and others, bad. The *sloka* (aphorism) says that however the people around us are, we need to choose to be happy for people who are doing well and compassionate for people not doing so well. Infusing the mind with friendliness, compassion, cheerfulness and uninvolved observation in relation to those living a happy, miserable, virtuous and non-virtuous life respectively, results in reclaiming a pristine state of mind.)

This sutra explains how to clear pollutants from the mind and make it serene by creating some virtues in relation to the people around us. This sutra is an example of the simple but immense knowledge which the *Yoga Sutra* contains.

> **The mind is both the source and solution of all problems. If the mind is agitated, distracted or conditioned by habit, then perception may be inaccurate, landing us in trouble. However, if the same mind is disciplined, focused and free from habits, perception is more accurate and therefore our actions based on this perception will not cause suffering. This is the crux of Patanjali's Philosophy of Yoga.**
>
> **— Guru T.K.V. Desikachar**

This emphasis on the mind is what makes the *Yoga Sutra* unique, meriting a timeless study. The mind plays a crucial role for everyone in any stage of life, no matter where you come from and whatever beliefs you hold dear. Everything starts in the mind and you have the power to change your circumstances with total awareness and knowledge. Yoga practice is the first step to achieve this goal.

Simple introduction to the Yoga Sutra

Who was Sage Patanjali?

Here's an interesting mythological story about this sage.

Have you seen the beautiful image of the Indian deity the mighty Vishnu and his two pets the Adi Shesha, the thousand-headed snake, and the great eagle Garuda?

Garuda is Vishnu's vehicle and Adi Shesha is the bed on which Vishnu sleeps.

One day, Adi Shesha expressed his desire to his master that he wanted to do something valuable for mankind. Vishnu agreed and asked him to go ahead.

At that time, on earth, a sage's wife who was bathing in a river was praying for a son. She lifted her hand up to seek blessings and a small snake landed on it. She closed her palms into an *anjali* (namaste) and a small snake fell into her arms making a 'pat' sound. She folded her hands into an *anjali* again. At home, when she opened her palms, there was a beautiful baby in her there. This is how the baby got the name Patanjali.

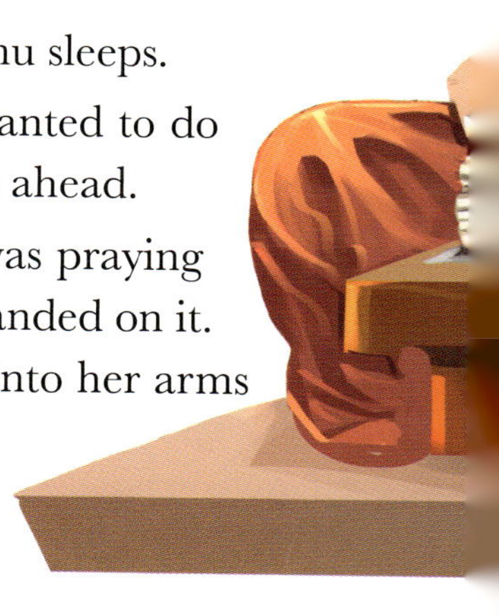

The baby grew up into the renowned sage Patanjali, the most knowledgeable sage ever. He was a master of all the scriptures. But he chose to do research and understand everything about human life. He wanted to get to the root of what exactly caused pain and sorrow. He knew that only if you understand the nature of problems could a viable solution be designed. He compiled all his research on the subject and arrived at a conclusion in one book called the *Yoga Sutra*.

Where Did Yoga Come From?

Legends say that yoga began with the gods. Yoga is a very ancient science. We can trace its origins to another ancient science – Ayurveda. Nobody knows for sure exactly when the practice of yoga began and who devised it. Ancient sculptures and paintings dating back to six thousand years show some signs of the practice of yoga.

The Four Padas (Chapters) of the Yoga Sutra

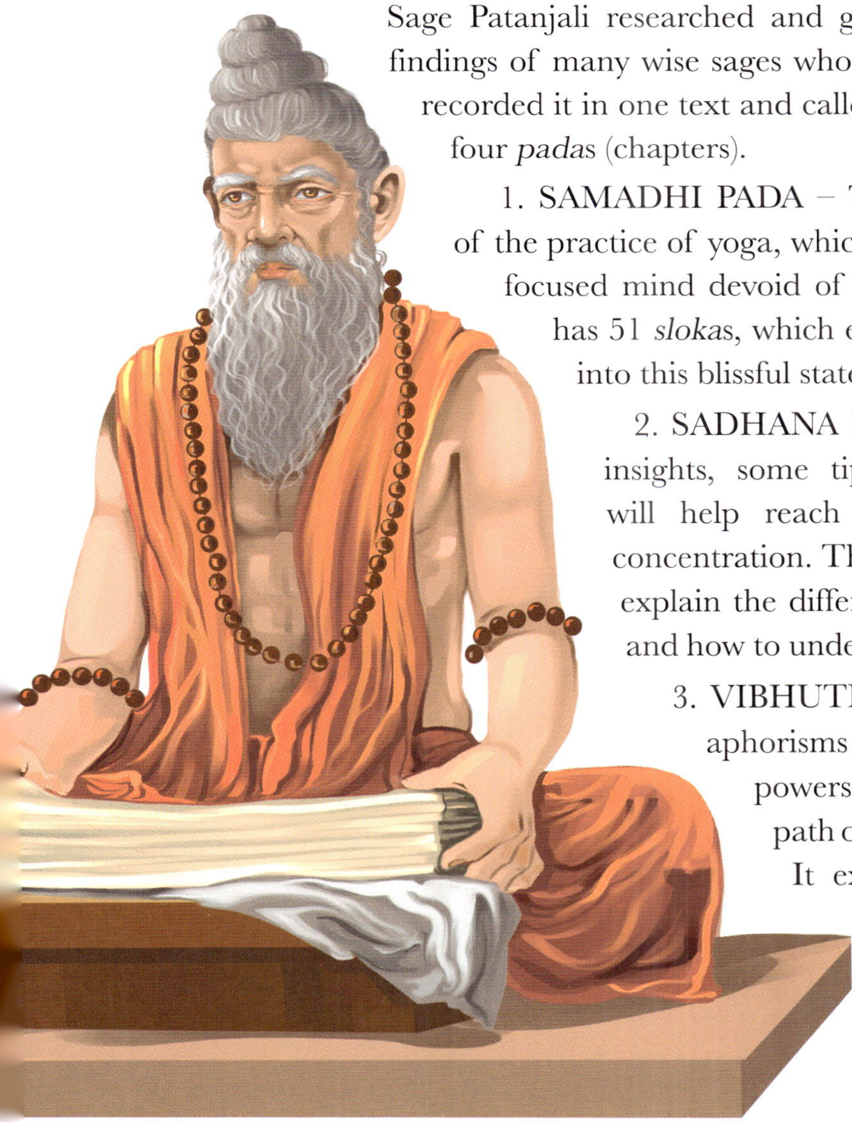

Sage Patanjali researched and gathered information from the findings of many wise sages who lived before his time. He then recorded it in one text and called it the *Yoga Sutra*, which has four *padas* (chapters).

1. SAMADHI PADA – This chapter explains the goal of the practice of yoga, which is to reach the state of a fully focused mind devoid of any distractions. This chapter has 51 *slokas*, which explains how to go about to get into this blissful state of mind.

2. SADHANA PADA – This chapter provides insights, some tips and practical tools which will help reach a state of a single-pointed concentration. This chapter has 55 *slokas*, which explain the different states of the human mind and how to understand them and sort them out.

3. VIBHUTI PADA – This chapter has 56 aphorisms and it explains the extraordinary powers which can be achieved if the path of yoga is followed and practised. It explains the powers which the mind can receive in a state of immense focus which is called siddhi in yogic terms. It is said that some of these

powers can defy the laws of science.

4. KAIVALYA PADA – The final chapter has only 34 aphorisms and explains the transformation of the mind and its progress towards freedom from suffering and attaining a state which is completely blissful.

Sage Patanjali's main definition in the *Yoga Sutra* is about how to train the mind to deal with fluctuations. After meticulous study of how the mind works, he elaborates on 8 steps called Ashtanga, which means 8 limbs.

They are: Yama, Niyama, Asana, Pranayama, Pratyaahara, Dharana, Dhyana and Samadhi.

Note to Parents

It should be understood that yoga is not merely restricted to breathing or physical exercises. Sage Patanjali explains that asanas or physical postures are one of the means to coordinate and train the mind. Patanjali's *Yoga Sutra* provides many such tools to bring about this one-pointed focus to lead a successful life. These tools can be studied eventually as the child matures in age and intellect.

THREE-LEVEL ADVANTAGE OF PATANJALI'S YOGA SUTRA

1. **Physical level**

- Helps you to be healthy and strong
- Builds up endurance and stamina
- Aids the growth and development of a healthy body

2. **Mental level**

- Helps you to remain calm and balanced
- Helps the mind stay peaceful and in harmony
- Builds up a sense of contentment as thoughts get tamed

3. **Spiritual level**

- Cultivates a sense of equanimity
  Increases focus and concentration in the mind
- Creates a positive approach to life

ASHTANGA PRINCIPLES

Chapter 2

Sutra II.29

||Yamaniyama Asana pranayama
pratyaaharadharanadhyanasamadhayo'stavangani ||

Sutra II.29 talks about the eight components that are important for the practice of yoga. The order in which the sutras are presented here starts from the outside and moves inward. The outside refers to the external perception of life or looking at one's life from the outside. Then it moves into introspection, the state of looking deep into the mind. Let's examine these eight components.

1. Yama – Our Cultural (Outward) Attitude

The five Yama principles indicated in the text are:

a. AHIMSA: Cultivate respect and love for everything around you. This is the best way to practise Ahimsa or non-violence. Respect nature, insects, animals, trees, your surroundings and that of your neighbours, your state, your country and your planet. The rule of Ahimsa is never to hurt anything on planet earth.

b. SATYA: Stay truthful to yourself and others. When you speak a lie, it is your feelings that suffer more than those of others. Stick to the truth as far as possible.

c. ASTEYA: Avoid being greedy. Greed is the main reason for the evil desire to steal. Someone else's possessions can never give joy. It will only cause suffering to you as well as suffering to the person who loses his/her possessions.

d. BRAHMACHARYA: 'Brahma' is God and 'acharya' means to follow. Following the path directed by God is what this Yama means. The scriptures say that there is God in all of us who always guides us. It is only when we get too busy and confident that we start ignoring this guidance given by our inner voice, which is God.

e. APARIGRAHA: Do not hoard or collect unnecessary things, thoughts and worries. This is like greed too, filling you with a desire to possess more than required. It is not exactly stealing but gathering more and more things and denying those possessions to others, an unhealthy practice that clutters the mind.

2. Niyama – Our Personal Conduct

a. SHOUCHA: This is about being clean externally and internally.

   i. Externally
      - Take a bath everyday
      - Clean eyes, ears and nails
      - Regulate bowel movement
      - Wear clean clothes

   ii. Internally

Keep thoughts clean. This is much harder but can be done with consistent practice.

b. SANTOSHA: This is a feeling of gratitude, satisfaction or contentment, a positive feeling. It is a state of mind that helps you to be satisfied with the work you have put in. It helps you to keep working towards progress.

c. TAPA: This involves working towards disciplining the mind to reach a point of calmness. Whether you win or lose, the mind should remain balanced.

d. SVADHYAHA: This is about self-study by focusing all concentration on your thoughts and actions. This is to make sure that you are moving in the right direction towards a successful and righteous life.

e. ISHWARA PRANIDHANA: Most of the ancient texts refer to a supreme power who guides and protects us all through life. Respecting and acknowledging this supreme power will bring freedom from the fear of the unknown.

3. Asana – The Practice of Exercise and Care for Physical Health

Asana practice is a physical practice. They are a set of postures which needs to be learnt, understood and practised. This practice helps us to overcome illness in the body (be it respiratory, digestive or nervous system issues) and dullness in the mind. By practising asanas daily, all the bones, muscles, blood vessels, glands, vital organs and body systems begin to function normally. Asanas also improve metabolism, enhance immunity, increase stamina and aid in the growth and development of the body.

Yoga helps improve stability of both the mind and the body. At the mental level, asanas help in overcoming distractions, greed, anger, lethargy, etc. Asanas purify the body and help generate healthy hormones and chemicals which are beneficial to the body.

An asana is a posture in which the practitioner is still, stable and in total equilibrium. Each asana is like a geometric pattern that needs to be carefully constructed. Each position positively affects a specific point in the body. To experience the effect and benefit of the asana, you should hold steady and be still, inhale and focus on what the asana is doing to the length of the body, exhale and observe the change it makes in your body. Initially, it will be difficult to observe the benefit and the effect. But, eventually, bodily awareness will improve and it will become easier.

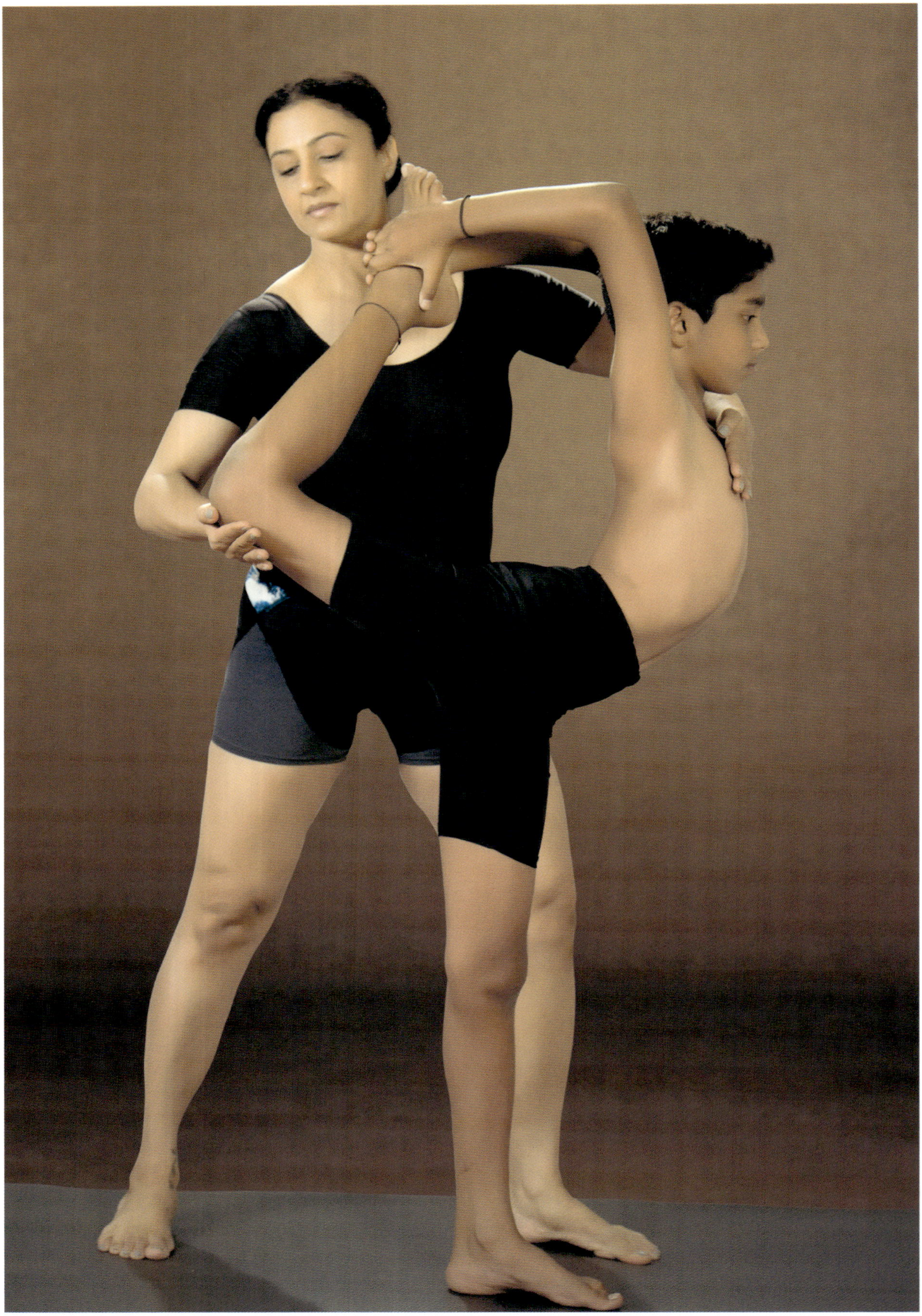

ASANAS

The Art of Physical Posture

Chapter 3

- Elaboration of the practice and introduction of methods of asana practice along with illustrated guidelines, benefits and caution are given here.
- Yoga asanas are specific physical postures. A posture is called an asana when the posture is steady and comfortable to breathe in. The main aim of practising asanas is to achieve a sound mind and a sound body. Yoga asanas are versatile in their benefits. The asanas mentioned in this chapter help in stimulating the body's functions, balance growth hormones, boost immunity and metabolism, and most importantly, work on the nervous system.
- A well-planned asana routine such as the ones in this chapter incorporates postures, breathing and cooling down techniques, which is ideal for a child to maintain good mental and physical health. In the initial stages, an asana can be done casually without challenging the body too much, and under the guidance of a yoga teacher or a parent. Eventually, as the practice progresses, the children will be able to do it on their own.
- Duration of practice: daily for half an hour, ideally in the morning after drinking a glass of water or in the evening with a two-hour gap after food.

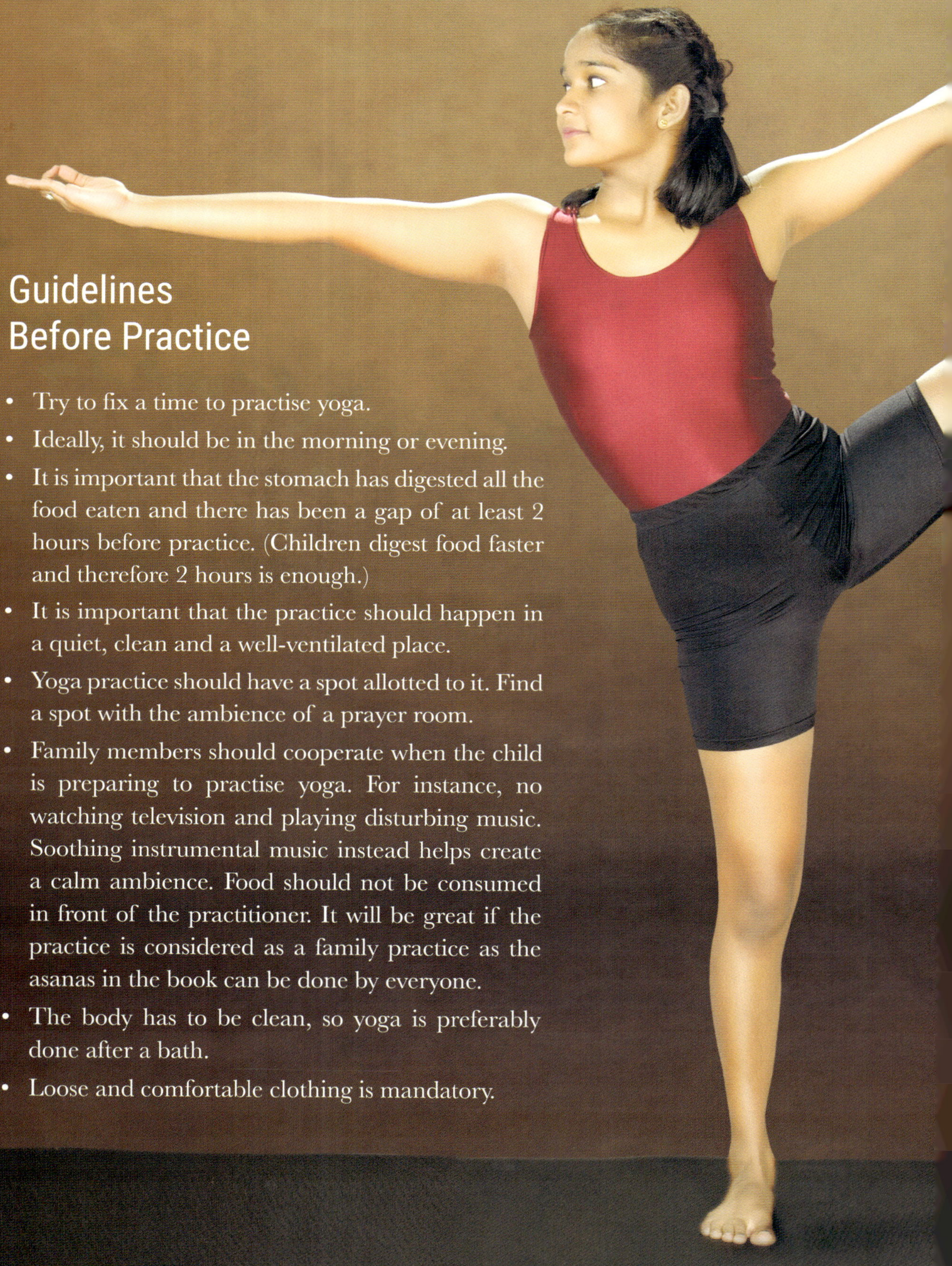

Guidelines Before Practice

- Try to fix a time to practise yoga.
- Ideally, it should be in the morning or evening.
- It is important that the stomach has digested all the food eaten and there has been a gap of at least 2 hours before practice. (Children digest food faster and therefore 2 hours is enough.)
- It is important that the practice should happen in a quiet, clean and a well-ventilated place.
- Yoga practice should have a spot allotted to it. Find a spot with the ambience of a prayer room.
- Family members should cooperate when the child is preparing to practise yoga. For instance, no watching television and playing disturbing music. Soothing instrumental music instead helps create a calm ambience. Food should not be consumed in front of the practitioner. It will be great if the practice is considered as a family practice as the asanas in the book can be done by everyone.
- The body has to be clean, so yoga is preferably done after a bath.
- Loose and comfortable clothing is mandatory.

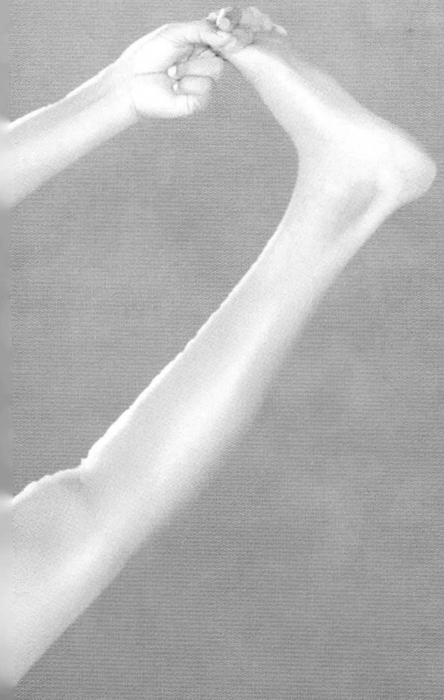

- Practice can be done on alternate days or every day.
- If a practice is done everyday then stick to a 30-minute routine, otherwise make it a 45-minute routine.
- Conversation should be avoided during the child's practice.
- Warming up the body with some gentle jogging and stretching is important. (Covered in the Warm Up section of the sequencing patterns.)
- A proper dedicated mat or a carpet is a must. This mat/ carpet should be clean and used only for yoga.
- Start with simple asanas and then only move to the advanced asana practice.
- Ideally, yoga practices should be learnt under the guidance of an experienced teacher.
- If the child is ill or recovering from an illness try to encourage him/her to get onto the mat. Refer to the sequencing section in Recovery Yoga. However, please go through the instructions and cautions carefully. It is important to consult a doctor and then decide whether to go ahead with the practice. A careful, gentle approach is important when the body is recovering from illness.
- Regularity in the practice is extremely beneficial.
- A sincere effort should be made while practising.
- Practising for half an hour during examination time will help kids settle down. (Refer to Exam Time Yoga sequence.)
- Do not ignore the philosophical importance of yoga. Understand the Yama, Niyama, Asana and Pranayama explained in Chapters 3 and 4.
- Understanding the Yoga Philosophy with respect to the circumstances of your nation, culture and traditions is a clever way of practising the principles.
- Yoga is not religious. It is a discipline which needs to be practised with understanding and respect.

NAMASKARAS

Guru Namaskara

A Guru is someone who imparts knowledge and leads us from the darkness of ignorance to the brightness of intelligence. Guru Namaskara is a series of asanas bowing in homage to the legacy of the Gurus. In Indian traditional practices, paying homage to the Guru is of utmost importance. This way we acknowledge knowledge.

The series of asanas are done keeping the mudra (hand gesture) of namaste, with both palms folded together.

Guru Namaskara can be done 2 or 4 times.

Facts

Yoga helps create an overall positivity that can eventually lead to excellence.

1 Samasthithi/Tadasana

1. Stand at the back end of the mat.
2. This is a point of being ready.
3. Exhale.

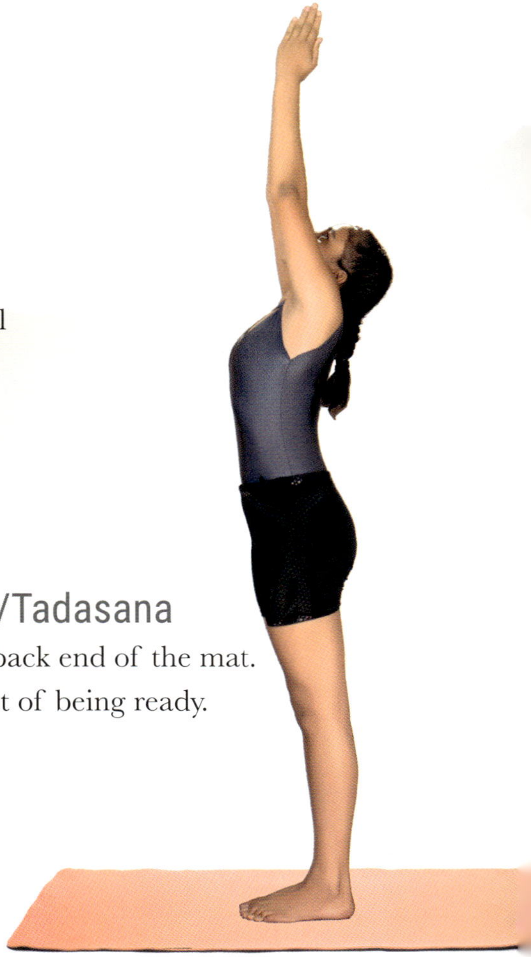

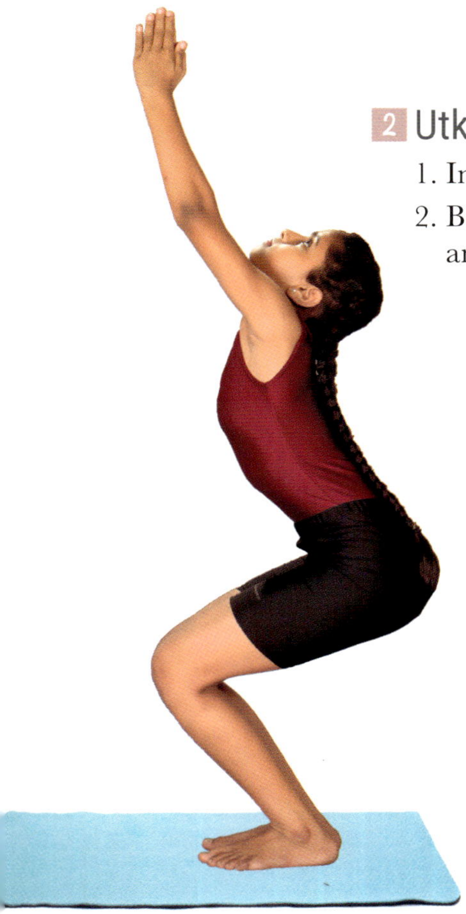

2 Utkattasana (Chair Pose)

1. Inhale
2. Bend knees, push hip back, expand chest and lift the hands up in a namaste.

3 Veerabadrasana – 3 (Right) – Warrior Pose 3

1. Exhale
2. Step forward into a lunge in a strong stance with arms stretched forward into a namaste.

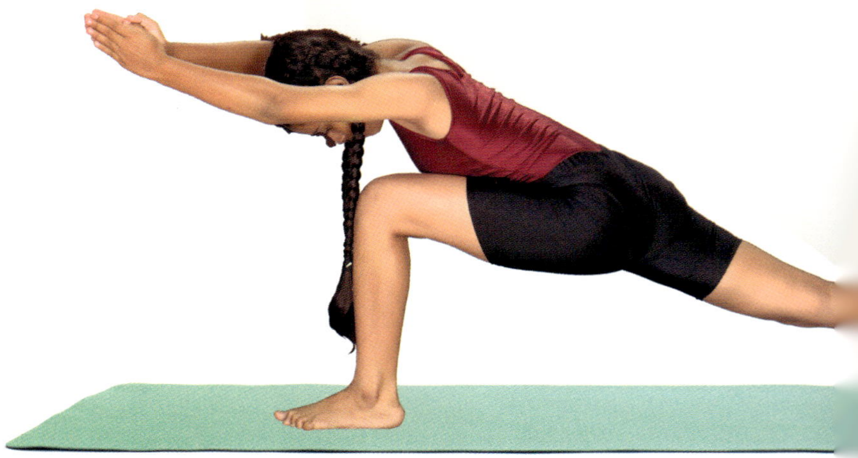

4 Veerabadrasana – 4 (Right) – Warrior Pose 4

1. Inhale
2. Lift the hands up.
3. Maintain the asana (lunge) with strength.

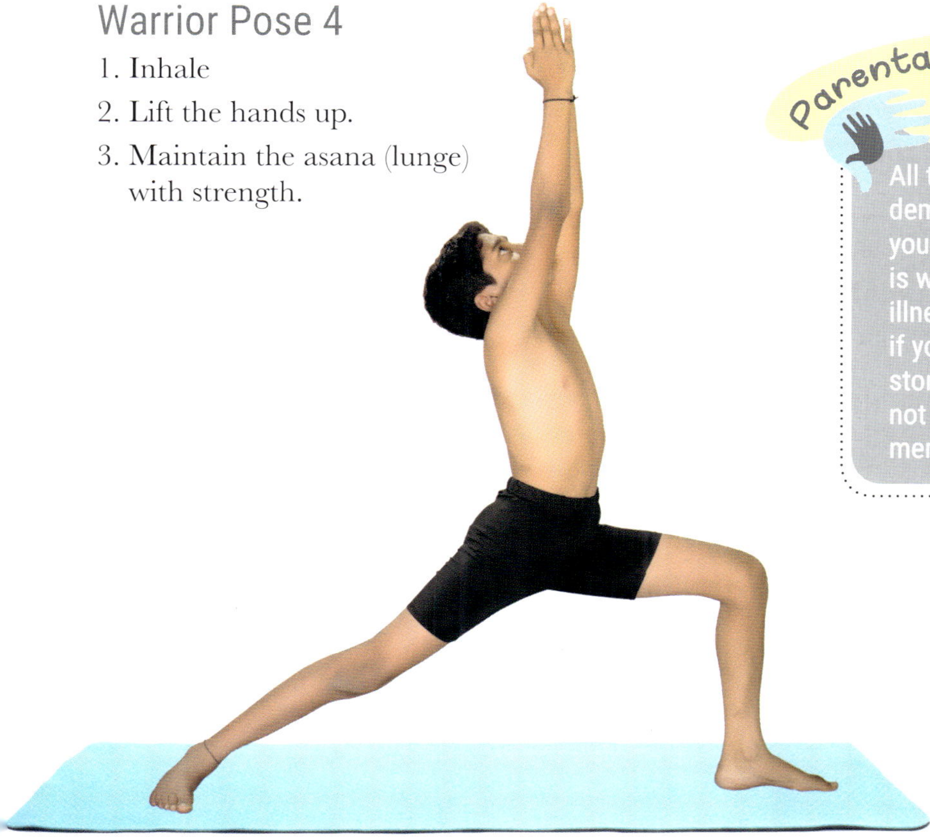

Parental guidance

All the asanas in this routine demand strength. Do not let your child practise if the body is weak and recovering from illness. Do not do this routine if you are recovering from stomach upset. Girls should not do this routine during menstruation.

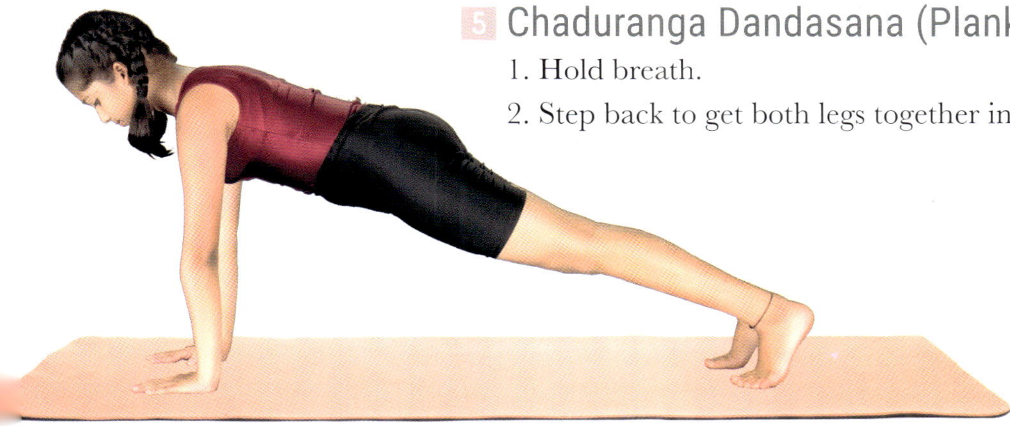

5 Chaduranga Dandasana (Plank Pose)

1. Hold breath.
2. Step back to get both legs together into a plank pose.

6 Shastanga Namaskara – Homage Namaskara

Exhale as the body drops down into a complete leg and arm stretch with the forehead pressed to the ground.

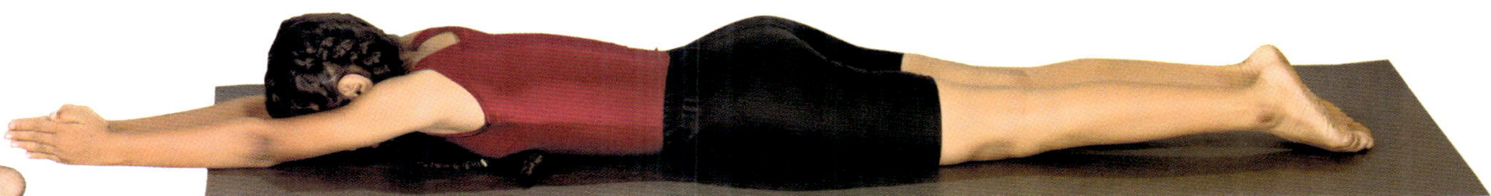

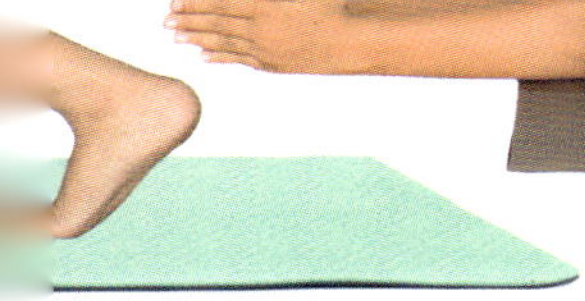

7 Chaduranga Dandasana (lift the body up) – Plank Pose

1. Inhale.
2. Lift the body up with strength and maintain a plank pose. Keep the shoulders strong.

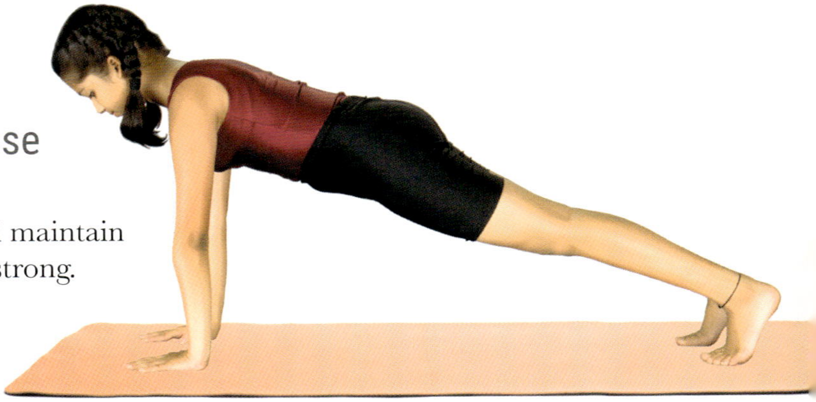

8 Step to Veerabadrasana – 3 (Left) – Warrior Pose 3

1. Exhale
2. Step forward into a lunge in a strong stance with arms stretched forward into a namaste.

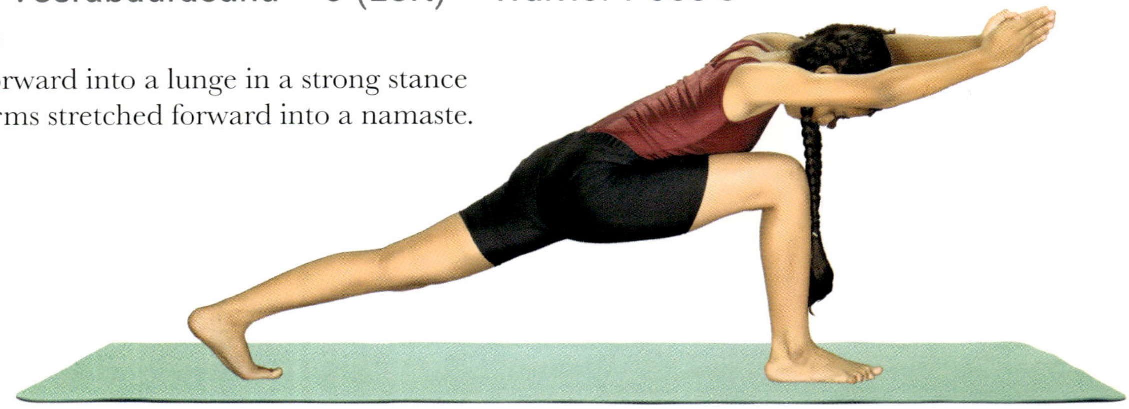

PRECAUTIONS

- All the asanas in this routine demand strength. Do not practise if the body is weak and recovering from illness.
- Do not do this routine if you are recovering from an upset stomach.
- Girls should not do this routine during menstruation

9 Veerabadrasana – 4 (Left) Warrior Pose 4

1. Inhale.
2. Lift the hands up. Maintain the asana (lunge) with strength.

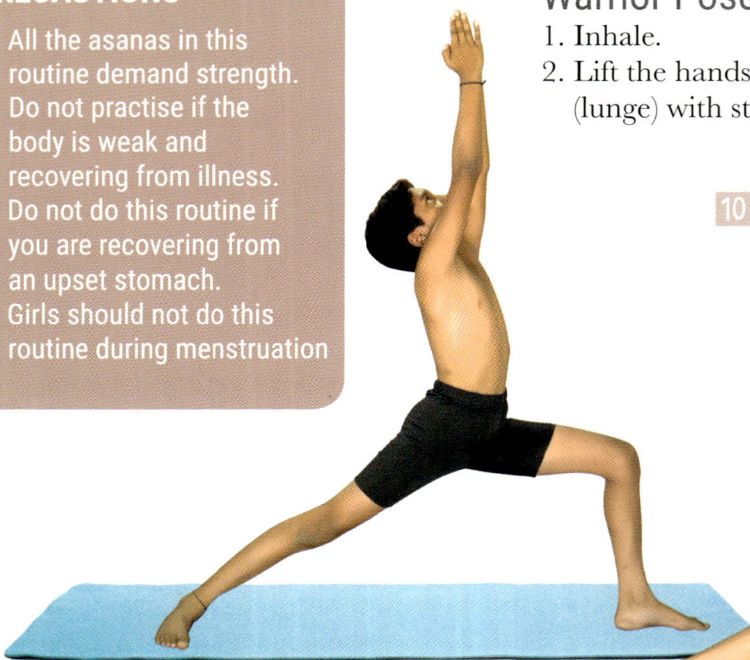

10 Chaduranga Dandasana (Plank Pose)

1. Hold breath.
2. Step back to get both legs together into a plank pose.

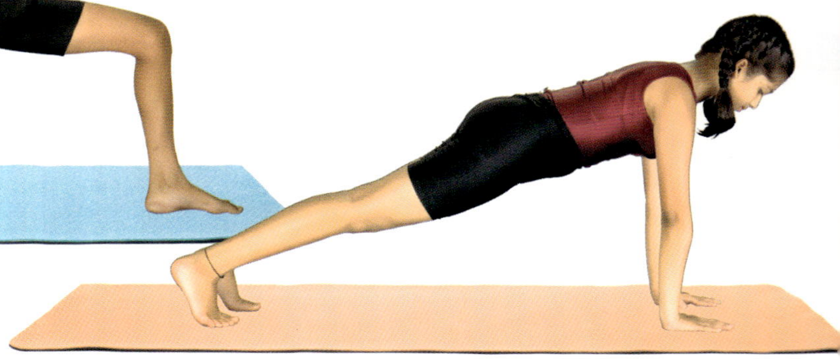

11 Shastanga Namaskara – Homage Namaskara

Exhale as the body drops down into a complete leg and arm stretch with the forehead pressed to the ground.

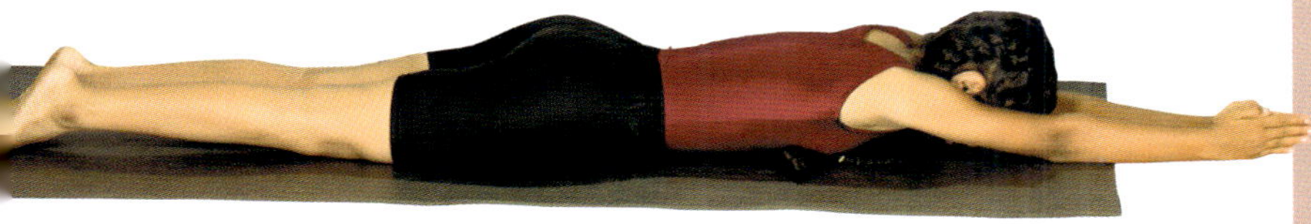

12 Balasana – Child's Pose

1. Inhale.
2. Slide the body to rest backwards and fold the body with strength along the thighs.

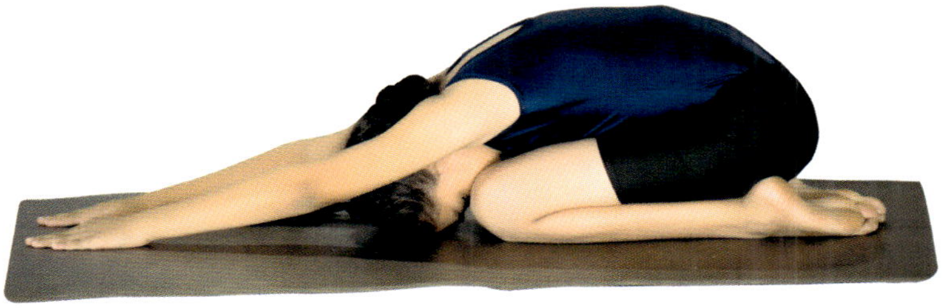

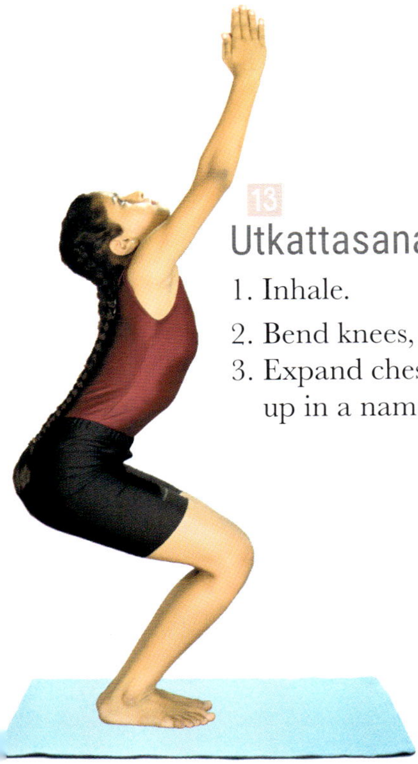

13 Utkattasana – Chair Pose

1. Inhale.
2. Bend knees, push hip back
3. Expand chest and lift the hands up in a namaste.

Samasthithi/Tadasana 14

1. Stand at the back end of the mat.
2. This is the point of readiness. Exhale.

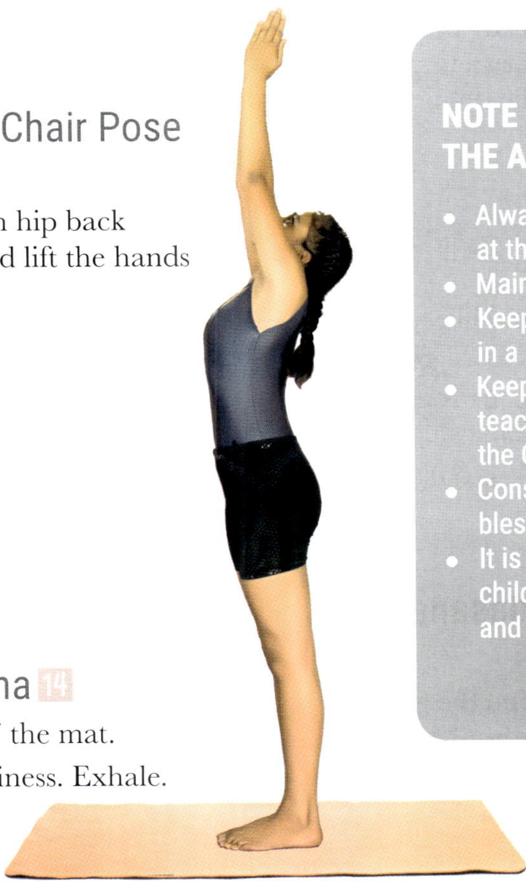

BENEFITS OF GURU NAMASKARA

- Brings in a feeling of humility and kindness
- Reduces the ego
- Enhances a sense of gratitude and surrender
- Brings in emotional strength,
- Builds up focus and concentration
- Helps steady the mind and body
- Readies the mind to learn and respect knowledge
- Acknowledges the presence of a higher intelligence
- Warms up the breathing
- Establishes stability and balance.
- Strengthens arms and legs
- Engages the entire body and warms the body

NOTE FROM THE ACHARYA

- Always do Guru Namaskara at the beginning of the practice.
- Maintain the breathing pattern.
- Keep the body strong and eyes in a straight line gaze.
- Keep in mind respect for all teachers and the lineage of the Guru from ancient times.
- Consider this a prayer seeking blessings from the Gurus.
- It is a good routine for children who are into sports and maritial arts.

SURYA NAMASKARA A

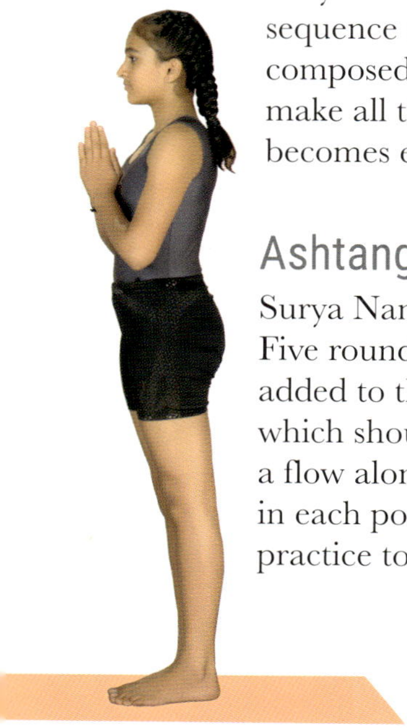

Surya Namaskara means paying salutations to the Sun and it is the most energising sequence of asanas. It is done with precision, technique and breathing. It is composed of several postures, which will help the working of the entire body. It helps make all the organs of the body efficient and enables proper breathing. The body becomes energetic and there is increased blood circulation.

Ashtanga Yoga Surya Namaskara

Surya Namaskara is usually done to warm up and prepare the body for the asanas. Five rounds of Variation A come first. Then Variation B comes with more asanas added to the sequence. In this method, each breath is accompanied by a movement, which should be in sync with the breath. Inhalations and exhalations happen in a flow along with the pose and not before or after. The number of breaths taken in each pose varies depending on the strength of the breathing. It takes time and practice to master this technique with proper breathing and body movements.

1 Samasthithi /Tadasana

1. Always begin the practice with this pose.
2. This is the way to ready the body for a series of asanas and remain mindful while doing the series of poses.

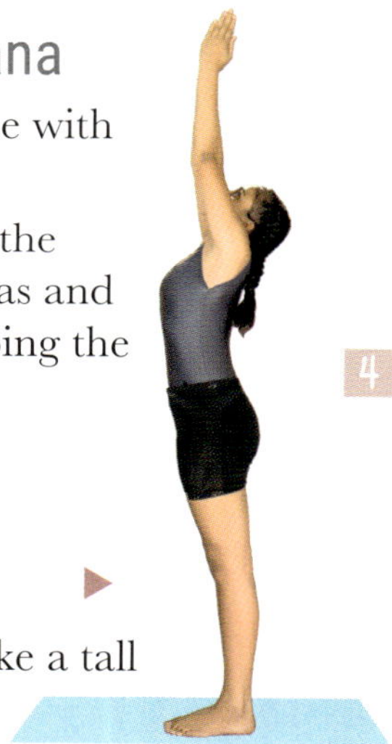

2 Urdwa Hastasana

1. Raise hands and stand like a tall pillar.
2. Inhale and bring the arms up over the head in a namaste.
3. Keep the shoulders relaxed.

3 Uttanasana – Head To Knee Pose

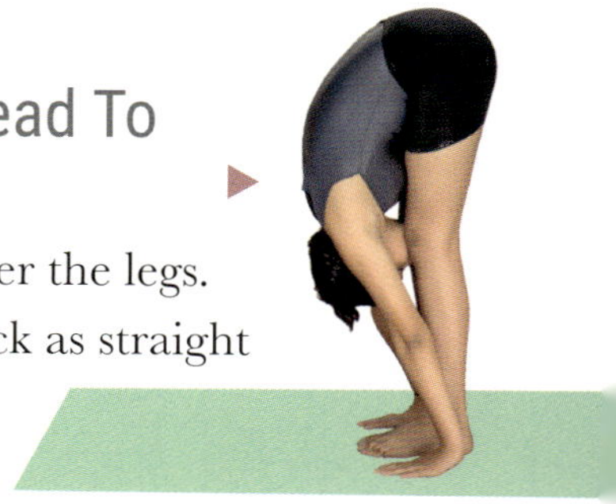

1. Exhale and fold over the legs.
2. Try to keep the back as straight as possible.

4 Chatushpadasana – Bear Pose

1. Inhale.
2. Look up keeping the back straight and jump or step back, holding inhaled breath for a second.

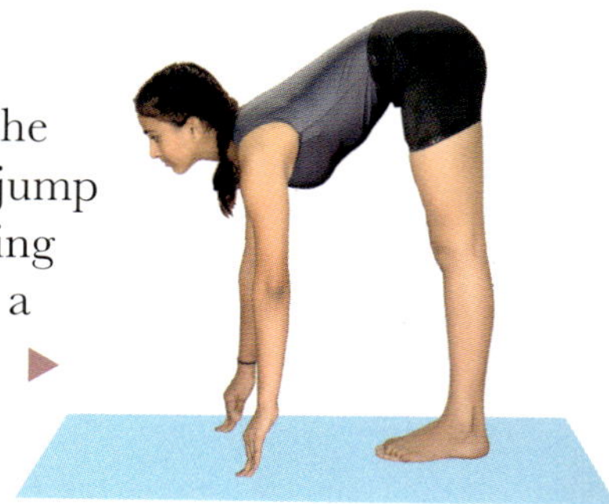

5 Chaduranga Dandasana – Plank Pose

1. Exhale.
2. Keep the palms flat on the ground and hold the pose with strength.
3. Then slide towards the floor.

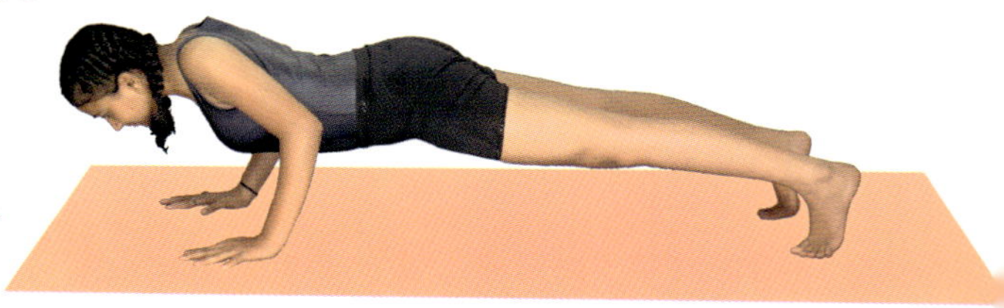

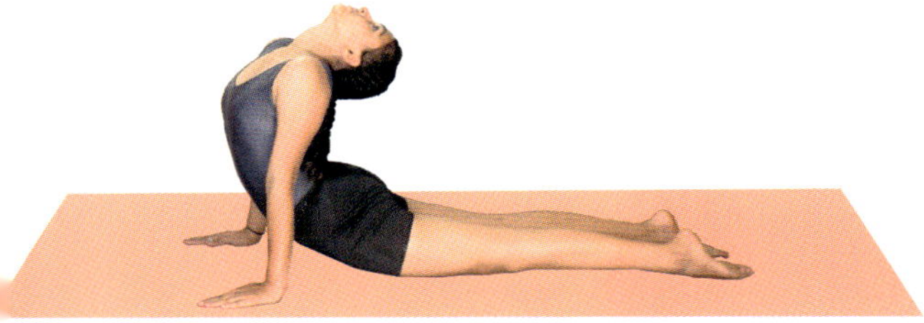

6 Urdwa Mukha Swanasana – Upward Facing Dog Pose

1. Inhale.
2. Now, slide forward and straighten the arms up and then lift the spine.
3. Keep the chest open towards the ceiling.

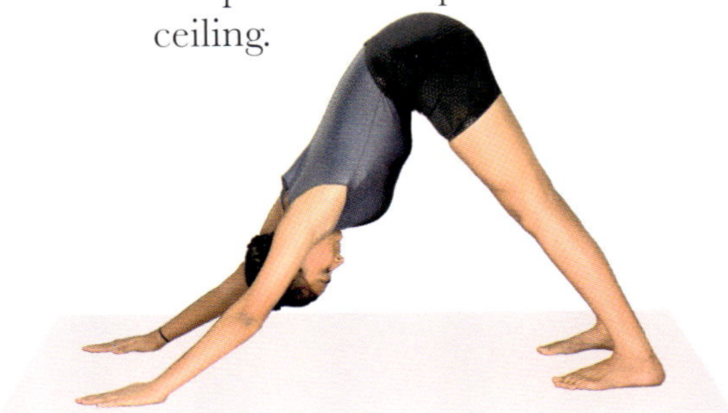

7 Adho Mukha Svanasana – Downward Facing Dog Pose

1. Exhale.
2. Roll back lifting the hip up towards the ceiling and with strength press the palms to the floor.
3. Let the head and length of the arms slide towards the hip.
4. Engage the thighs and observe the weight of the body move away from the arms.

8 Uttanasana – Move Forward Head To Knee Pose

1. Exhale.
2. Jump or step forward.
3. Try to keep the back and knees as straight as possible.

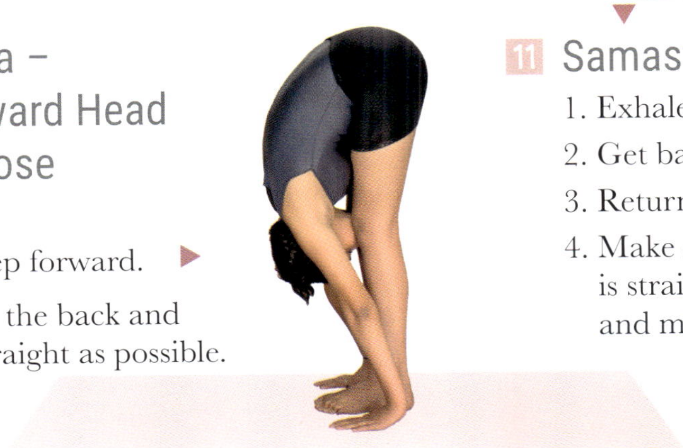

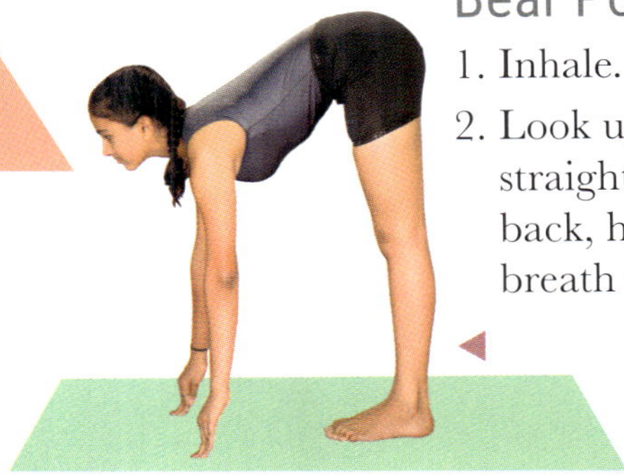

9 Chatushpadasana – Bear Pose

1. Inhale.
2. Look up keeping the back straight and jump or step back, holding the inhaled breath for a second.

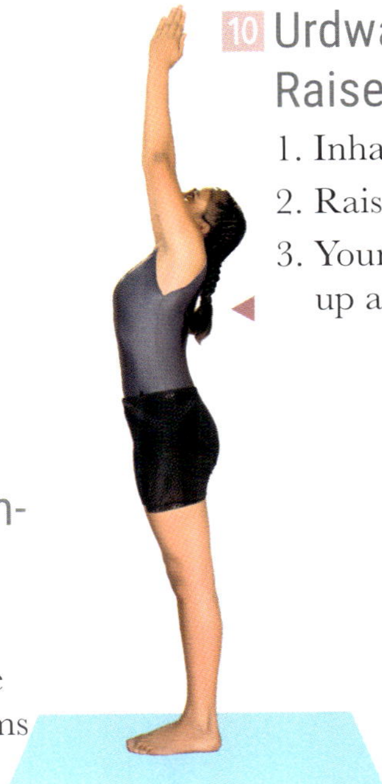

10 Urdwa Hastasana – Raised Hands Tall Pillar

1. Inhale
2. Raise hands.
3. Your gaze should be looking up at your namaste.

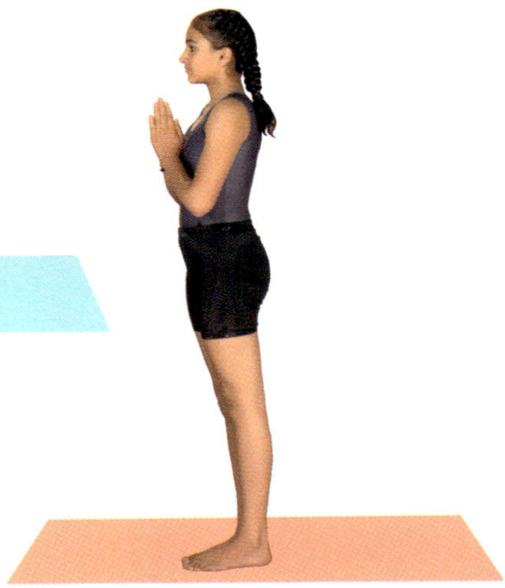

11 Samasthithi /Tadasana

1. Exhale.
2. Get back to pose number one.
3. Return the arms to the sides.
4. Make sure every part of the body is straight and the mind is alert and mindful.

SURYA NAMASKARA B

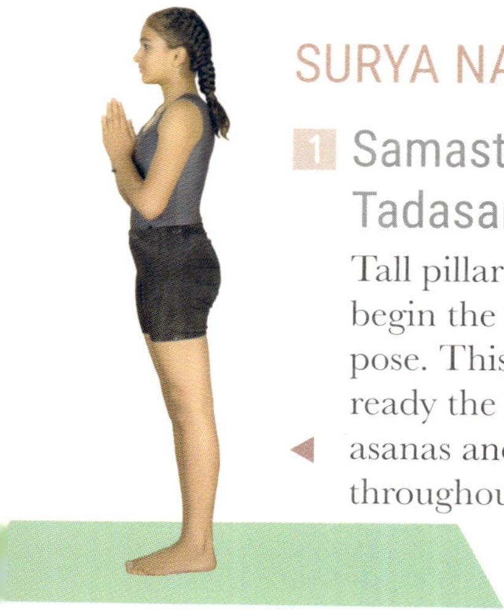

1 Samasthithi / Tadasana

Tall pillar pose. Always begin the practice with this pose. This is the way to ready the body for a series of asanas and remain mindful throughout.

2 Utkatasana – Chair Pose

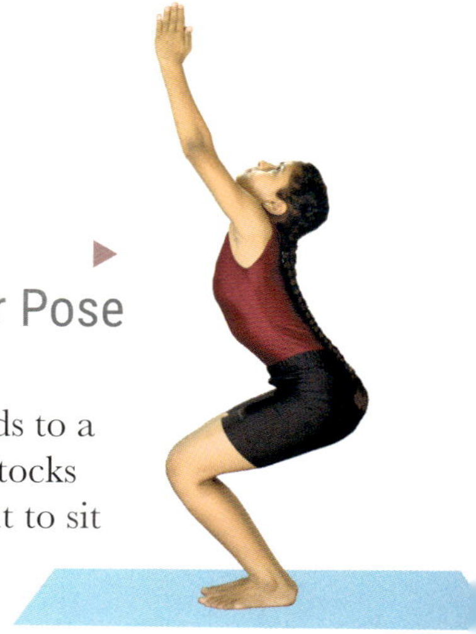

1. Inhale.
2. Bend knees, raise hands to a namaste and push buttocks back like you are about to sit on a chair.

3 Pada Hastasana – Head To Knee Pose

1. Exhale and fold over the legs.
2. Try to keep the back as straight as possible.

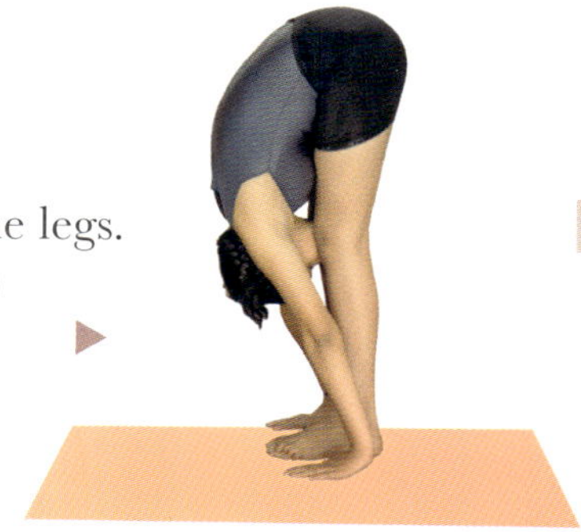

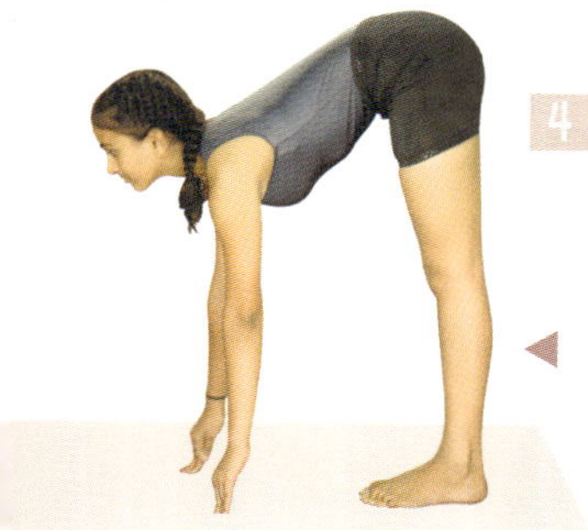

4 Chatushpadasana – Bear Pose

1. Inhale.
2. Look up keeping the back straight and jump or step back, holding inhaled breath for a second.

5 Chaduranga Dandasana – Plank Pose

1. Exhale.
2. Keep the palms flat on the ground and hold the pose with strength. Then slide towards the floor.

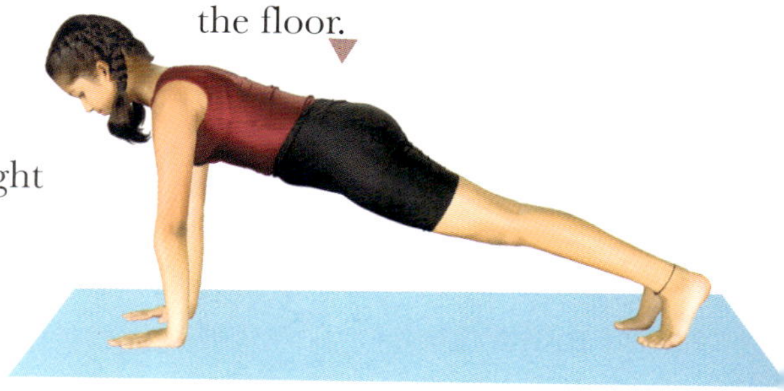

6 Urdwa Mukha Swanasana – Upward Facing Dog Pose

1. Inhale.
2. Now, slide forward and straighten the arms up and then lift the spine. Keep the chest open towards the ceiling.

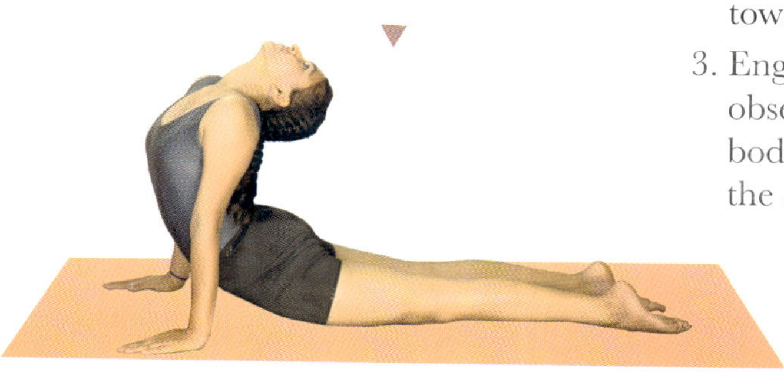

7 Adho Mukha Svanasana – Downward Facing Dog Pose

1. Exhale. Roll back lifting the hip up towards the ceiling and pressing the palms with strength to the floor.
2. Let the head and length of the arms slide towards the hip.
3. Engage the thighs and observe the weight of the body move away from the arms.

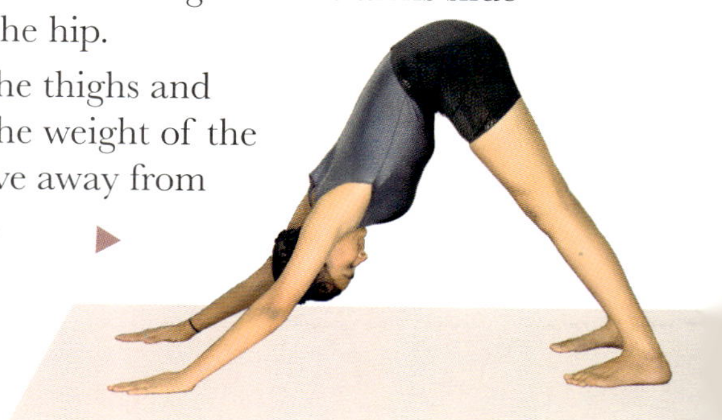

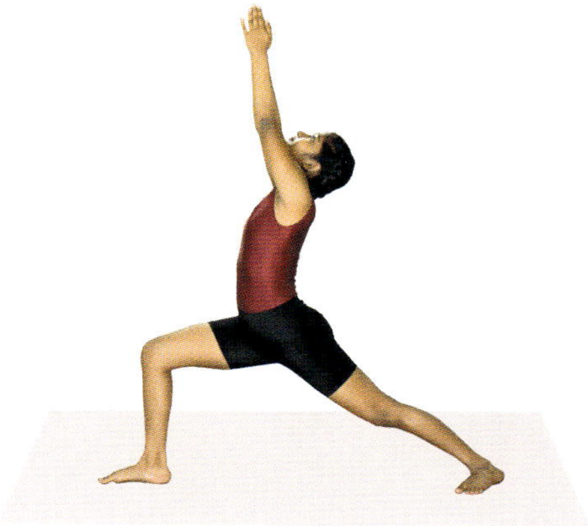

8 Veerabadhrasa – Warrior 3 Pose (Right)

1. Put the right leg forward next to the right hand. Bend the right leg so that the thigh is parallel to the floor.
2. Drop both the heels firmly to the floor and lift the hands above the head in a namaste.

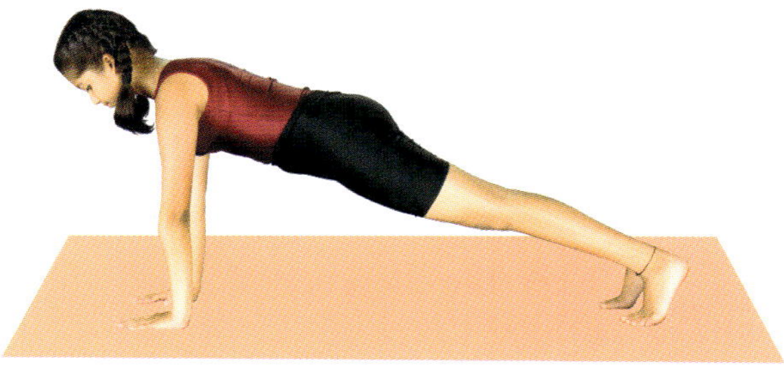

9 Chaduranga Dandasana – Plank Pose

Exhale. Keep the palm flat on the ground and hold the pose with strength and slide towards the floor.

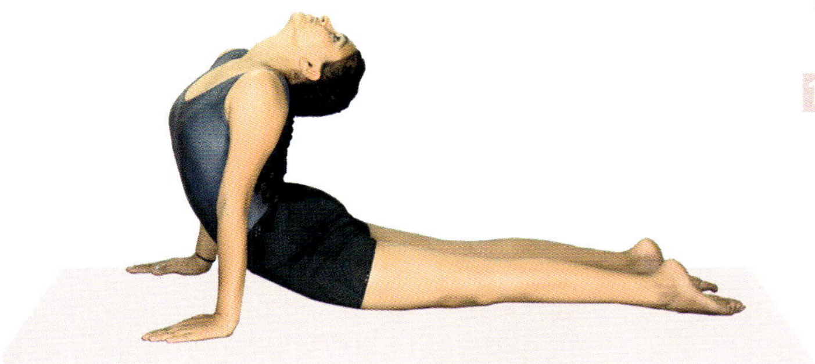

10 Urdwa Mukha Swanasana – Upward Facing Dog Pose

1. Inhale.
2. Now, slide forward and straighten the arms up and the lift the spine.
3. Keep the chest open towards the ceiling.
4. Shoulders should stay over the wrists.

11 Adho Mukha Svanasana – Downward Facing Dog Pose

Exhale. Roll back, lifting the hip up towards the ceiling and pressing the palms with strength to the floor. Let the head and length of the arms slide towards the hip. Engage the thighs and observe the weight of the body move away from the arms.

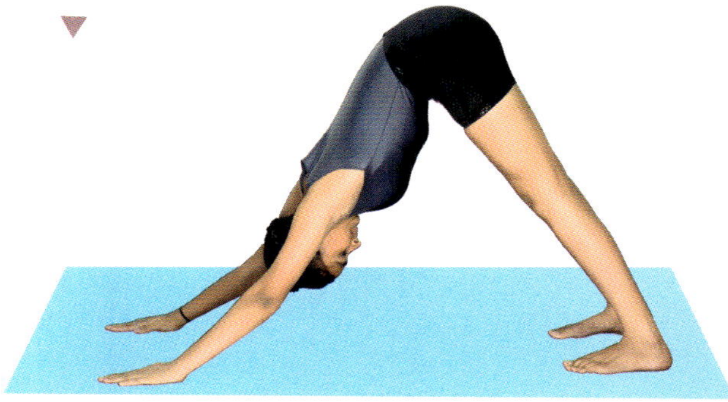

12 Veerabadhrasa – Warrior 3 Pose (Left)

1. Put the left leg forward next to the left hand. Bend the left leg so that the thigh is parallel to the floor.
2. Drop both the heels firmly to the floor and lift the hands above the head in a namaste.

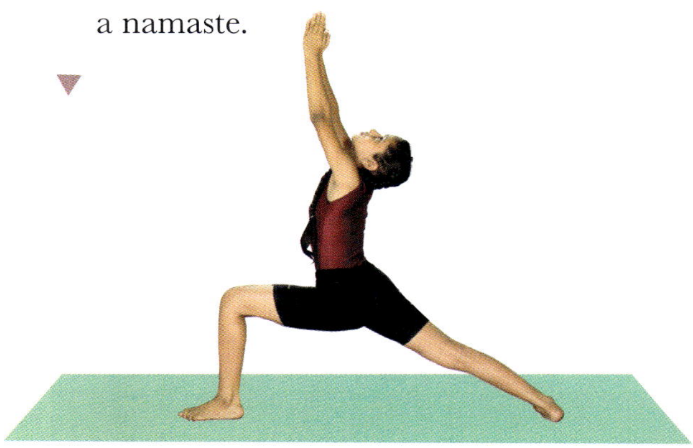

13 Chaduranga Dandasana – Plank Pose

Exhale. Keep the palms flat on the ground and hold the pose with strength and slide towards the floor.

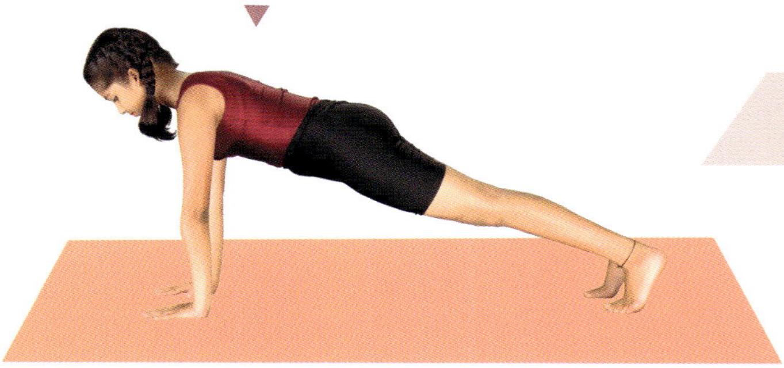

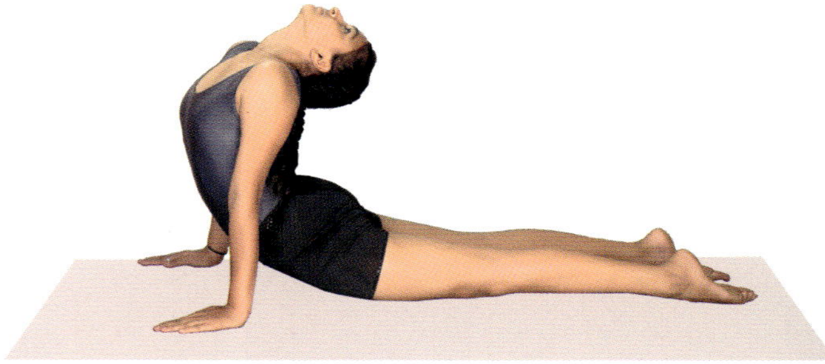

14 Urdwa Mukha Swanasana – Upward Facing Dog Pose

1. Inhale.
2. Now, slide forward and straighten the arms up and the lift the spine.
3. Keep the chest open towards the ceiling.
4. Shoulders should stay over the wrists.

15 Adho Mukha Svanasana – Downward Facing Dog Pose

Exhale. Roll back, lifting the hip up towards the ceiling and pressing the palms with strength to the floor. Let the head and length of the arms slide towards the hip. Engage the thighs and observe the weight of the body move away from the arms.

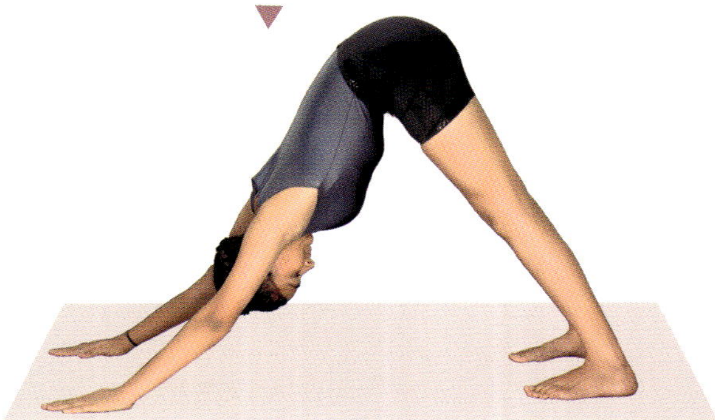

16 Chatushpadasana – Bear Pose

1. Inhale.
2. Look up keeping the back straight and jump or step back, holding inhaled breath for a second.

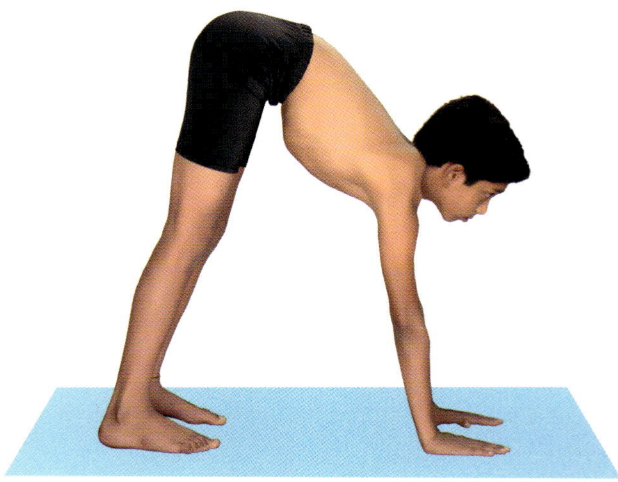

PRECAUTIONS

Surya Namaskara should be skipped if:

- The body is strained with fever.
- The body is recovering from fever.
- The body is recovering from an upset stomach.
- During menstruation.

17 Pada Hastasana – Head To Knee Pose

1. Exhale and fold over the legs.
2. Try to keep the back as straight as possible.

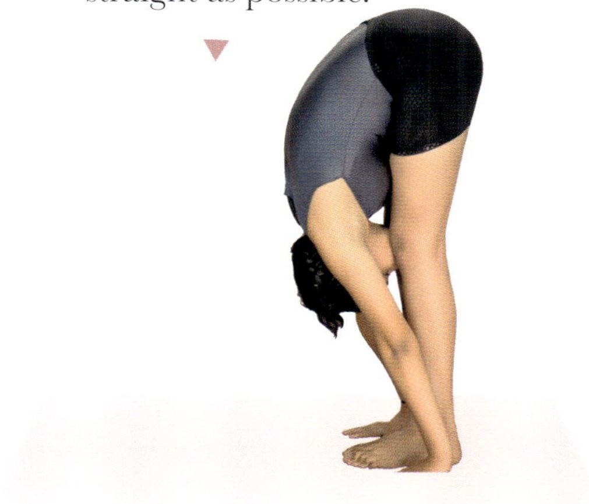

18 Utkatasana – Chair Pose

1. Inhale.
2. Bend knees, raise hands to a namaste and push buttocks back like you are about to sit on a chair.

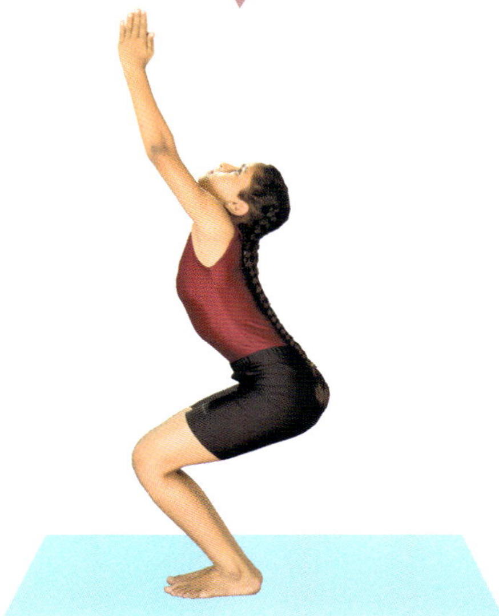

19 Urdwa Hastasana – Raised Hands Tall Pillar

1. Inhale
2. Raise your hands. Your gaze should be looking up at your namaste.

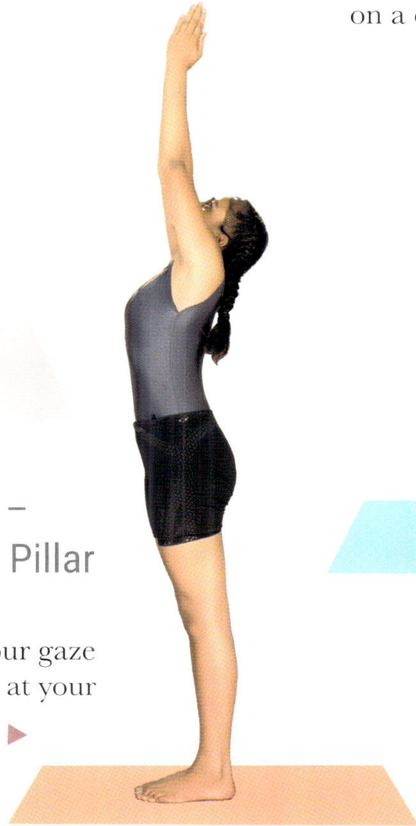

NOTE FROM THE ACHARYA

- Surya Namaskara is best done during sunrise and sunset.
- It should be done on an empty stomach.
- The body should be warmed up well. For warm ups you can do the following:

1. Soft jumps like you are skipping – 60 times.
2. Sit ups – 20 times.
3. Swinging arms from left to right – 10 times.
4. Circling arms like swimming (Breast stroke style) – 10 times.
5. Circling hips clockwise 10. times and anti-clockwise 10 times
6. Spot jogging 30 times.

20 Samasthithi /Tadasana

1. Exhale.
2. Get back to pose number one.
3. Return the arms to the sides.
4. Make sure every part of the body is straight and the mind is alert.

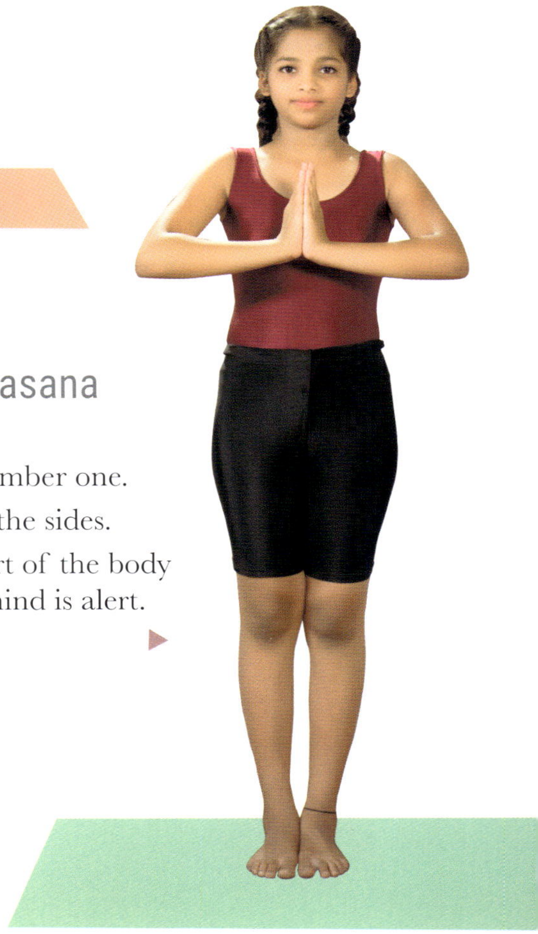

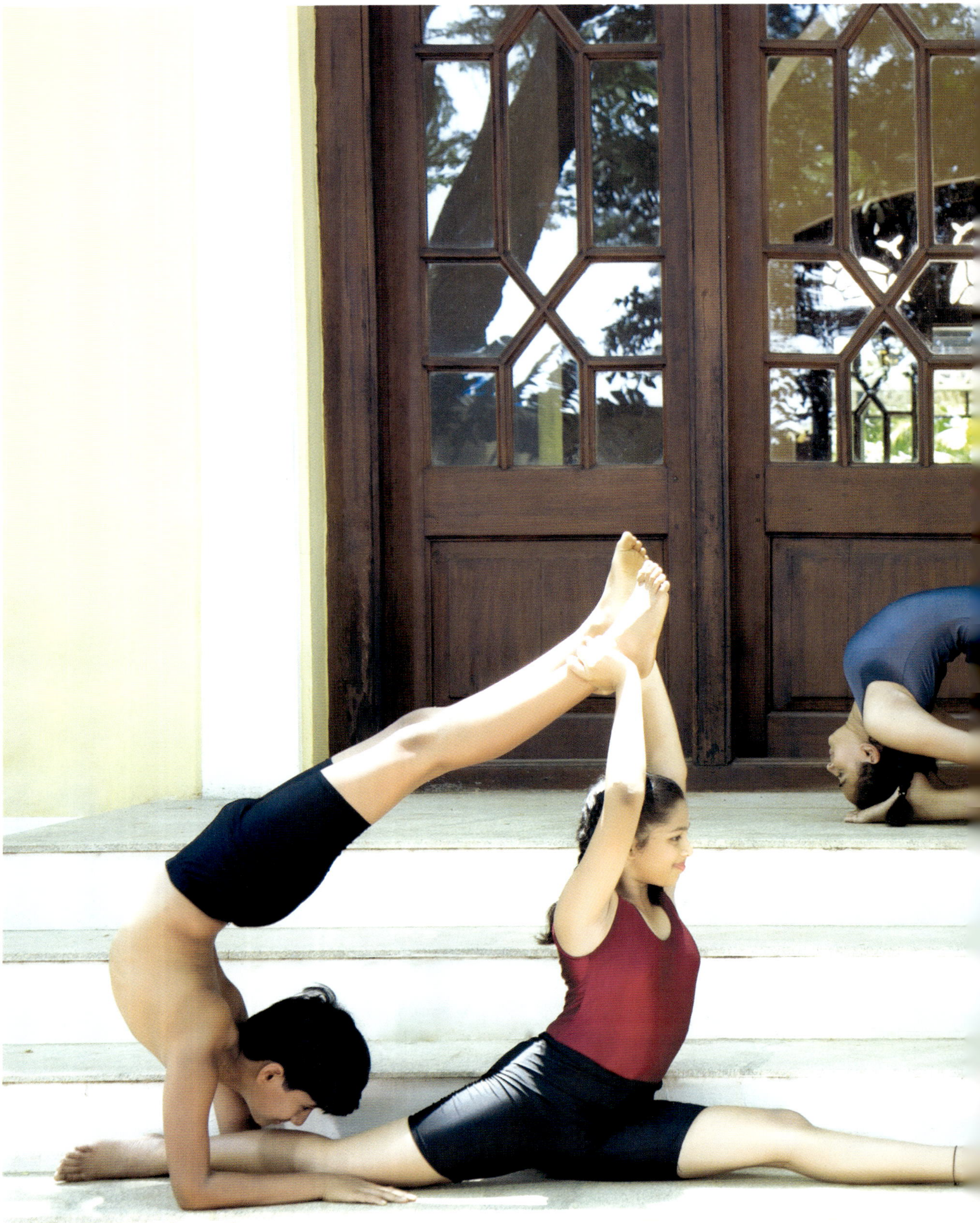

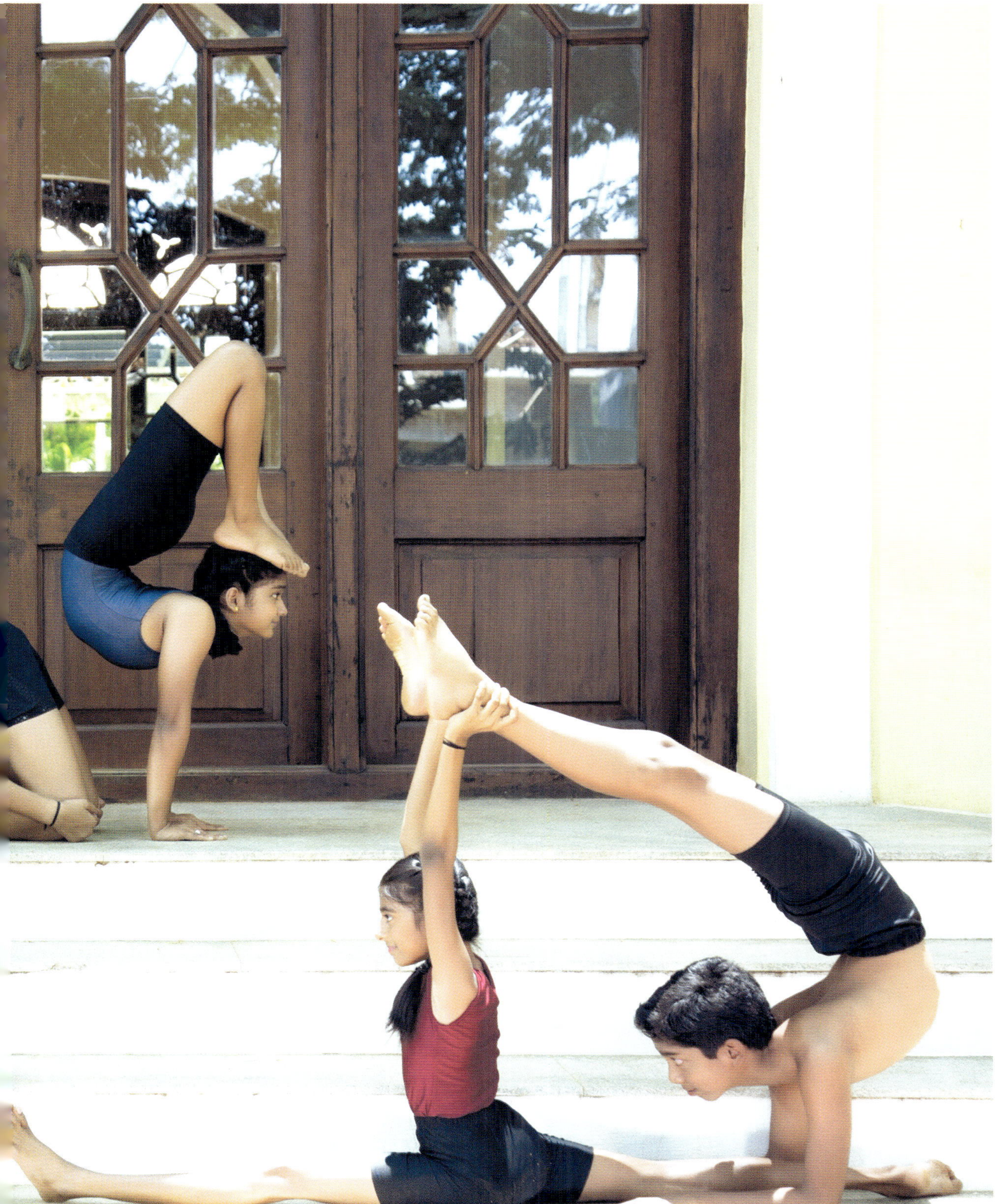

GROUP VRICHIKASANA

TADASANA/SAMASTHITHI (Pillar Pose)

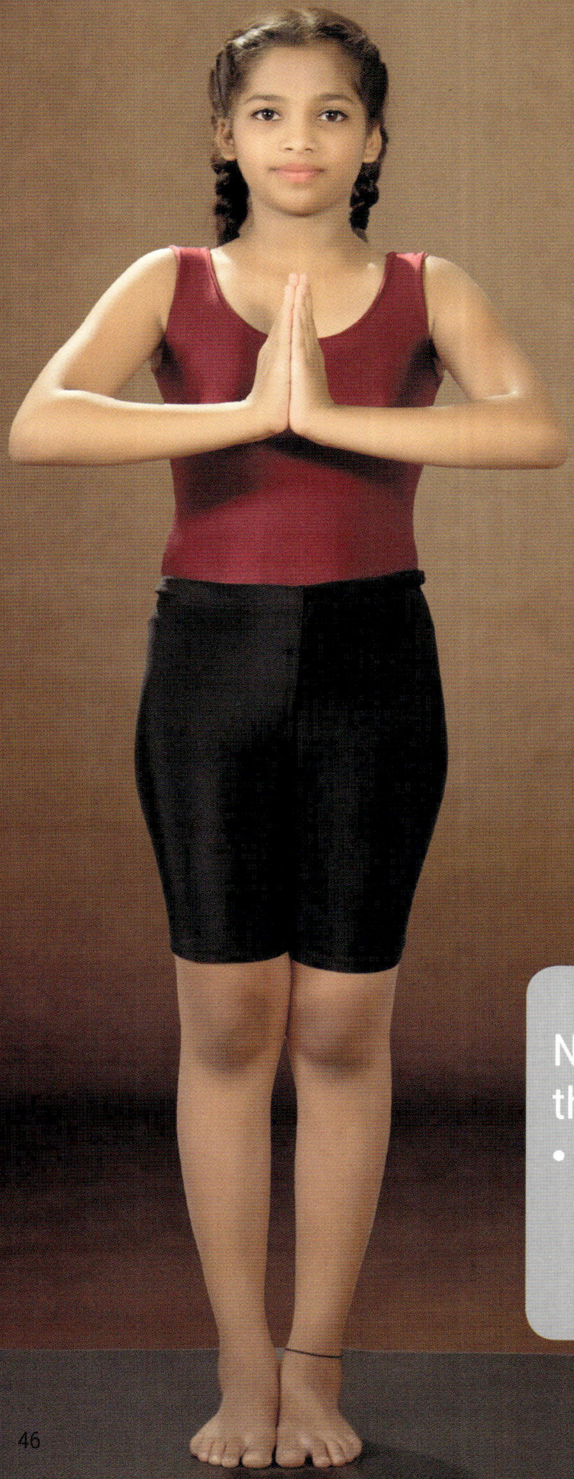

PREPARE – Ready!

- Keep the body straight and look straight ahead.
- Keep the eyes calm and fix the gaze to a point in the front.

CONSTRUCT – Steps

1. Start by paying attention to the toes.
2. Make sure the big toe is touching the ground.
3. Raise the body up on to the toes and open up the toes like a paper fan.
4. Rotate the thighs inwards which will open up the hips.
5. Keep the buttocks pressed tight.

BENEFITS – WOW!

- Builds up intention for the practice
- Helps focus on breathing and asanas to follow
- Aligns posture and makes the body feel calm and strong

Note from the Acharya

- Always begin any asana routine from a Samasthithi.

Relax–Steps

- Release muscular tension from the length of the body.
- Relax the gaze.

URDWA HASTASANA (Tall Pillar Pose)

PREPARE – READY!

- Keep the body straight and look straight ahead.
- Keep the eyes calm and fix the gaze to a point in the front.

BENEFITS – WOW!

- Helps maintain posture
- Lifts the midriff up and creates space and movement for the diaphragm
- Expands the chest and allows deep breathing
- Lengthens the spine and aids growth

CONSTRUCT – Steps

1. Start by paying attention to the toes.
2. Make sure the big toe is touching the ground.
3. Raise the body up on to the toes and open up the toes like a paper fan.
4. Rotate the thighs inwards which will open up the hips.
5. Keep the buttocks pressed tight.

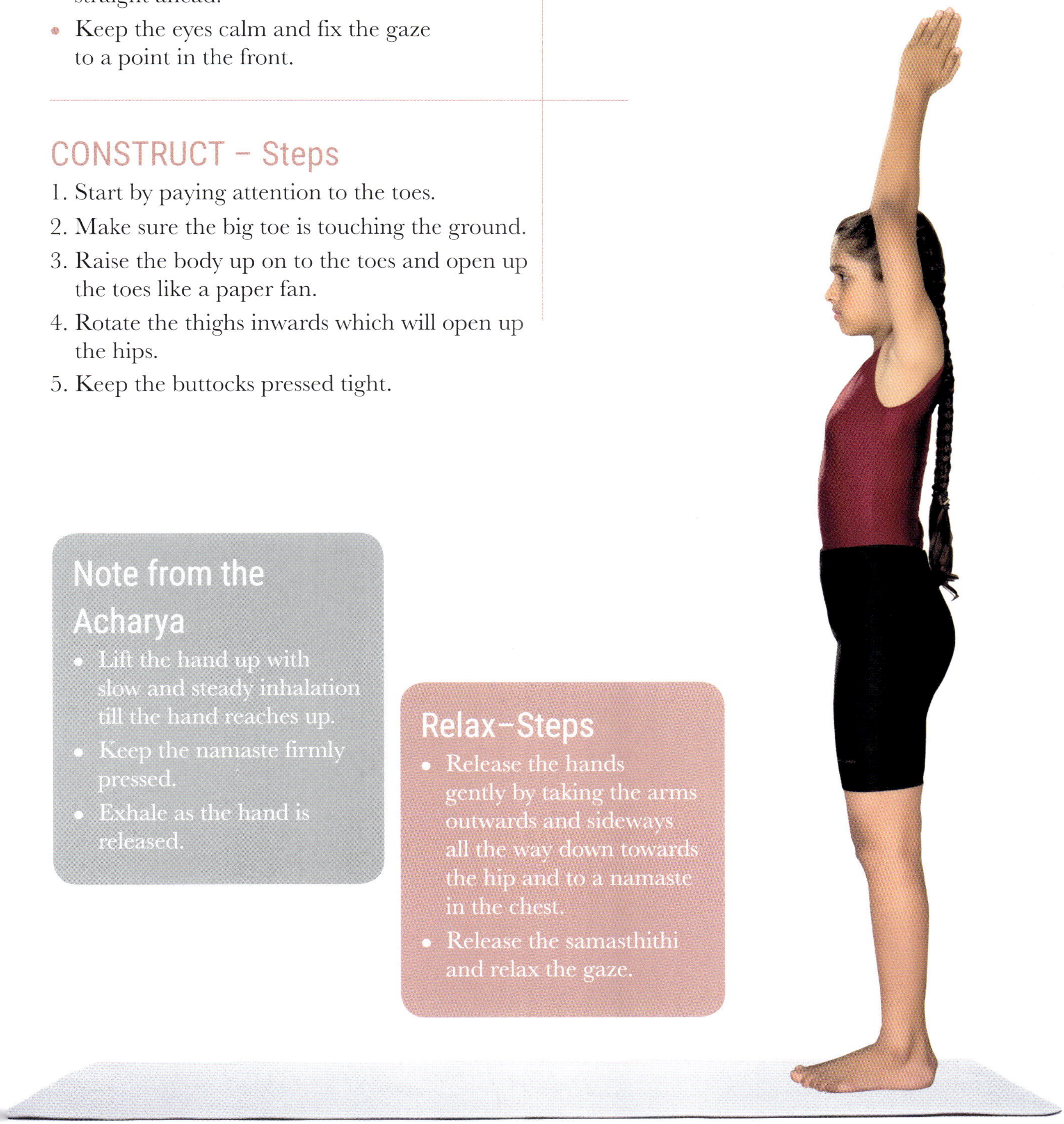

Note from the Acharya

- Lift the hand up with slow and steady inhalation till the hand reaches up.
- Keep the namaste firmly pressed.
- Exhale as the hand is released.

Relax–Steps

- Release the hands gently by taking the arms outwards and sideways all the way down towards the hip and to a namaste in the chest.
- Release the samasthithi and relax the gaze.

PURVA HASTASANA (Backward Namaste Pose)

PREPARE – Ready!

- Keep the body straight and look straight ahead.
- Keep the eyes calm and fix the gaze to a point in the front.

CONSTRUCT – Steps

1. Start by paying attention to the toes.
2. Make sure the big toe is touching the ground.
3. Raise the body up on to the toes and open up the toes like a paper fan.
4. Rotate the thighs inwards which will open up the hips.
5. Keep the buttocks pressed tight.

BENEFITS – WOW!

- Opens chest and lifts the midriff up
- Expands the diaphragm and aids deep breathing
- Keeps the shoulders and wrists flexible and strong

Note from the Acharya

- Do not hunch the back.
- Keep the abdominal length pulled in.
- Keep the spine straight and tall with tailbone tucked in.
- Keep the chest lifted up and breathe deep.
- Feel the chest expand as you breathe in and try not to drop the chest down as you breathe out.

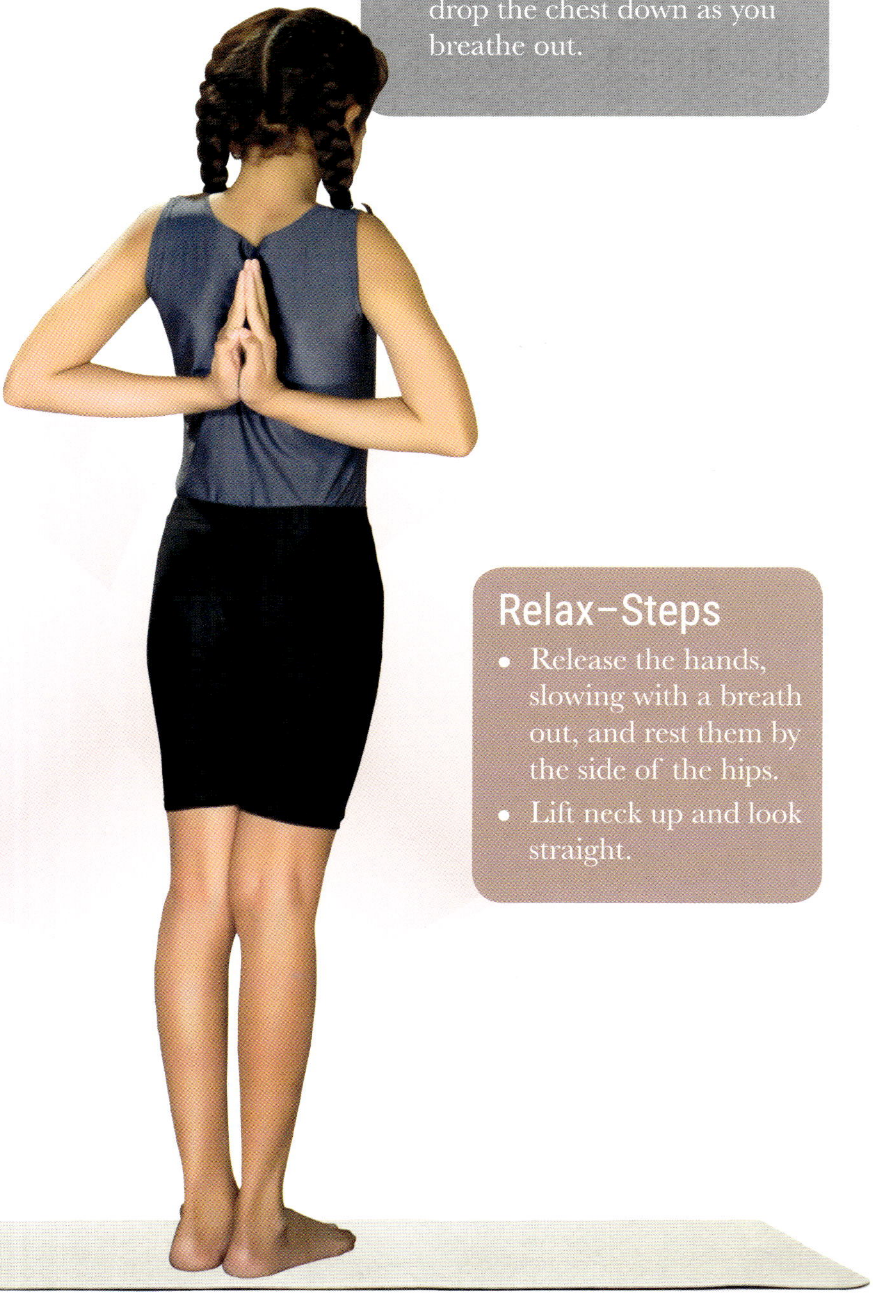

Relax–Steps

- Release the hands, slowing with a breath out, and rest them by the side of the hips.
- Lift neck up and look straight.

URDWA TADASANA (Lifted Pillar Pose)

PREPARE – Ready!

- Samasthithi
- Stand straight with feet together and pressed to the ground.
- Stomach pulled in and buttocks tucked in.
- Shoulders open and chest relaxed.
- Head in line with the shoulders.
- *Drishti* (gaze): Calmly look straight and fix your eyes to a point in front of you.
- Smile calmly and enjoy.

CONSTRUCT – Steps

- Slowly and steadily lift your heels off the floor and focus on balance.
- When you are balanced, open your arms from the sides and join your palms into a namaste above the head towards the ceiling.
- Keep your eyes focused to a straight point and hold the position.
- Breathe 3 times.

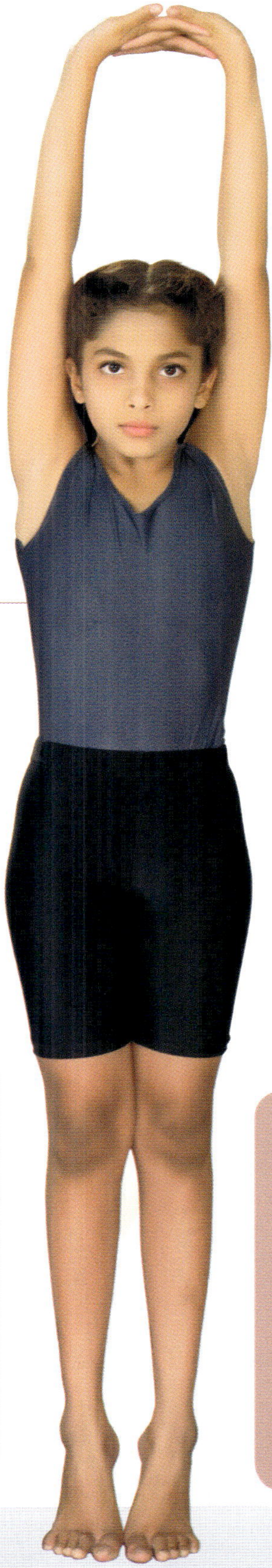

BENEFITS – WOW!

- Helps build strong legs and feet
- Lengthens the body and spine
- Helps in the overall growth of the body
- Improves focus and balance
- Engages the core for support
- Establishes balance in the right and left hemisphere of the brain

Note from the Acharya

- Keep your gaze fixed to a point even if you are losing balance.
- Do not let go the asana at least for a count of 30.
- Challenge yourself to hold the asana for a longer time.
- Stay tall and don't hunch the back or push the stomach forward.

Relax–Steps

- Gently drop the heels to the ground still with eyes focused to a point.
- Bring arms down around the sides of the body into a namaste.

ARDHACHAKRASNA (Half Wheel Pose)

PREPARE – Ready!

- Samasthithi
- Stand straight with feet together and pressed to the ground.
- Pull stomach in and tuck buttocks in.
- Open shoulders and relax chest.
- Keep head in line with the shoulders.
- Keep your *drishti* straight by fixing your eyes to a point in front of you.
- Smile calmly and enjoy.

CONSTRUCT – Steps

1. Keep looking straight as you curve the spine into a backward movement.
2. Slowly and steadily expand the chest and stretch the neck backward.
3. Press the back with hands and look upwards.
4. Gaze should be looking backwards with neck completely stretched.
5. Breathe deep 3 times.

BENEFITS – WOW!

- Helps increase the height of the body
- Expands chest and increases diaphragm strength
- Helps deep breathing
- Increases heart rate and relaxes it
- Benefits the organs around the chest area
- Strengthens the spine

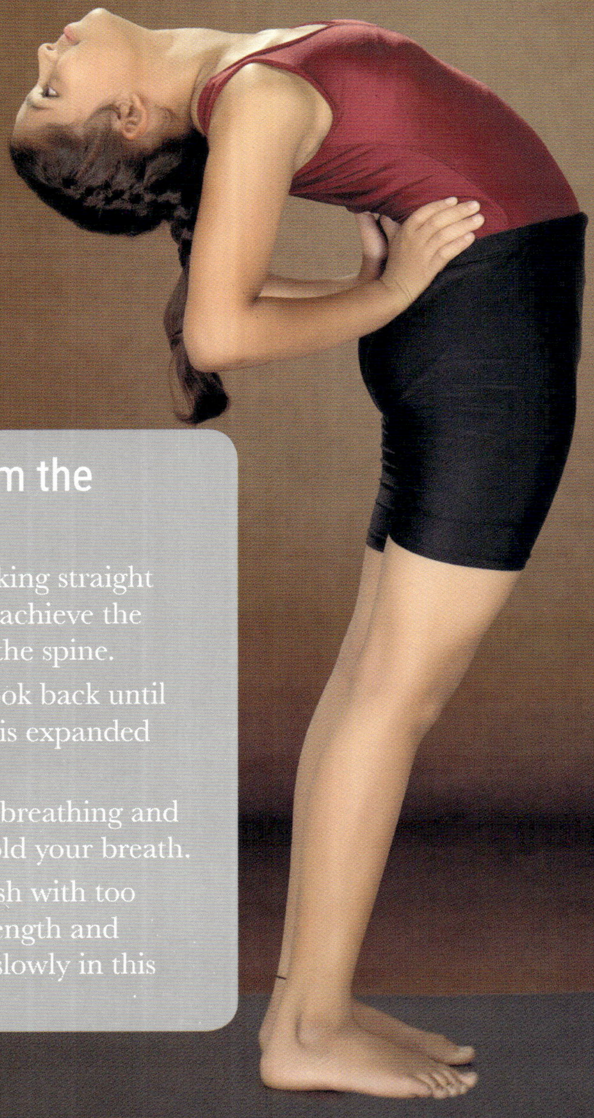

Note from the Acharya

- Keep looking straight until you achieve the curve of the spine.
- Do not look back until the chest is expanded fully.
- Focus on breathing and do not hold your breath.
- Don't push with too much strength and progress slowly in this asana.

Relax–Steps

- Release the neck position, lift the head up and point chin towards the neck.
- Slowly straighten the spine from top of the spine to the bottom.
- When the spine feels straight lift the head up to Samasthithi.

ARDHA KATI CHAKRASANA
Half-side Wheel

PREPARE – Ready!

- Samasthithi
- Stand straight with feet together and pressed to the ground.
- Pull stomach in and tuck in buttocks.
- Keep your shoulders open and chest relaxed.
- Your head should be in line with the shoulders.
- Keep your *drishti* straight by fixing your eyes to a point in front of you.
- Smile calmly and enjoy.

BENEFITS – WOW!

- Makes the spine strong and flexible
- Lengthens the spine to benefit growth
- Helps maintain strong posture.
- Helps align hips and corrects postural defects from the hips

CONSTRUCT – Steps

1. Rise hands up to do a namaste.
2. Curve trunk and extend the namaste to the right.
3. Drop the left hand to rest on the thigh.
4. Stay for 3 deep breathing.
5. Get hands back to namaste and to the centre.
6. Repeat to the other side.

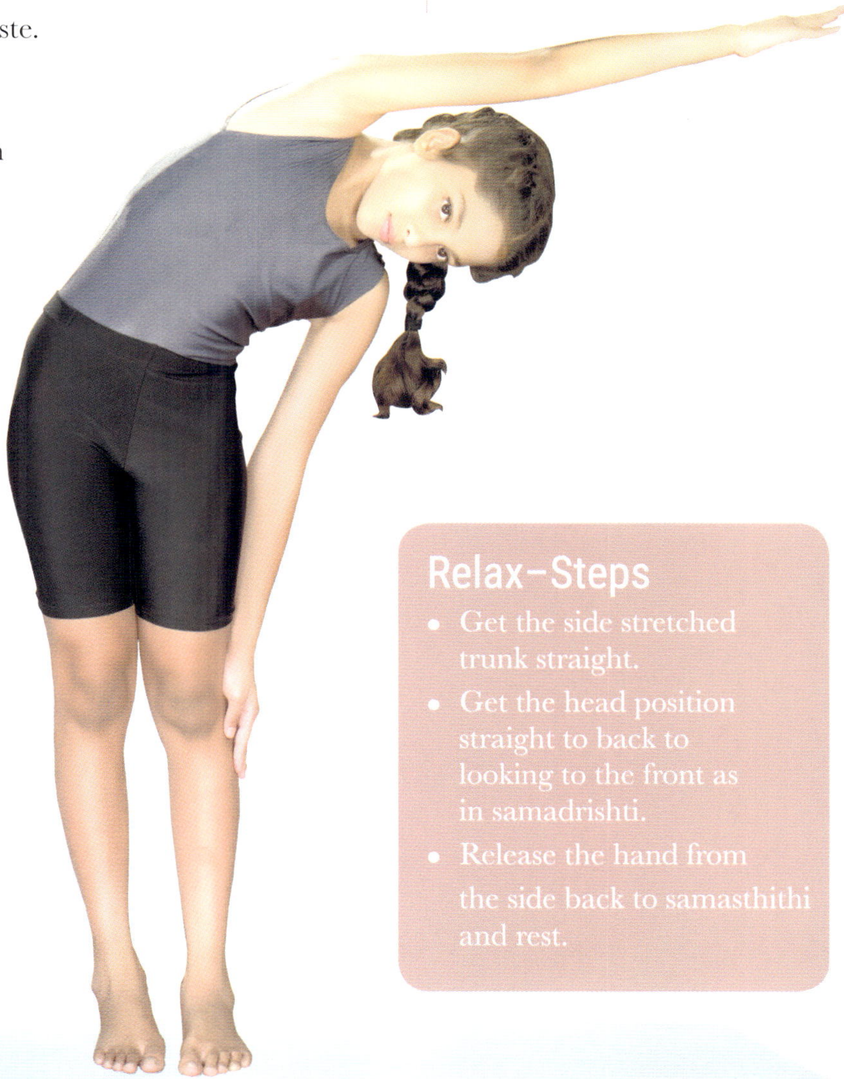

Note from the Acharya

- Do not bend forward.
- Stay comfortable, only then breathing will be easy.
- If breathing gets difficult, release the stretch and focus on breathing.

Relax–Steps

- Get the side stretched trunk straight.
- Get the head position straight to back to looking to the front as in samadrishti.
- Release the hand from the side back to samasthithi and rest.

PADA HASTASANA (Toe Hold)

PREPARE – Ready!

- Samasthithi
- From a straight line position start folding the length of the body forward.
- Keep the body parallel to the ground as far as comfortable and possible.

BENEFITS – WOW!

- Makes the body super flexible
- Engages the spine and makes it supple and strong
- Reduces baby fat around the waist and stomach
- Increases blood supply to the brain and relaxes the back
- Keeps the brain alert and sharp

CONSTRUCT – Steps

1. Stretch the hands towards the ground while pulling the stomach.
2. Try to reach the head to the knee while breathing out.
3. Keep the chest and shoulders open and press the chest towards the knees.

DID YOU KNOW

Yoga was compiled and documented only 3,000 years ago by a great Rishi called Patanjali

Note from the Acharya

- Please do not do this asana if you have a headache or pain in the back.
- Do not do this asana if your stomach is upset.
- If the blood rush into the head is too much and you feel that you are losing balance, then keep your eyes open and stay fixed until you feel better.

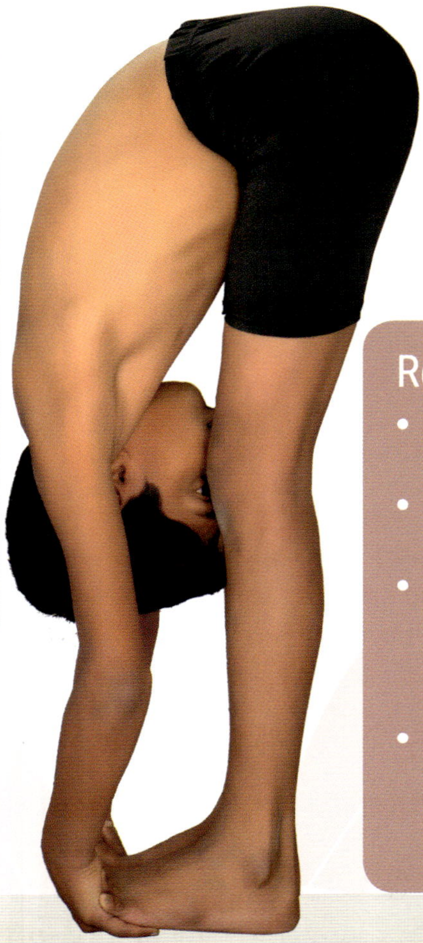

Relax–Steps

- Keep the position for 3 deep breaths.
- Relax the back and shoulders.
- Lift the body using the strong abdominal muscle while the back should remain relaxed.
- Once the entire length of the spine is up then open the shoulder and raise the head up.

Uttanasana (Head To Knee)

PREPARE – Ready!

- Samasthithi.
- Keep the feet slightly apart.
- Fold the body forward as far as possible.

BENEFITS – WOW!

- Improves flexibility of the lower spine and benefits the length of the legs
- Relaxes a tired body and rejuvenates it with fresh energy
- Activates the brain and makes it alert
- Helps remove baby fat from around the abdomen and aids digestion

CONSTRUCT – Steps

1. Get a grip of the toes.
2. Pull abdominal length in as much as possible to create a space to fold further.
3. Keep the neck relaxed.
4. Hold the position comfortably for 3 deep breaths.

Facts

The information of the practice of yoga comes from the ancient texts of the Vedas

Note from the Acharya

- This asana will progress gradually so do not push or impose too much to reach the head towards the knees.
- Do not suddenly lift the body up from the position to avoid feeling disoriented.

Relax-Steps

- Start by relaxing the back and slowly rolling up while breathing in.
- Gradually lift the head up to avoid feeling giddy.

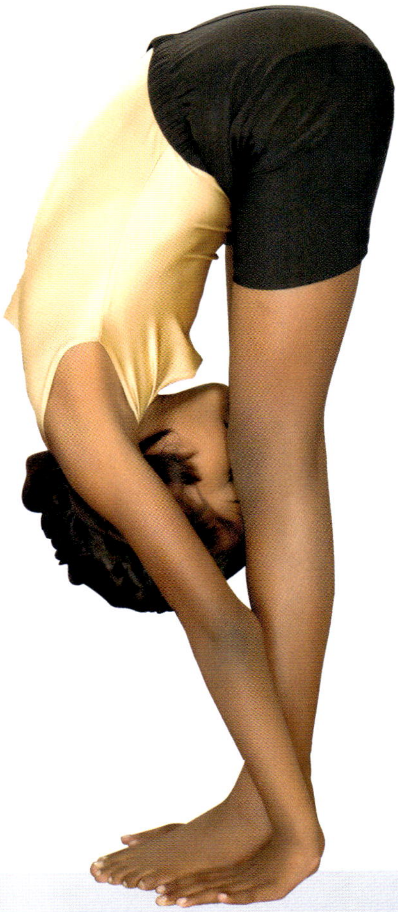

CHATUSHPADASANA (Bear Pose)

PREPARE – Ready!

- Samasthithi
- Keep the feet slightly apart.
- Fold the body forward and reach the ground.

CONSTRUCT – Steps

1. Walk the palms forward till the body is parallel to the ground.
2. Pull your abdominal length in and keep it strong.
3. Keep the neck relaxed and gaze on the ground.
4. Hold the position comfortably for 3 deep breaths.

BENEFITS – WOW!

- Improves flexibility of the lower spine and benefits the length of the legs
- Relaxes the tired body and rejuvenates it with fresh energy
- Activates the brain and makes it alert
- Helps remove baby fat from around the abdomen and aids digestion
- Strengthens back

Relax–Steps

- Start by relaxing the back and slowly roll up while breathing in.
- Gradually lift the head up to avoid feeling giddy.

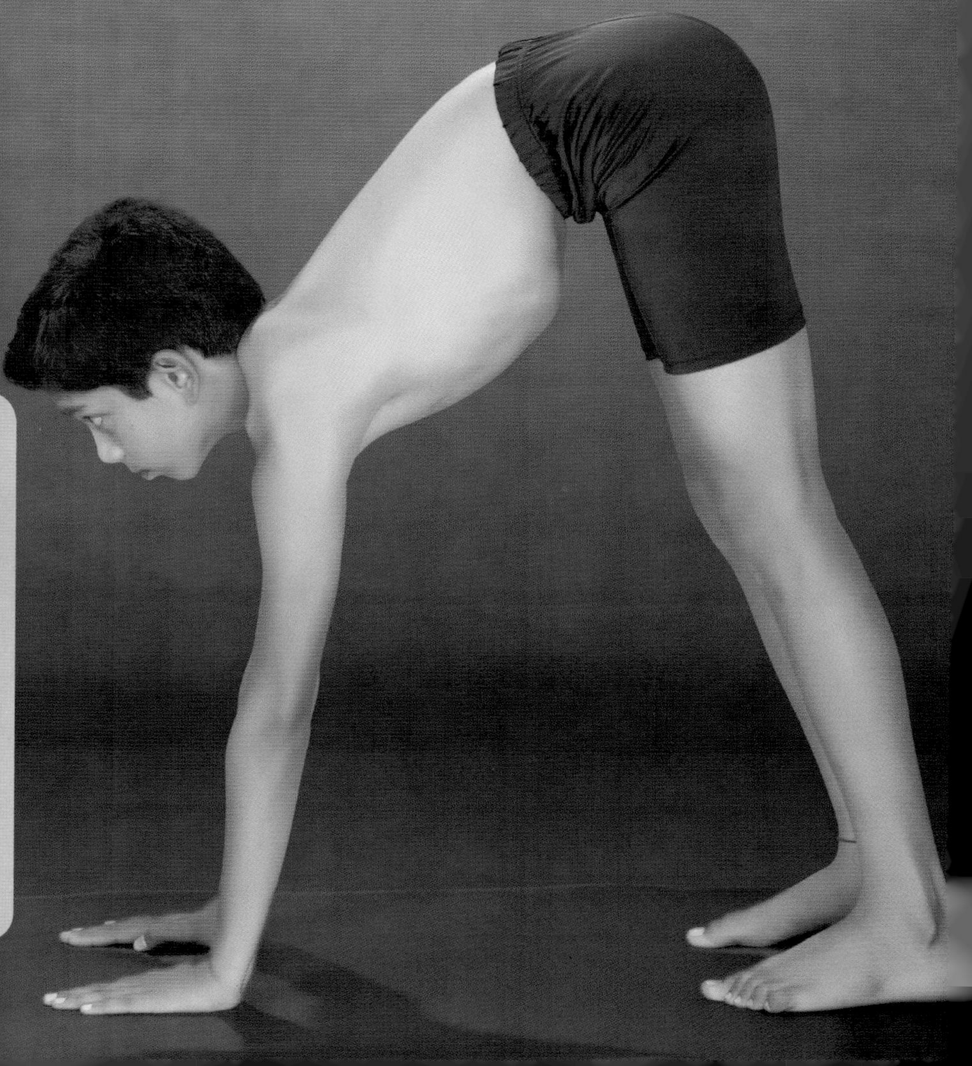

Note from the Acharya

- This asana will progress gradually.
- If it is difficult to reach the hand to the floor, slightly bend the knees but keep the back straight.
- Keep the spine steady without moving.

UTKATTASANA1 - Chair Pose

PREPARE – Ready!

- Samasthithi.
- Stand straight with feet together and pressed to the ground.
- Pull stomach in and tuck in buttocks.
- Keep your shoulders open and chest relaxed.
- Your head should be in line with the shoulders.
- Keep your *drishti* straight by fixing your eyes to a point in front of you.
- Smile calmly.

BENEFITS – WOW!

- Strengthens abdominal muscles
- Strengthens the legs
- Lengthens the spine and trims the waist
- Builds balance and focus
- Expands the chest for efficient respiration
- Benefits the abdominal organs

CONSTRUCT – Steps

1. Keep the feet firmly on the ground with your gaze straight.
2. Start bending the knees keeping the abdominal length strong.
3. Keep the heels pressed to the ground and thighs strong.
4. Establish a good balance without curving the spine.
5. Stay in position for 30 seconds.

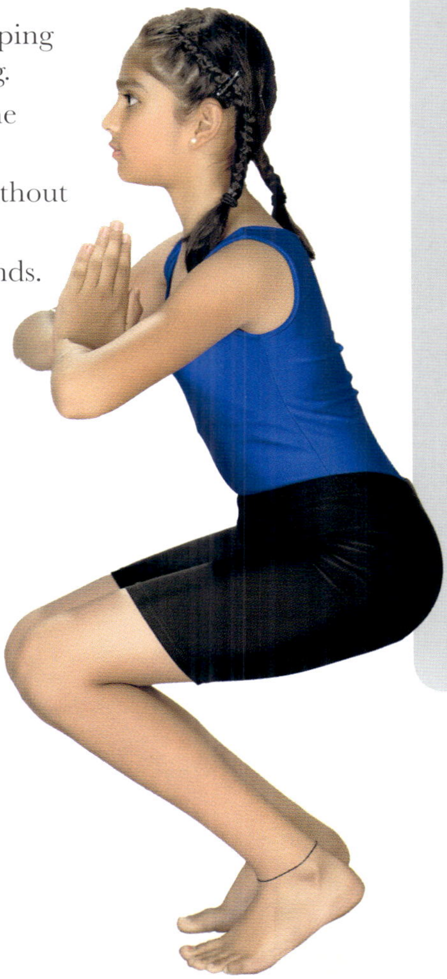

Note from the Acharya

- This asana is slightly painful.
- Do not snap or suddenly come out of the asana.
- Release the pain slowly and enjoy the feel of blood circulation along the length of the legs.
- It helps if you keep smiling and enjoy the challenge of holding this highly beneficial stretch for growing kids.

Relax–Steps

- Slowly relax the abdominal hold.
- Release the thighs and gently straighten the knees.

UTKATTASANA 2 and 3 – Chair Pose 2, Chair Pose 3

PREPARE – Ready!

- Samasthithi
- Stand straight with feet together and pressed to the ground.
- Pull stomach in and tuck buttocks.
- Keep your shoulders open and chest relaxed.
- Your head should be in line with the shoulders.
- Keep your *drishti* straight by fixing your eyes to a point in front of you.
- Smile calmly and enjoy.

BENEFITS – WOW!

- Strengthens abdominal muscles
- Strengthens the legs
- Lengthens the spine and trims the waist
- Builds balance and focus
- Expands the chest for efficient respiration
- Benefits the abdominal organs

CONSTRUCT – Steps

1. Keep the feet firmly on the ground with the gaze straight.
2. Start bending the knees keeping the abdominal length strong.
3. Keep the heels pressed to the ground and thighs strong.
4. Establish a good balance without curving the spine.
5. Stay in position for 30 seconds.

Note from the Acharya

- This asana is slightly painful.
- Do not snap or suddenly come out of the asana.
- Release the pain slowly and enjoy the feel of blood circulation along the length of the legs.
- It helps if you keep smiling and enjoy the challenge of holding this highly beneficial stretch for growing kids.

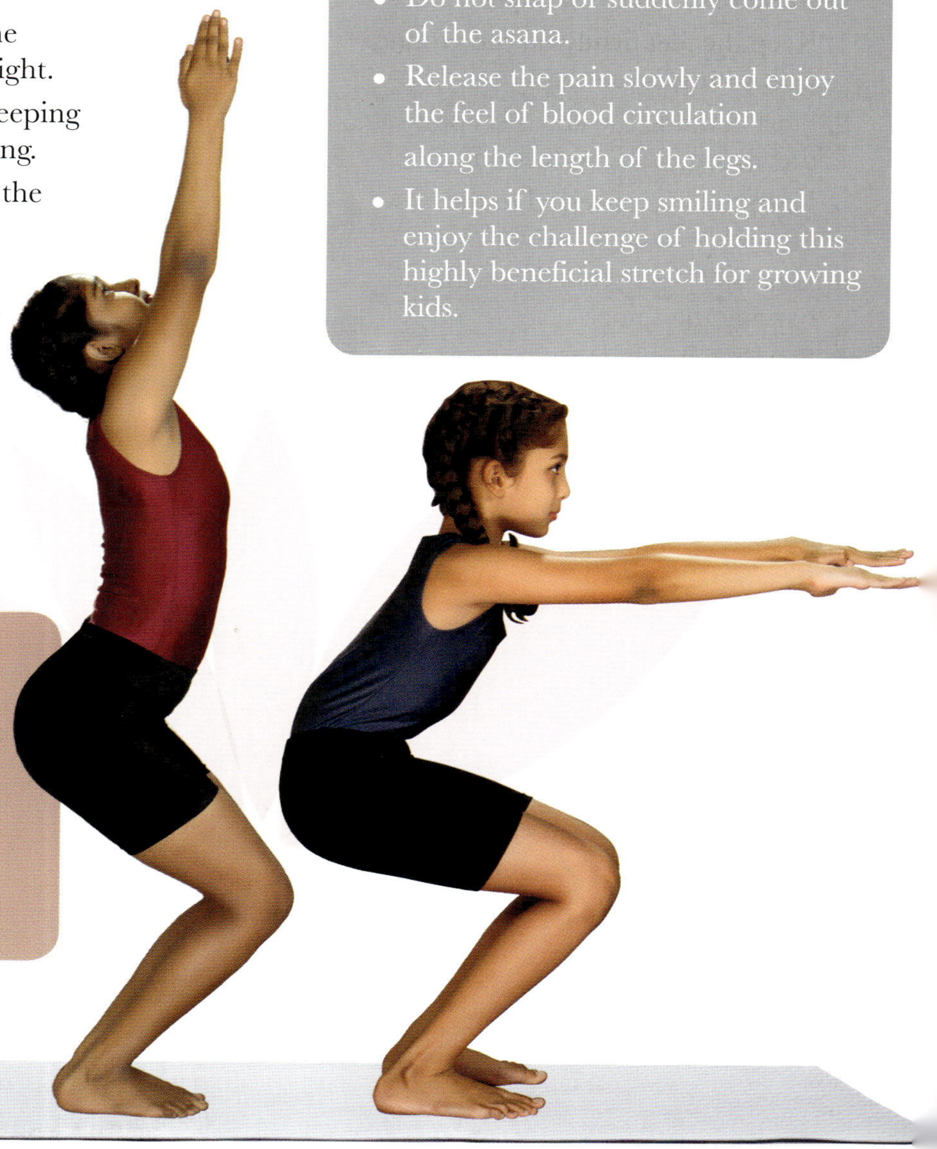

Relax–Steps

- Slowly relax the abdominal hold.
- Release the thighs and gently straighten the knees.

PARIVRITTI UTKATTASANA – (Twisted Chair Pose)

PREPARE – Ready!

- Samasthithi
- Stand straight with feet together and pressed to the ground.
- Pull stomach in and tuck in buttocks.
- Keep your shoulders open and chest relaxed.
- Your head should be in line with the shoulders.
- Keep your *drishti* straight by fixing your eyes to a point in front of you.
- Smile calmly and enjoy.

CONSTRUCT – Steps

1. Keep the feet firmly on the ground with gaze straight.
2. Start bending the knees keeping the abdominal length strong.
3. Keep the heels pressed to the ground and thighs strong.
4. Establish a good balance without curving the spine.
5. Stretch the hand in line with the shoulders and twist the waist.
6. Extend the opposite palm towards the ground across both the thighs.
7. Rest the length of the waist along the length of the thighs.
8. Stay in position for 30 seconds breathing comfortably.

Relax–Steps

- Slowly relax the abdominal hold.
- Release the twist in the waist.
- Release the thighs and gently straighten the knees.

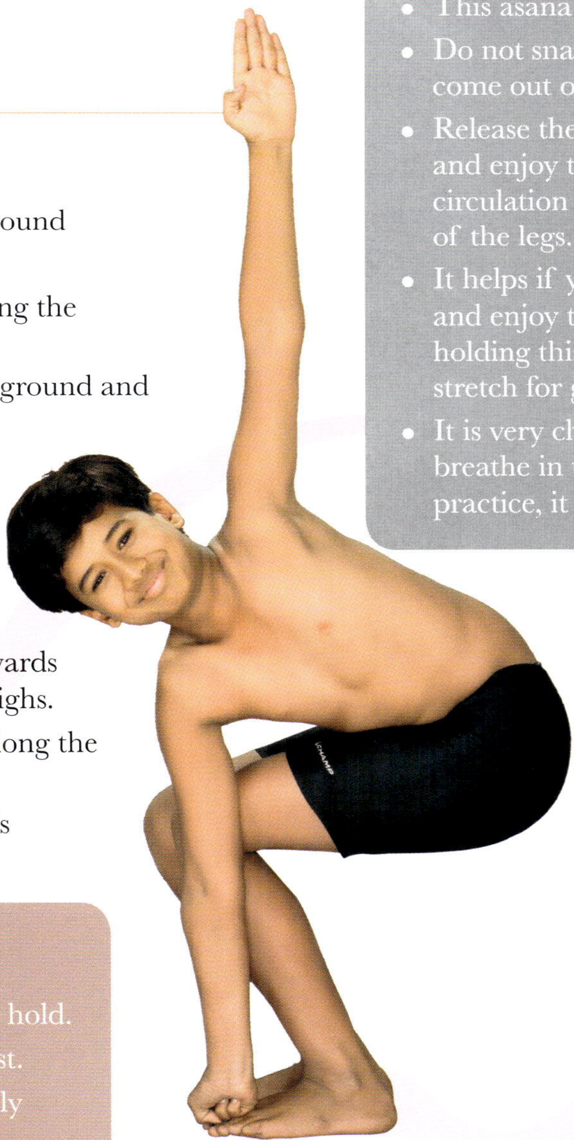

BENEFITS – WOW!

- Strengthens abdominal muscles
- Strengthens the legs
- Lengthens the spine and trims the waist
- Builds balance and focus
- Expands the chest for efficient respiration
- Benefits the abdominal organs

Note from the Acharya

- This asana is slightly painful.
- Do not snap or suddenly come out of the asana.
- Release the pain slowly and enjoy the feel of blood circulation along the length of the legs.
- It helps if you keep smiling and enjoy the challenge of holding this highly beneficial stretch for growing kids.
- It is very challenging to breathe in this asana. With practice, it will get easy.

VRIKSHASANA – (Tree Pose)

BENEFITS – WOW!

- Helps build focus and concentration in everything you do
- Helps you get stable hips, strong legs and stable feet
- Shapes your muscles and makes you grow tall
- Helps you establish a good balance in everything you do

Prepare – Ready!

- Samasthithi
- Stand straight with feet together and pressed to the ground.
- Pull stomach in and tuck buttocks.
- Keep your shoulders open and chest relaxed.
- Your head should be in line with the shoulders.
- Keep your *drishti* straight by fixing your eyes to a point in front of you.
- Smile calmly and enjoy.

Construct – Steps

1. Fold your right leg and hold your ankle with your right hand.
2. Place the feet at the top of your right thigh and place it firm. (Lift it as high as possible. Initially it is difficult and eventually with practice it gets easy.)
3. Fold hands in a namaste and wait for balance.
4. Slowly lift hands up towards the ceiling.
5. Stay and count to 20.
6. Breathe (3 times)…That's it! Done!
7. Don't forget the other side!

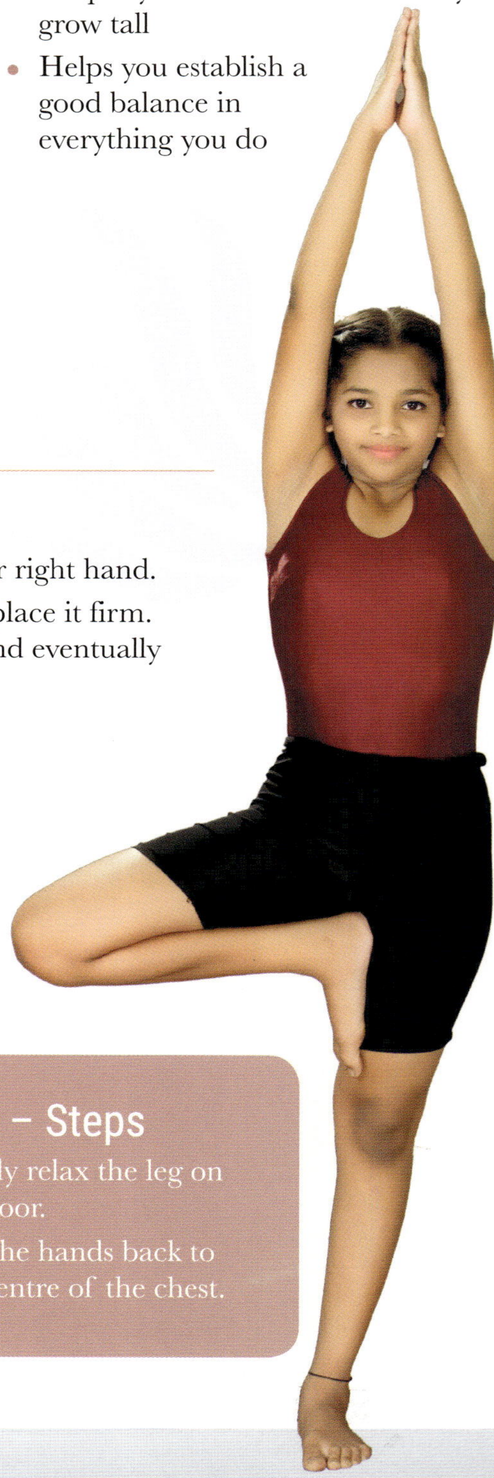

Note from the Acharya

- It's a fun asana. Can be done anywhere any time!
- Don't fall! Take support initially.
- Challenge to hold the position for 1 minute.
- Keep smiling and enjoy!

Relax – Steps

- Slowly relax the leg on the floor.
- Get the hands back to the centre of the chest.

BHADRASANA (Goddess Pose)

PREPARE – Ready!

- Samasthithi
- Stand straight with feet together and pressed to the ground.
- Pull stomach in and tuck in buttocks.
- Keep your shoulders open and chest relaxed.
- Your head should be in line with the shoulders.
- Keep your *drishti* straight by fixing your eyes to a point in front of you.
- Smile calmly and enjoy.

BENEFITS – WOW!

- Improves flexibility of the hips and increases circulation around the area
- Releases tightness in the lower back area
- Strengthens knees and legs.
- Improves digestion and assimilation of food
- Builds focus and concentration
- Helps children sit for long hours comfortably

CONSTRUCT – Steps

1. Open both feet outwards as much as possible.
2. Lift heels up and start folding the knees to squat down.
3. Half way through the squat, open up the thighs as wide as possible.
4. Let the hips sit on the heels.
5. Hold balance in this position.
6. Keep the eyes calm and focus on breathing.

Relax – Steps

- Slowly lift the hips up from the heels.
- When it is comfortable, press the feet to the ground.
- Slowly straighten the knees.
- Stand straight and work on relaxing the knees.

Note from the Acharya

- Challenging asana to hold one's balance.
- With practice, it will progress.
- Can be done any time when the back is feeling stiff after long hours of sitting or sports.
- Helps girls during menstruation to relieve stiff back and relieve cramps in the abdominal area.

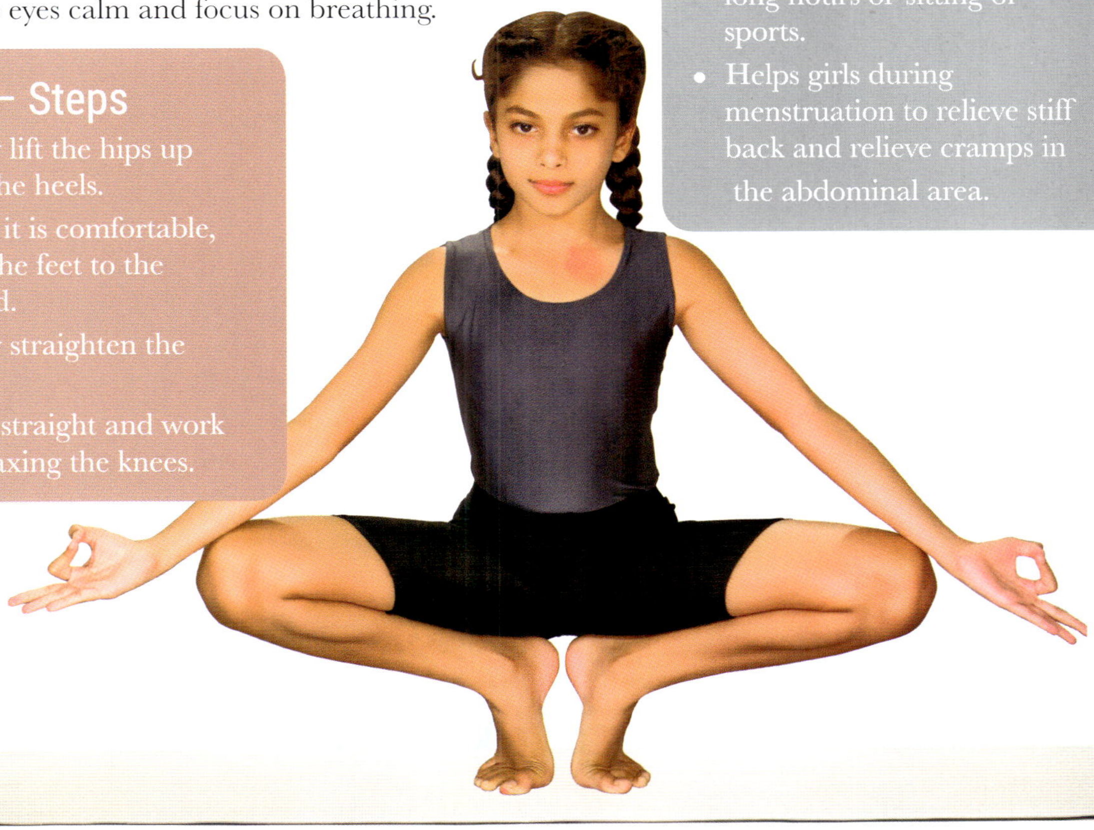

MANIPURASANA – Deep Squat Pose

PREPARE – Ready!

- Samasthithi
- Stand straight with feet together and pressed to the ground.
- Pull stomach in and tuck in buttocks.
- Keep your shoulders open and chest relaxed.
- Your head should be in line with the shoulders.
- Keep your *drishti* straight by fixing your eyes to a point in front of you.
- Smile calmly and enjoy.

BENEFITS – WOW!

- Improves flexibility of the hips and increases circulation around the area
- Releases tightness in the lower back area
- Strengthens knees and legs
- Improves digestion and assimilation of food
- Builds focus and concentration
- Helps children sit for long hours comfortably

CONSTRUCT – Steps

1. Open both feet outwards as wide as possible.
2. Fold at the knees and squat with heels pressed to the ground.
3. Halfway through the squat open up the thighs as wide as possible.
4. Let the hips sit on the calves.
5. Hold balance in this position.
6. Keep the eyes calm and focus on breathing and hands folded.

Relax – Steps

- Slowly lift the hips.
- Slowly straighten the knees and relax.

Note from the Acharya

- Keep the back straight as possible.
- With practice, it will progress.
- Can be done any time when the back is feeling stiff after long hours of sitting or after sports.
- Helps girls during menstruation to relieve stiff back and relieve cramps in the abdominal area.

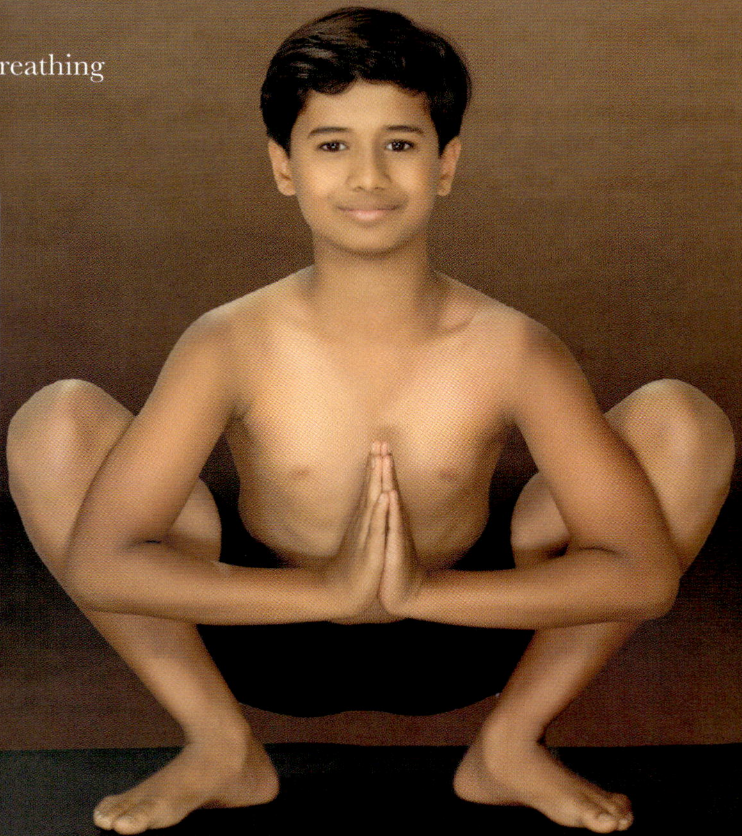

MALASANA (Garland Pose)

PREPARE – Ready!

- Squat down with thighs as open as possible. If the heels feel lifting up place a cushion under the heels.
- Keep the spine and back straight and open.
- Keep shoulders open and chest relaxed.
- Head in line with the shoulders.
- Keep your *drishti* straight by fixing your eyes to a point in front of you.
- Smile calmly and maintain deep breathing.

BENEFITS – WOW!

- Improves flexibility of the hips and increases circulation around the area
- Releases tightness in the lower back area
- Strengthens knees and legs.
- Improves digestion and assimilation of food
- Builds focus and concentration
- Helps children sit for long hours comfortably

CONSTRUCT – Steps

1. Keep feet open.
2. Keep the hips steady in a balance and open as wide as possible.
3. Keep the hands in a namaste, with elbows pushing open the thighs to the maximum.
4. Keep the chest lifted up and each time you breathe feel the chest expand strong.
5. Keep the eyes calm and focus on breathing as deep as possible.
6. Stay strong in the position.

Relax – Steps

- Relax the back and release the namaste. Let the arms rest on the floor.
- Slowly lift the hips.
- Slowly straighten the knees and relax.

Note from the Acharya

- Keep the shoulders relaxed but chest open and lifted up.
- Can be done any time, especially when the back is feeling stiff after long hours of sitting or after sports.
- Girls should not do this asana during menstruation.
- Do not do this asana while recovering from an upset stomach, indigestion or even constipation.

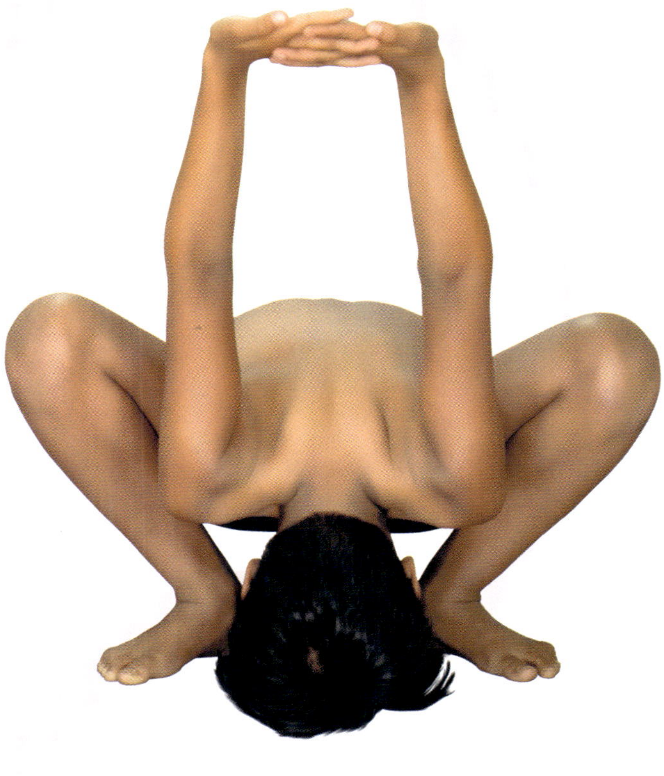

MALASANA PARIVRITTI (Twisted Garland Pose)

PREPARE – Ready!

- Samasthithi Malasana
- Stay in Malasana.
- Keep shoulders open and chest relaxed.
- Keep head in line with the shoulders.
- Keep your *drishti* straight by fixing your eyes to a point in front of you.
- Smile calmly and maintain deep breathing.

BENEFITS – WOW!

- Improves flexibility of the hips and increases circulation around the area.
- Releases tightness in the lower back area.
- Strengthens knees and legs.
- Improves digestion and assimilation of food.
- Builds focus and concentration.
- Helps children sit for long hours comfortably.

CONSTRUCT – Steps

1. Keep feet open.
2. Keep the hips steady in balance and open as wide as possible.
3. Bend forward and take the right hand around the right knee and wrap the left hand around the back and reach to hold the right palm.
4. Keep the chest turned towards the left and look backwards.
5. Keep the eyes calm and focus on breathing as deep as possible. Repeat to the other side.

Relax – Steps

- Release the clasp of the hands.
- Slowly lift the hips.
- Slowly straighten the knees and relax.

Note from the Acharya

- Keep the shoulders relaxed and in line with each other making sure that one shoulder is not lifted up and other dropped down.
- Can be done any time when the back is feeling stiff after long hours of sitting or after sports.
- Girls should not do this asana during menstruation.
- Do not do this asana while recovering from an upset stomach, indigestion or even constipation.

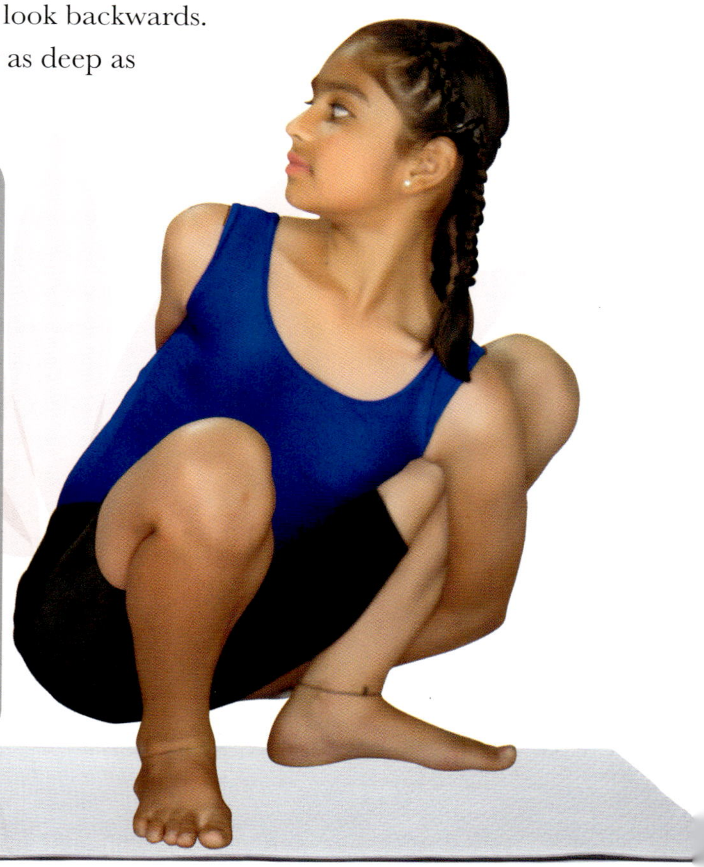

TRIKONASANA (Triangle Pose)

PREPARE – Ready!

- Samasthithi
- Stand straight with feet together and pressed to the ground.
- Pull stomach in and tuck buttocks.
- Keep your shoulders open and chest relaxed.
- Your head should be in line with the shoulders.
- Keep your *drishti* straight by fixing your eyes to a point in front of you. Smile calmly and enjoy.

CONSTRUCT – Steps

1. From the centre, jump keeping arm distance apart.
2. Turn right feet 90 degrees pointing out while the left leg is pointing 90 degrees in front.
3. Keep the arms stretched in a straight line along the side length of the shoulders.
4. Stretch the body towards the right length as far as the stretch can go.
5. Stretch the arm downward towards the knee and stop when the stretch feels like a pull.
6. Stay in position and establish balance.
7. Then look up and stare at the palm.
8. Breathe comfortably and enjoy.
9. Do not forget to do the other side.

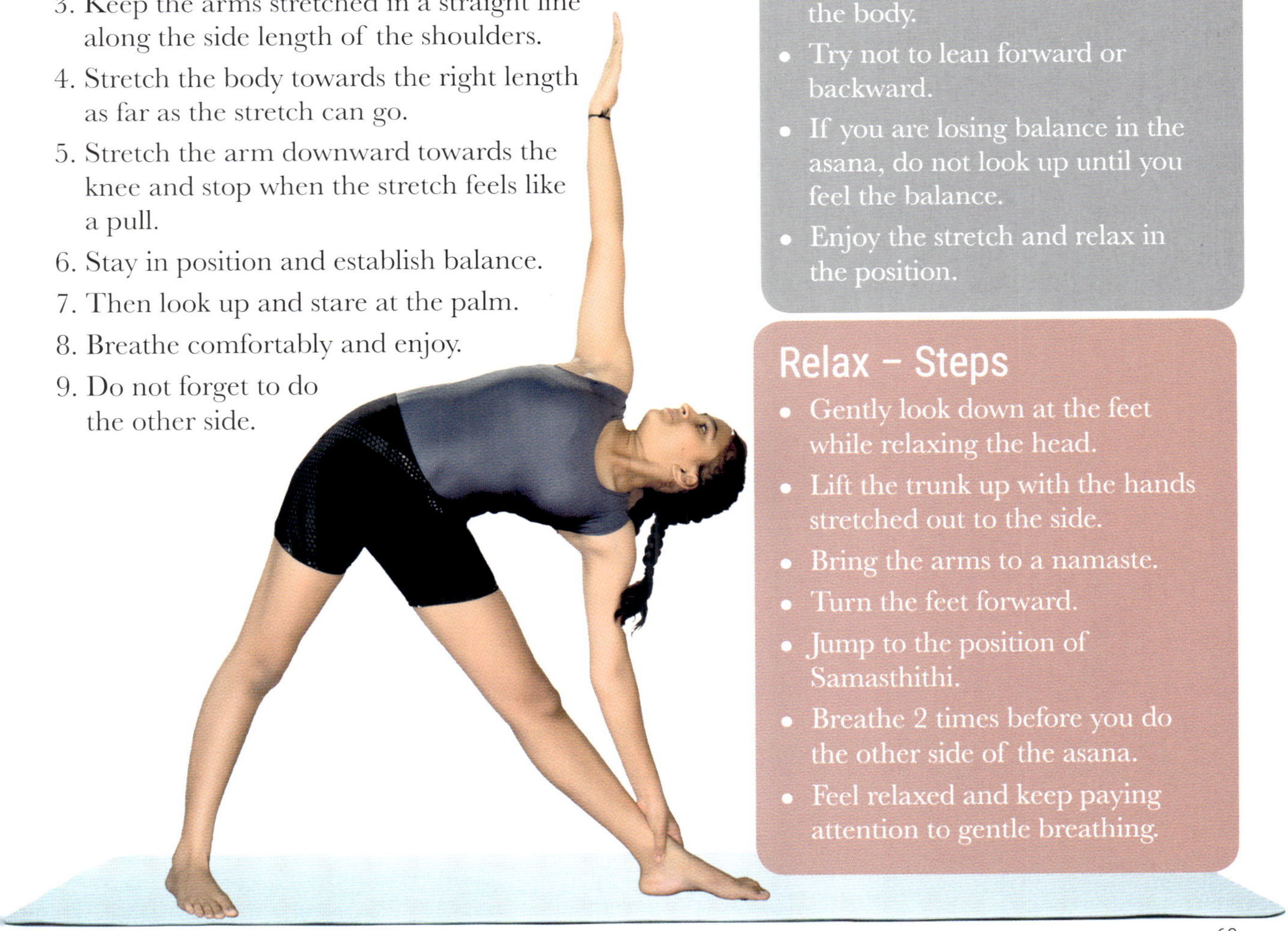

BENEFITS – WOW!

- Strengthens and stretches the shoulders, arms, trunk, hips, thighs and legs
- Makes the body flexible and lengthens it
- Stabilises the hips and roots the feet to the floor
- Helps remove baby fat from waist and thighs
- Cures indigestion
- Improves eyesight
- Improves balance and increases concentration

Note from the Acharya

- Do not force the stretch to reach the floor. That's not the aim!
- Maintain the straight lines of the body.
- Try not to lean forward or backward.
- If you are losing balance in the asana, do not look up until you feel the balance.
- Enjoy the stretch and relax in the position.

Relax – Steps

- Gently look down at the feet while relaxing the head.
- Lift the trunk up with the hands stretched out to the side.
- Bring the arms to a namaste.
- Turn the feet forward.
- Jump to the position of Samasthithi.
- Breathe 2 times before you do the other side of the asana.
- Feel relaxed and keep paying attention to gentle breathing.

PARIVRITTI TRIKONASANA (Twisted Triangle)

PREPARE – Ready!

- Samasthithi
- Stand straight with feet together and pressed to the ground.
- Pull stomach in and tuck buttocks.
- Keep your shoulders open and chest relaxed.
- Your head should be in line with the shoulders.
- Keep your *drishti* straight by fixing your eyes to a point in front of you. Smile calmly and enjoy.

CONSTRUCT – Steps

1. From the centre, jump with one arm distance apart.
2. Turn your right foot at a 90 degree angle pointing outwards, while the left leg points 90 degrees in the front.
3. Keep the arms stretched in a straight line along the side length of the shoulders.
4. Twist the body towards the right side as far as possible.
5. Stretch the left arm downward towards the knee and if possible towards the floor.
6. Stay in position and establish balance.
7. Then look upwards at the left palm.
8. Breathe comfortably and enjoy.
9. Do not forget to do the other side.

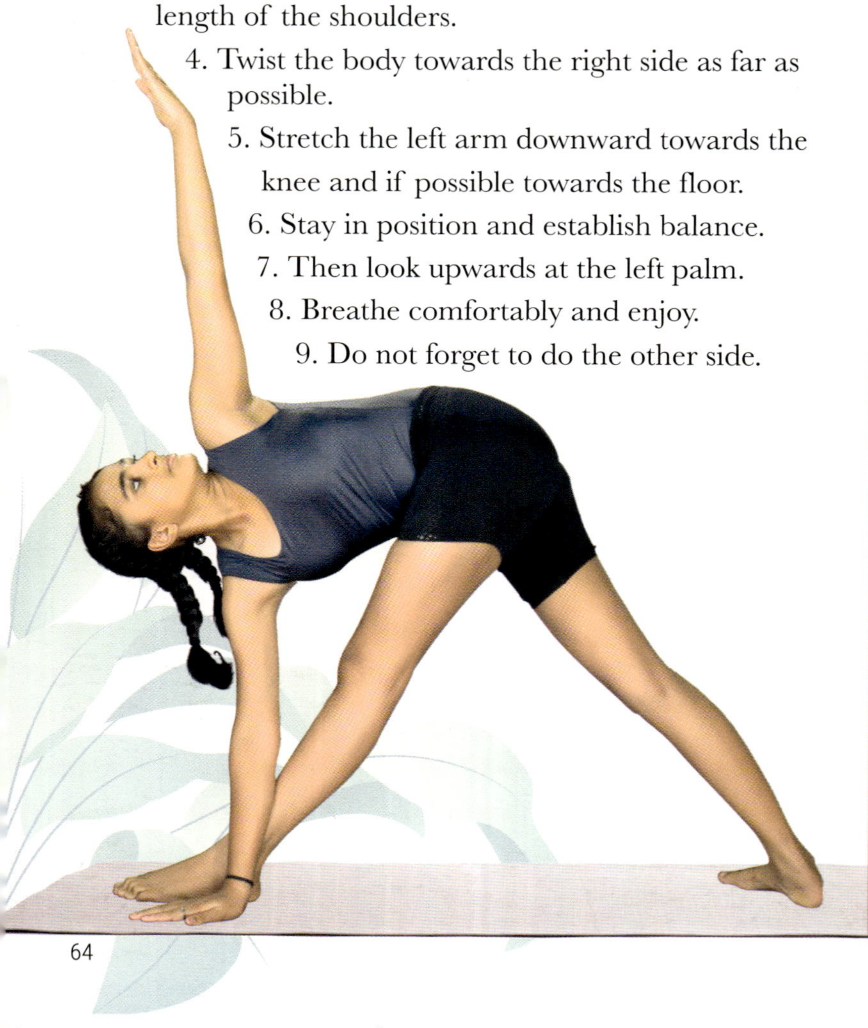

BENEFITS – WOW!

- Strengthens and stretches the shoulders, arms, trunk, hips, thighs and legs
- Makes the body flexible and lengthens it
- Stabilises the hips and roots the feet to the floor
- Helps remove baby fat from waist and thighs
- Improves hip flexibility
- Improves balance and increases concentration

Note from the Acharya

- Do not force a stretch to reach the floor. That's not the aim!
- Maintain balance for which the back has to be straight.
- If you are losing balance in the asana do not look up until you feel the balance.
- Enjoy the stretch and relax focusing on the breathing.

Relax – Steps

- Gently look down towards the right hand while relaxing the head.
- Lift the trunk up with the hands stretched out to the side.
- Bring the arms to a namaste.
- Turn the feet forward 90 degrees.
- Jump to the position of Samasthithi.
- Breathe 2 times before you do the other side of the asana.
- Feel relaxed and keep paying attention to your gentle breathing.

PARSHVAKONASANA (Stretched Angle Pose)

PREPARE – Ready!

- Samasthithi
- Stand straight with feet together and pressed to the ground.
- Pull stomach in and tuck buttocks.
- Keep your shoulders open and chest relaxed.
- Your head should be in line with the shoulders.
- Keep your *drishti* straight by fixing your eyes to a point in front of you.
- Smile calmly and enjoy.

CONSTRUCT – Steps

1. From the centre of the mat jump as far as possible.
2. Turn the right feet 90 degrees out towards the right and bend the knee while the left leg and knee stay straight.
3. Keep the body straight and arms stretched outwards.
4. Fix the feet firmly on the floor and bend the trunk to the right side.
5. Stretch the right arm over the head along the length of the ears.
6. Keep the chest open strong and comfortable
7. Hold the position and breathe for 3 breaths.
8. Enjoy and keep the face calm and smiling.
9. Come out of the position back to Samasthithi.
10. Then repeat on the other side.

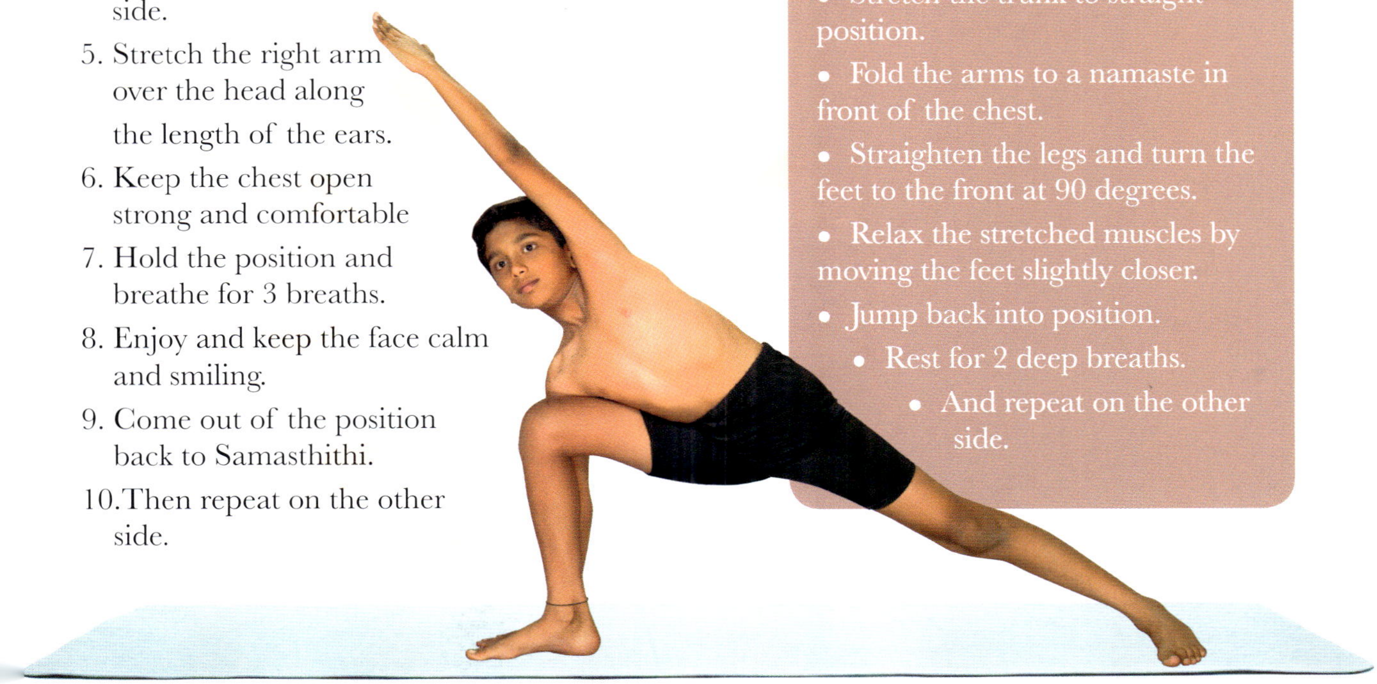

BENEFITS – WOW!

- A complete body stretch which fills up the body with strength
- Prepares the body for strong physical activities
- Strengthens the lower back and keeps the hamstrings supple
- For girls, it releases menstrual discomfort

Note from the Acharya

- The stretch should not be too much that your heels are unsteady.
- Keep the thighs strong and feet firm.
- If reaching the floor with the right palm is difficult, place your right elbow on the right knee and stretch the left arm out from above the head. Practise this way until the flexibility of your trunk increases.
- Do not drop the hip to the floor.
- Keep smiling.

Relax – Steps

- Stretch the trunk to straight position.
- Fold the arms to a namaste in front of the chest.
- Straighten the legs and turn the feet to the front at 90 degrees.
- Relax the stretched muscles by moving the feet slightly closer.
- Jump back into position.
- Rest for 2 deep breaths.
- And repeat on the other side.

PARIVRITTI PARSHVAKONASANA (Twisted Stretched Angle Pose)

PREPARE – Ready!

- Samasthithi
- Pull stomach in and tuck in buttocks.
- Keep your shoulders open and chest relaxed.
- Keep your *drishti* straight by fixing your eyes to a point in front of you.
- Smile calmly and enjoy.

CONSTRUCT – Steps

1. From the centre of the mat, jump as far as possible.
2. Turn the right feet 90 degree out towards the right and bend the knee while the left leg and knee stay straight.
3. Twist the body towards the right knee with arms stretched along the shoulder line.
4. Fix the feet firmly on the floor and bend forward towards the right knee until the length of the abdomen feels is along the length of the knee.
5. Stretch the left arm over the head along the length of the ears.
6. Come out of the position back to samasthithi.
7. Then repeat to the other side.

Relax – Steps

- Release the hand and neck.
- Lift the chest away from the right knee.
- Gently release the fold of the legs and bring it together.
- Jump back into position.
- Rest for 2 deep breathing.
- And repeat to the other side.

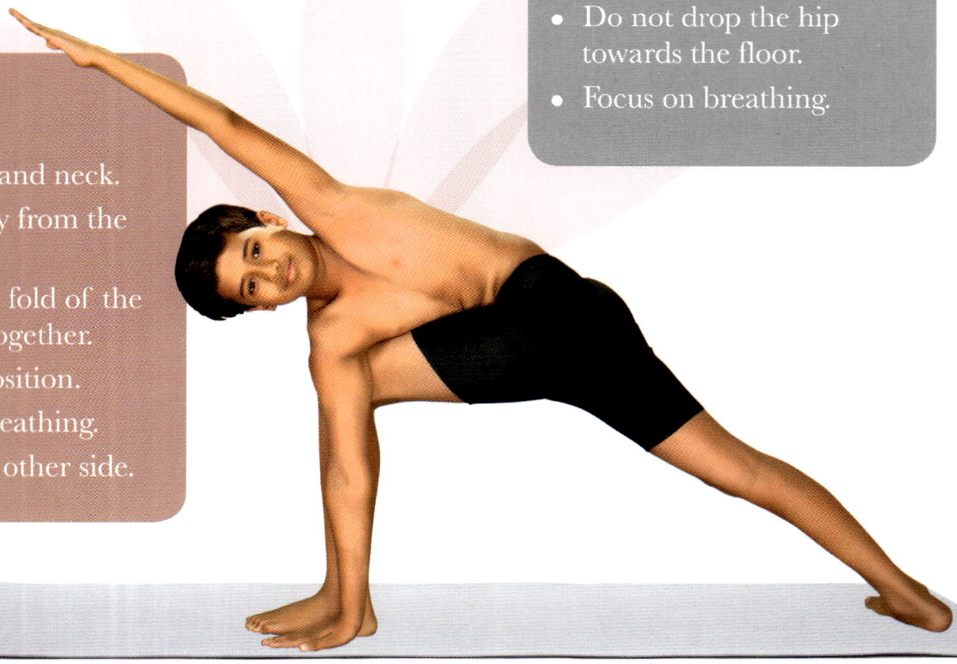

BENEFITS – WOW!

- This is a challenging stretch which fills up the body with strength and energy.
- It prepares the body for strong physical activities.
- Increases flexibility in the hips.
- Improves the stamina and challenges breathing thus works on developing diaphragm strength.
- Lengthens the spine and aids in growth of the body.

Note from the Acharya

- Keep the thighs strong and feet firm.
- If reaching the floor with the right palm is difficult, place your left elbow on the right knee and stretch the left arm out from above the head. Practise this way until you progress in flexibility of the trunk.
- Do not drop the hip towards the floor.
- Focus on breathing.

SHIRASAPARSHVAKONASANA (Head Down Stretched Angle)

PREPARE – Ready!

- Samasthithi
- Pull stomach in and tuck in buttocks.
- Keep your shoulders open and chest relaxed.
- Keep your *drishti* straight by fixing your eyes to a point in front of you. Smile calmly and enjoy.

CONSTRUCT – Steps

1. From the centre of the mat, jump as far as possible.
2. Turn the right feet 90 degrees out towards the right and bend the knee while the left leg and knee stay straight.
4. Twist the waist and place the left arm on the outer side of the knee and lift the right hand up towards the ceiling.
5. Stretch the right arm over the head along the length of the ears.
6. Enjoy and keep the face calm and smiling.

Relax – Steps

- Stretch the trunk back into a straight position.
- Fold the arms to a namaste in front of the chest.
- Straighten the legs and turn the feet to the front at 90 degrees.
- Relax the stretched muscles by getting the feet slightly closer.
- Jump back into position.
- And repeat on the other side.

BENEFITS – WOW!

- A complete body stretch which fills the body with strength
- Prepares the body for strong physical activities
- Strengthens the lower back and keeps the hamstrings supple
- Trims the waist and lengthens the trunk. Lengthens the spine and increases the flow of the spinal fluid into the brain
- Sharpens the brain and keeps the spine healthy

Note from the Acharya

- A challenging asana which will get easy with practice.
- The stretch should not be too much that the heels get unsteady.
- Keep the thighs strong and feet firm.
- If reaching the floor with the right palm is difficult, place your right elbow on the right knee and stretch the left arm out from above the head.
- Try to keep the hips lifted up and steady, and keep smiling.

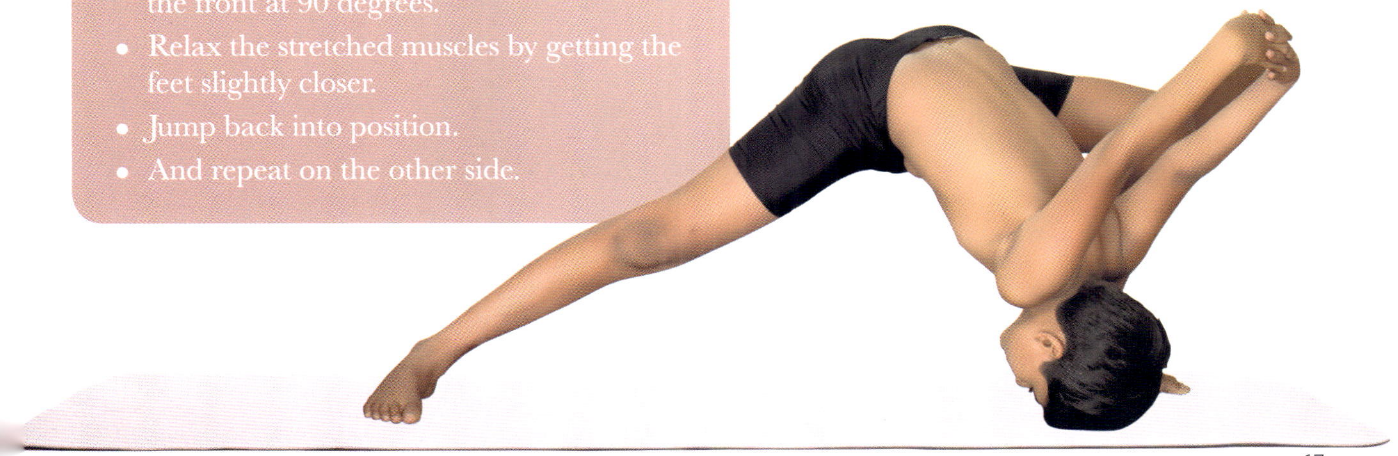

ANJANEYASANA – Monkey God Pose

PREPARE – Ready!

- Samasthithi
- Stand straight with feet together and pressed to the ground.
- Pull stomach in and tuck buttocks.
- Keep your shoulders open and chest relaxed.
- Your head should be in line with the shoulders.
- Keep your *drishti* straight by fixing your eyes to a point in front of you.
- Smile calmly and enjoy.

BENEFITS – WOW!

- A complete and a powerful body stretch which fills the body with strength.
- Prepares the body for strong physical activities
- Helps build a strong back and hip muscles
- Releases back strain after sports
- Strengthens the lower back and keeps the hamstrings supple
- For girls, releases menstrual discomfort

CONSTRUCT – Steps

1. From the centre of the mat, jump as far as possible
2. Turn the right foot 90 degrees out and bend the knee while the left leg and knee stay straight.
3. Fix the feet firmly on the floor.
4. Raise arms upwards towards the ceiling and drop the left arm along the left length of the leg.
5. Stretch the neck upwards towards the ceiling.
6. Keep the chest open strong and comfortable.
7. Hold the position and breathe thrice.
8. Enjoy and keep the face calm and smiling.
9. Come out of the position back to Samasthithi.

Note from the Acharya

- Keep the leg position steady and strong.
- Do not drop the hips to the floor.
- Keep the hands strong and stretched towards the ceiling.
- Keep the chest open and strong with deep breathing.
- Keep smiling and enjoy the challenge.

Relax – Steps

- Release the left hand from the thigh and raise it up in line with the right lifted hand.
- Fold the arms to a namaste in front of the chest.
- Straighten the legs.
- Relax the stretched muscles by getting the feet slightly closer.
- Jump back into position.
- Rest for 2 deep breaths.
- And repeat on the other side.

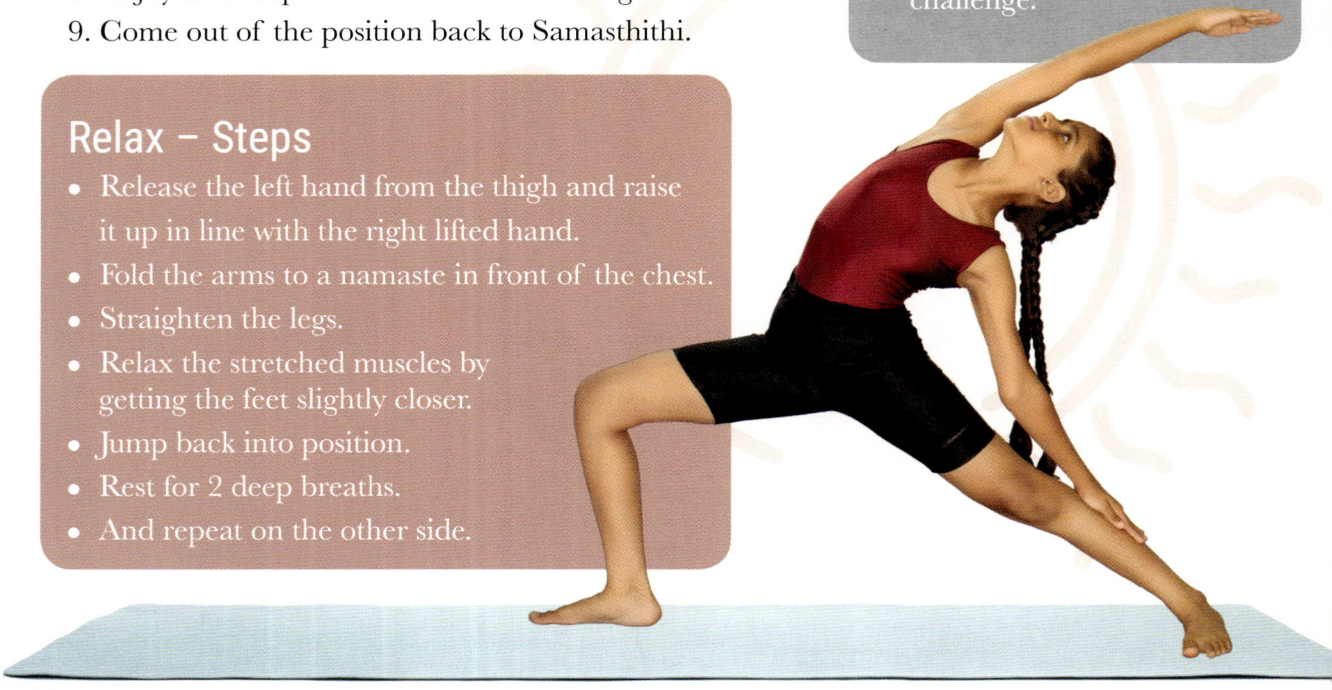

PRASARITHAPADOTTANASANA (Pyramid Pose)

PREPARE – Read!

- Samasthithi
- Stand straight with feet together and pressed to the ground.
- Pull stomach in and tuck in buttocks.
- Keep your shoulders open and chest relaxed.
- Your head should be in line with the shoulders.
- Keep your *drishti* straight by fixing your eyes to a point in front of you.
- Smile calmly and enjoy.

BENEFITS – WOW!

- Relaxes the mind
- Good for eyes and ears as the position is almost inverted
- Increases blood circulation around the brain
- Strengthens the legs and spine
- Increases flexibility around the hips

CONSTRUCT – Steps

1. From the centre of the mat, jump a comfortable distance.
2. Keep hand on the waist and fold forward till the head reaches the ground.
3. Or fold forward till where it is comfortable.
4. Breathe 5 times in this pose.

Relax – Steps

- Place hands on the floor.
- Slowly lift the body up.
- Lift the head up.
- Get feet together and relax.

Note from the Acharya

- Practise this asana with patience.
- Wait for the spine to slowly lengthen instead of imposing with too much strength.
- Relax the breathing and the spine with a gradual stretch.
- Practise this asana on an empty stomach
- This exercise can be done after sports activities to relax the body and provide an overall stretch.

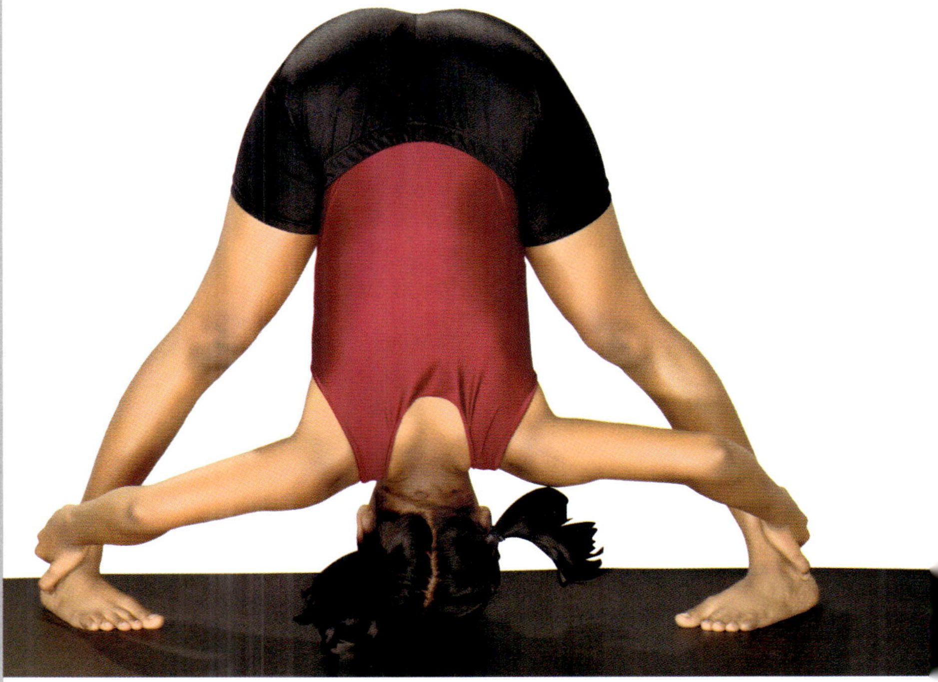

TANDAVASANA (Dancing Lord)

PREPARE – Read!

- Samasthithi
- From the position of feet apart from the previous asana (Prasarithapadotanasana), stand with feet turned outwards completely.

CONSTRUCT – Steps

1. Bend the knees with thighs strongly open and feet rooted to the ground.
2. Thighs are to be parallel to the ground and the body straight.
3. Stretch the hand outwards with the abdominal muscles pulled in.
4. Stabilise the hips and stay in balance for 3 deep breaths.

BENEFITS – WOW!

- Helps build focus and concentration
- Strengthens legs, arms, hips, waist and trunk
- Has an overall benefit
- Builds up stamina and strength

Note from the Acharya

- This is a challenging asana.
- Try to stay in position in spite of the pain it sends through the body.
- Do not let the knees beyond the ankle limit.
- Keep the feet pressed to the ground.
- Stay with deep breathing as it relaxes the pain.

Relax – Steps

- Relax the breathing and straighten the legs.
- Rotate the feet forward and relax the knees.
- Get the feet together and relax the muscles of the legs.

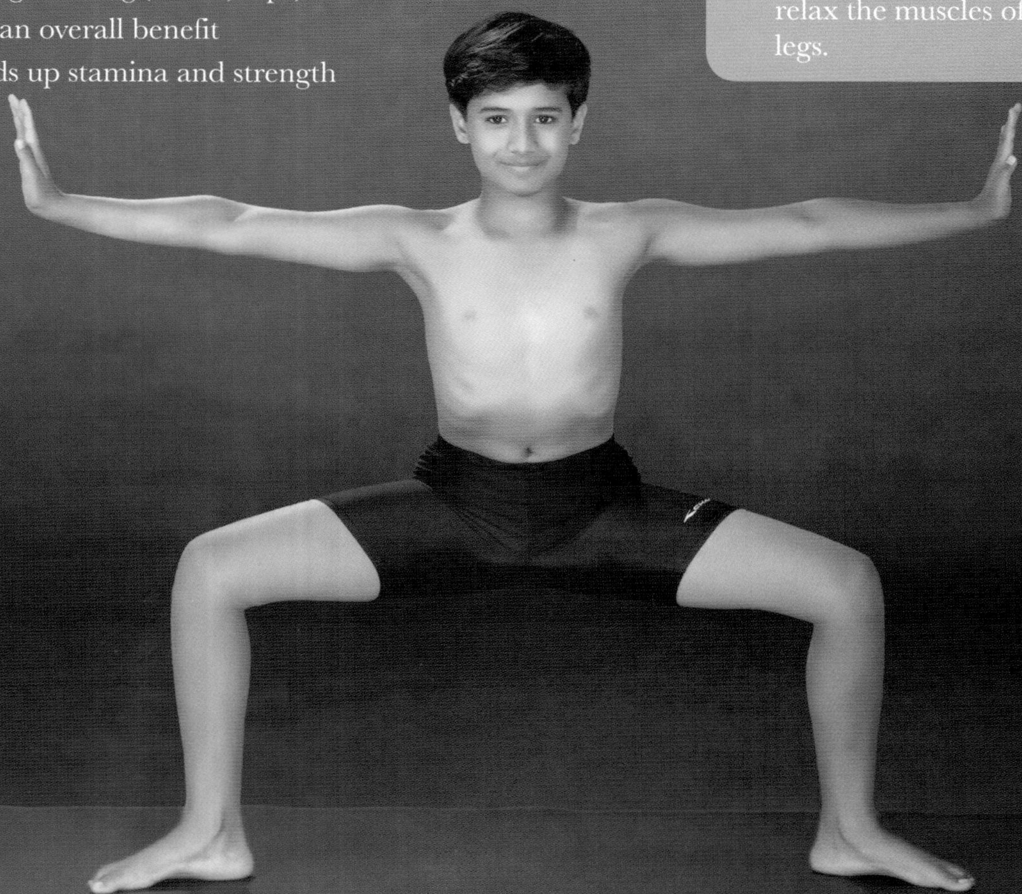

PARSHVATTANASANA (Forward Fold)

PREPARE – Ready!

- Samasthithi
- Stand straight with feet together and pressed to the ground.
- Pull stomach in and tuck buttocks.
- Keep the shoulders open and chest relaxed.
- Your head should be in line with the shoulders.
- Keep your *drishti* straight by fixing your eyes to a point in front of you.
- Smile calmly and enjoy.

CONSTRUCT – Steps

1. Stand in the front of the mat and step back to a comfortable distance.
2. Keep both the feet pointing forward.
3. Keep the hand in a namaste behind the back and lean backwards stretching the chest upwards.
4. Look straight.
5. Lean forward without hunching the back and folding the legs.
6. Reach the head towards the right knee or as far comfortable.

Relax – Steps

- Lift the chest upwards and get the shoulders in line with the hip bones.
- Keep looking straight and maintain balance.
- Step forward and get the feet in line with each other.

BENEFITS – WOW!

- Builds focus and concentration
- Lengthens the hamstrings and increases its flexibility
- Kids interested in sports like athletics will benefit from this asana
- Reduces injuries in the muscles for sporty kids
- Reduces baby fat around the hip area
- Helps maintain balance

Note from the Acharya

- Initially, this asana may seem difficult but with patience and regular practice this asana can be achieved.
- If the pull of the hamstring, i.e. the back of the thigh is too strong, keep the knee relaxed and do not force yourself to go lower.
- This asana will eventually progress.

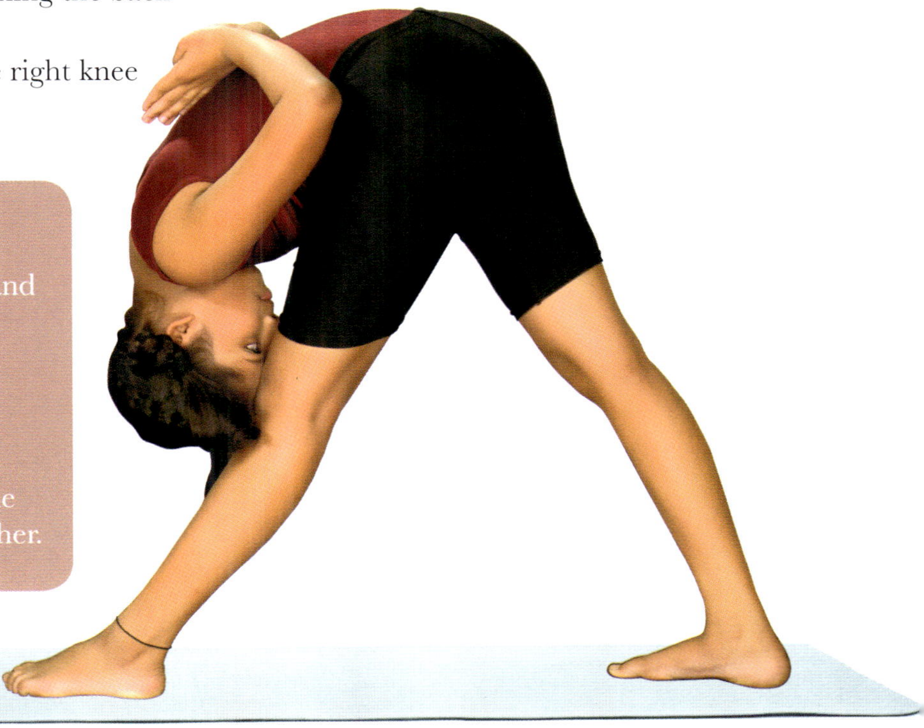

VEERABADRASANA (Warrior Sequence)

PREPARE – Ready!

- Samasthithi
- Stand straight with feet together and pressed to the ground.
- Pull stomach in and tuck in buttocks.
- Keep your shoulders open and chest relaxed.
- Your head should be in line with the shoulders.
- Keep your gaze straight by fixing your eyes to a point in front of you.
- Smile calmly and enjoy.

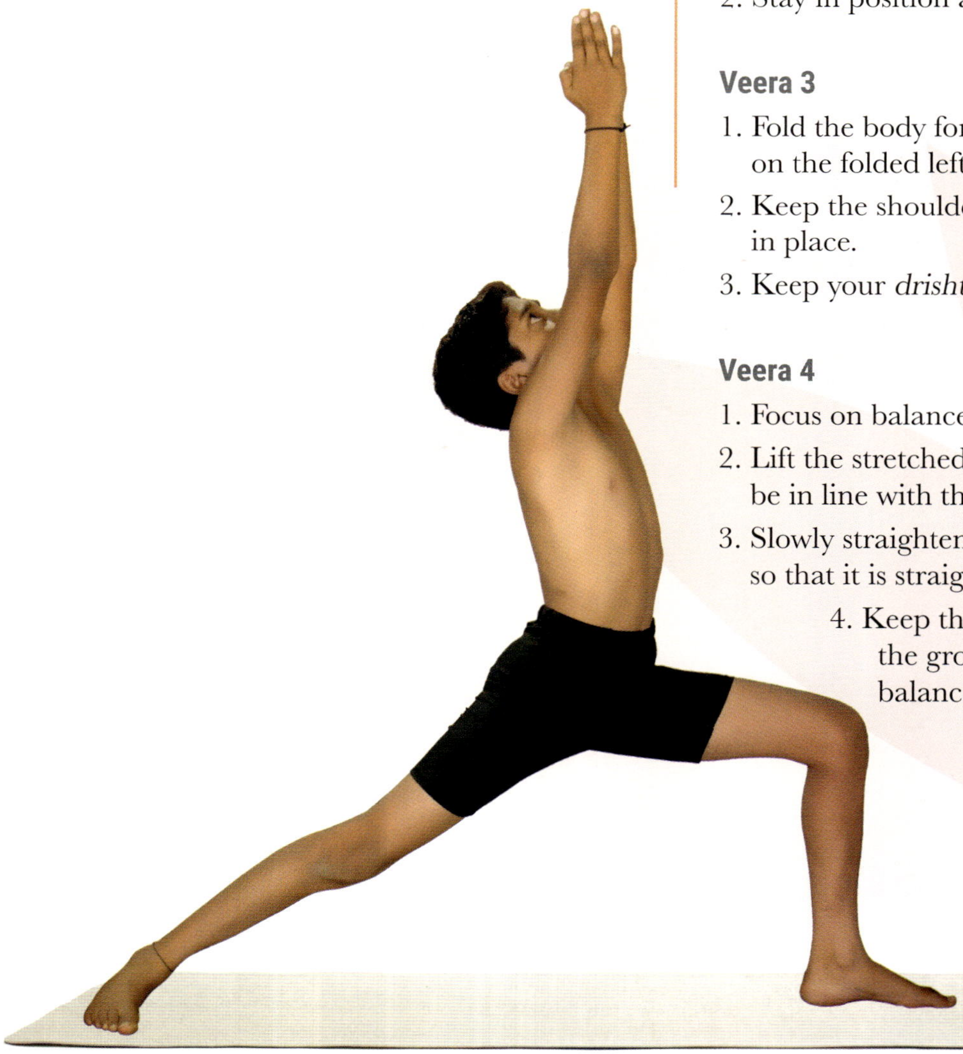

CONSTRUCT – Steps

Veera 1

1. Stand at the centre of the mat and step back to a comfortable distance
2. Make sure both the feet are in line with each other.
3. Lift the hand in a namaste in line with the head.
4. Keep the chest relaxed and make sure the shoulders are in line with the hip bones.
5. Keep looking straight and maintain balance.

Veera 2

1. Stretch the right leg backward into a lunge with the left knee folded.
2. Stay in position and maintain balance.

Veera 3

1. Fold the body forward so that it rests on the folded left knee.
2. Keep the shoulders strong and namaste in place.
3. Keep your *drishti* and look at the feet.

Veera 4

1. Focus on balance.
2. Lift the stretched back right leg up to be in line with the hip.
3. Slowly straighten the folded left knee so that it is straight.
4. Keep the left feet pressed to the ground and work on balance.

Facts

Vedic texts say that the source of light and breath which brings life to all beings on earth is God.

BENEFITS – WOW!

- Increases focus and concentration
- Lengthens the hamstrings and increases its flexibility.
- Kids interested in sports like athletics will benefit from this asana.
- Reduces injuries in the muscles for sporty kids
- Keeps the hips strong and flexible
- Strengthens the legs and shoulders
- Helps maintain balance

Note from the Acharya

- Initially, this asana may seem difficult but with patience and regular practice it can be achieved.
- It is a difficult balancing asana, but once achieved, it is very beneficial for the overall growth and development of the body.
- If the pull of the hamstring, i.e., the back of the thigh is too strong, keep the knee steady and do not force to go lower.
- This asana will eventually progress.

Relax – Steps

- Gently get arms back by the side of the hips.
- Carefully bring the lifted leg down to place it on the floor.
- Bend knees for balance and bring the leg forward to Samasthithi.
- Repeat on the other side.

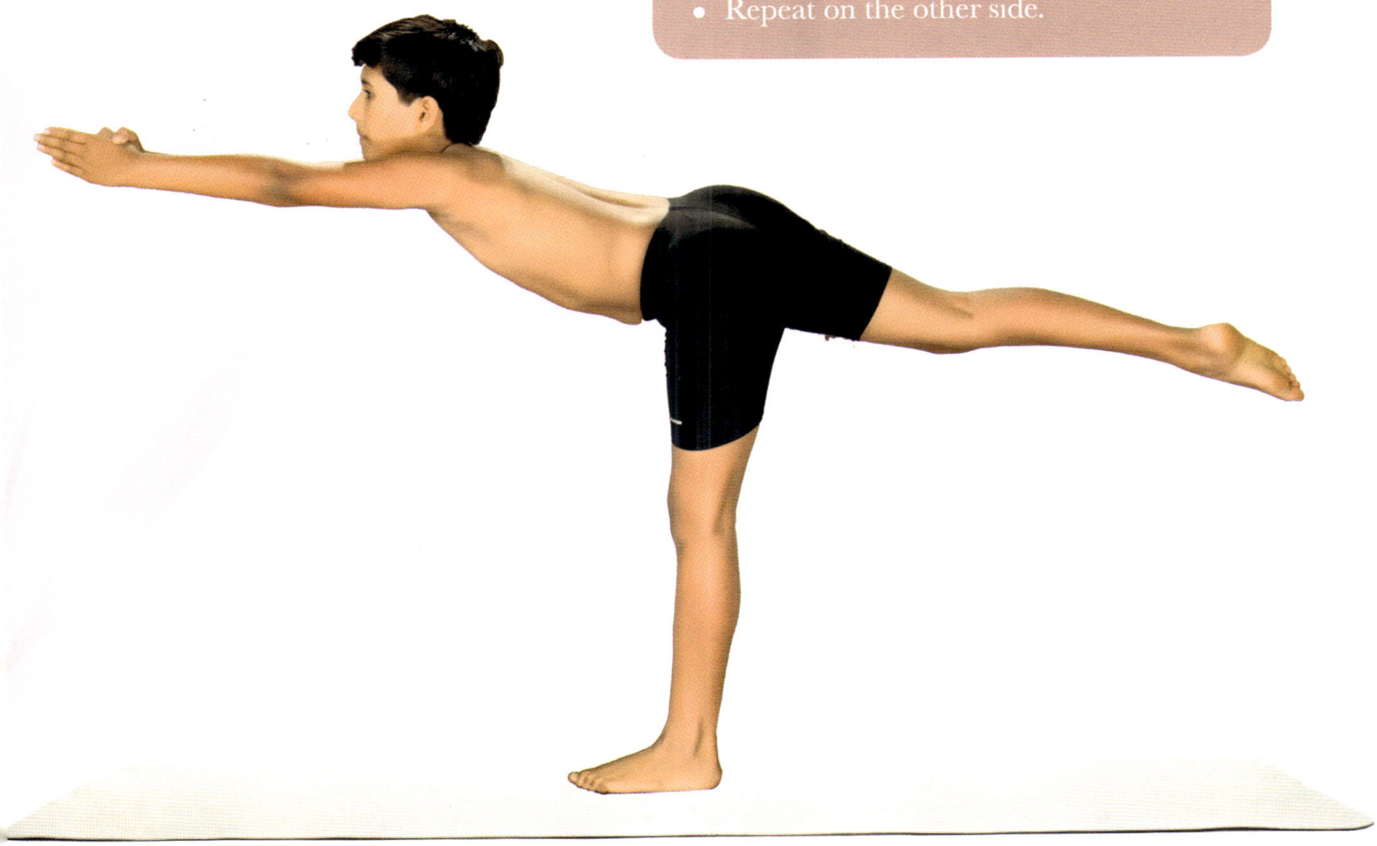

UTHITHA HASTHAPADANGUSTASANA (Toe Hold Pose)

PREPARE – Ready!

- Samasthithi
- Stand straight with feet together and pressed to the ground.
- Pull stomach in and tuck buttocks.
- Keep your shoulders open and chest relaxed.
- The head should be in line with the shoulders.
- Keep your *drishti* straight by fixing your eyes to a point in front of you.
- Smile calmly and enjoy.

BENEFITS – WOW!

- Increases hip flexibility and mobility
- Helps maintain balance
- Aligns the hips and strengthens the thighs and stretches the glutes
- Helps get a good shape for the legs for sports activities

Relax – Steps

- Release the leg to the floor and breathe.
- Stand straight and repeat on the other side.

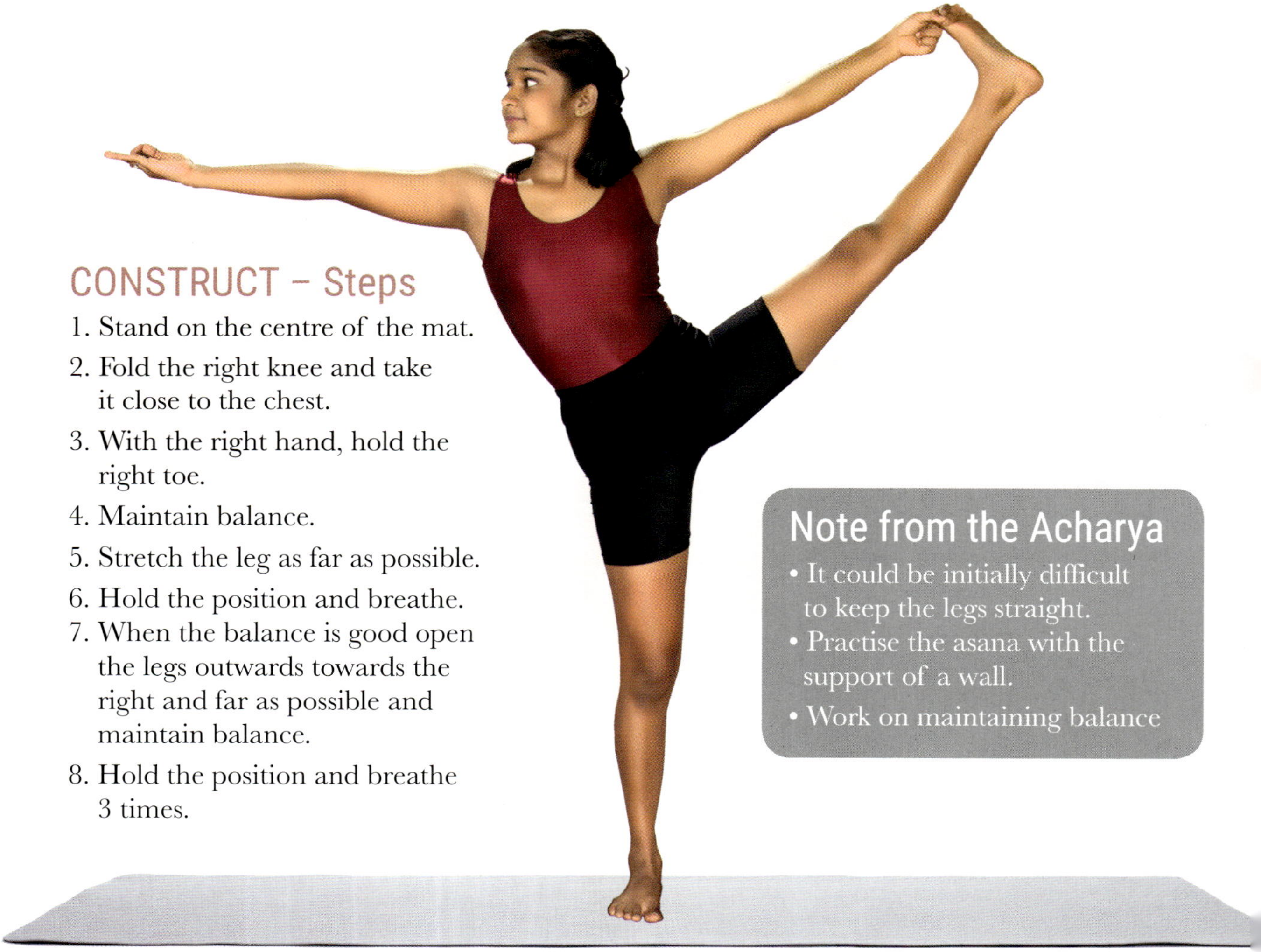

CONSTRUCT – Steps

1. Stand on the centre of the mat.
2. Fold the right knee and take it close to the chest.
3. With the right hand, hold the right toe.
4. Maintain balance.
5. Stretch the leg as far as possible.
6. Hold the position and breathe.
7. When the balance is good open the legs outwards towards the right and far as possible and maintain balance.
8. Hold the position and breathe 3 times.

Note from the Acharya

- It could be initially difficult to keep the legs straight.
- Practise the asana with the support of a wall.
- Work on maintaining balance

ARDHABADHA PADMOTTANASANA (Half Lotus Toe Hold)

PREPARE – Ready!

- Samasthithi
- Stand straight with feet together and pressed to the ground.
- Pull stomach in and tuck in buttocks.
- Keep your shoulders open and chest relaxed.
- Your head should be in line with the shoulders.
- Keep your *drishti* straight by fixing your eyes to a point in front of you.
- Smile calmly and enjoy.

CONSTRUCT – Steps

1. Fold the right knee and place the feet close to the thighs.
2. Look straight and maintain balance.
3. Take the left hand around the back and hold the right toe.
4. Fold forward till the head reaches the standing left knee.
5. Hold in position and breathe 3 times.
6. Repeat to the other side.

Note from the Acharya

- It could be difficult to hold on to the toes initially. With consistent practice it can be achieved.
- Keep the knee bent and if the back of the knees is very tight, eventually attempt to straighten the knees.

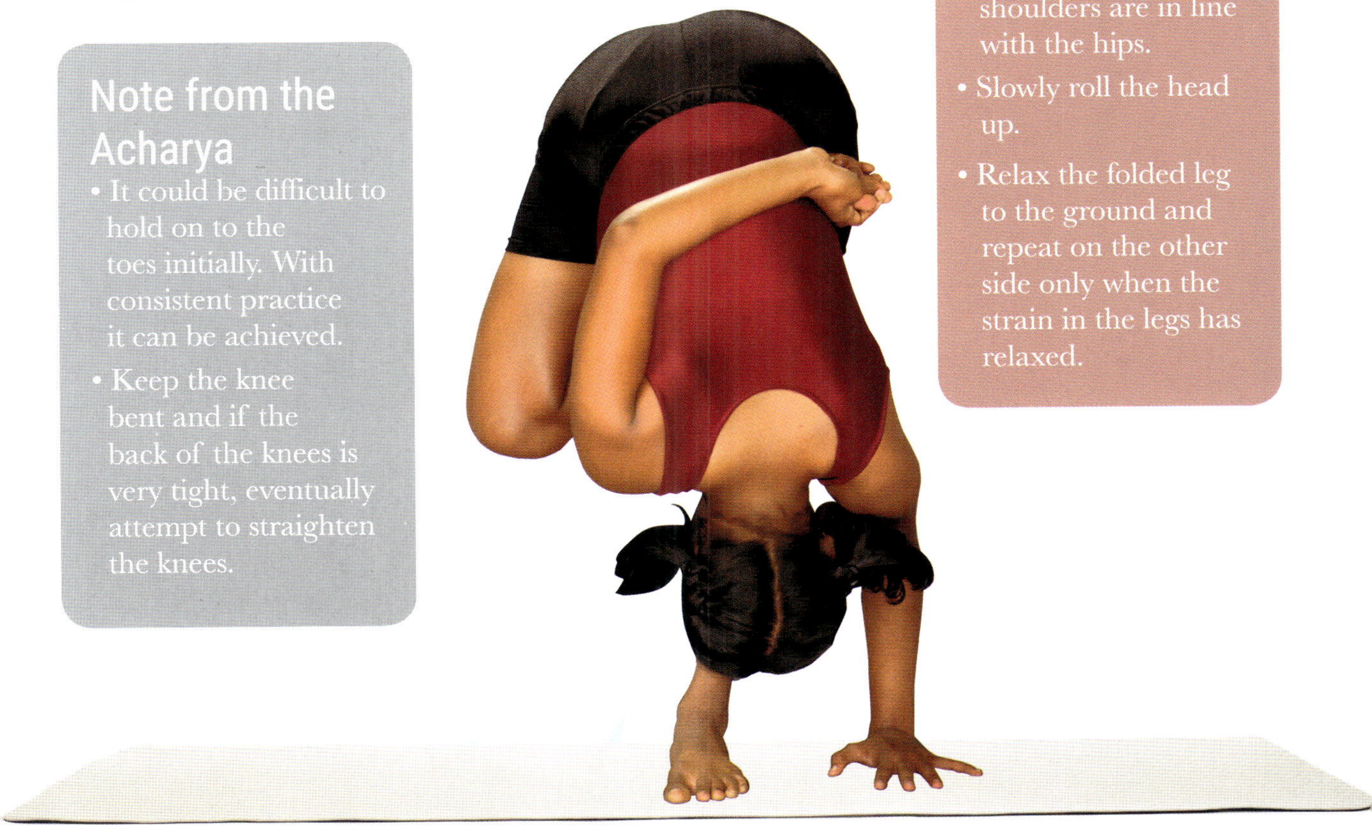

BENEFITS – WOW!

- Strengthens the legs and feet
- Increases flexibility in the hips
- Increases balance and concentration
- Keep the mind alert
- Forward bend increases circulation into the brain

Relax – Steps

- Slowly release the left hand and place it on the floor.
- Slightly bend the left standing leg before rolling the body upwards.
- Keep the head looking downward till the shoulders are in line with the hips.
- Slowly roll the head up.
- Relax the folded leg to the ground and repeat on the other side only when the strain in the legs has relaxed.

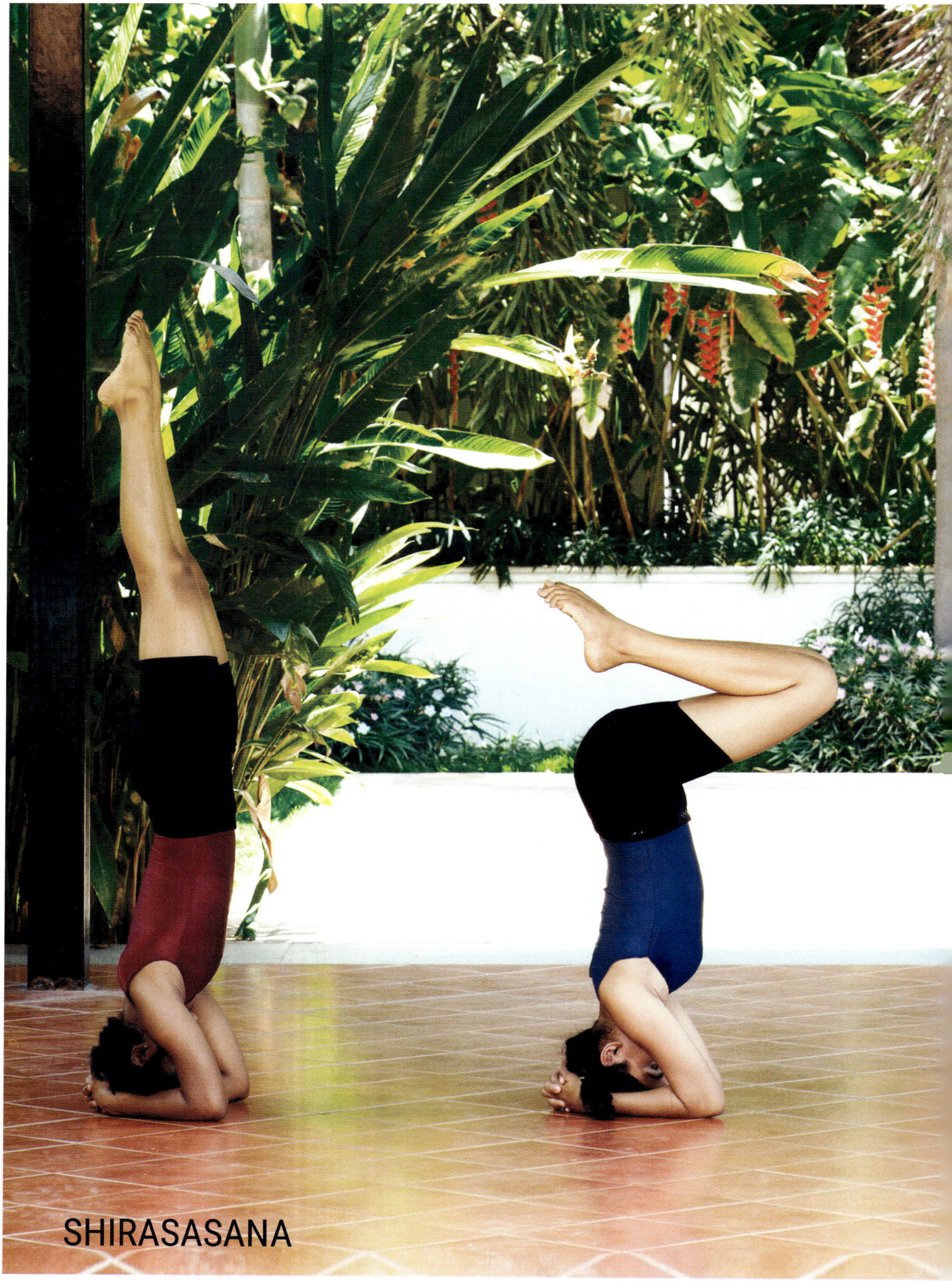

SHIRASASANA

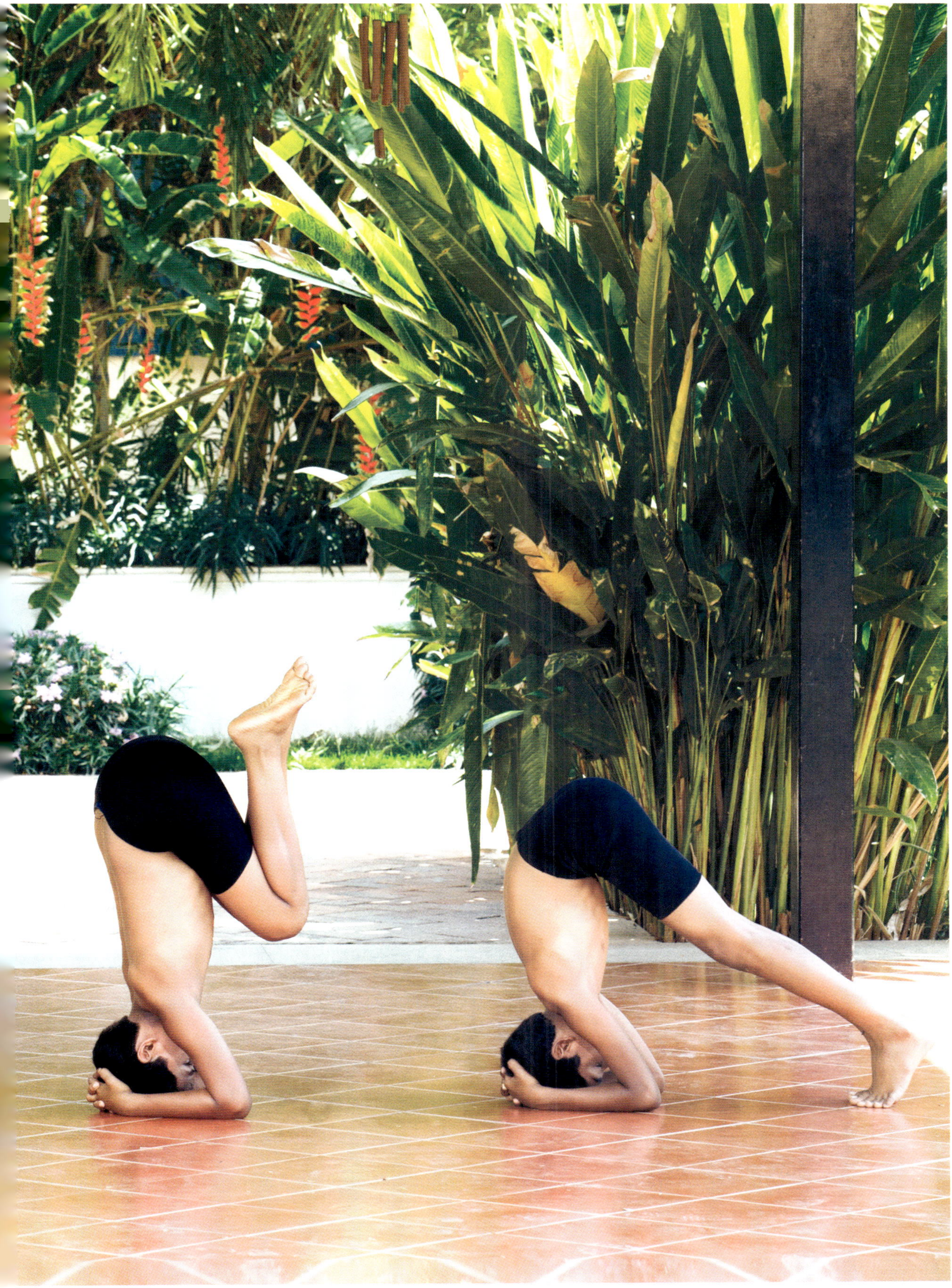

VAJRASANA (Diamond Pose)

PREPARE – Ready!

- Sit with legs folded backwards.
- Head relaxed and spine straight.
- Keep eyes closed and relax.

BENEFITS – WOW!

- Helps blood circulation along the length of the body
- Increases blood flow to the digestive organs
- Relaxes lower back tightness
- Helps lose belly fat
- Relaxes the nerves and calms the mind

CONTRUCT – Steps

1. Keep the toes together and sit on the heels.
2. Keep the thighs together and rest on the calves.
3. Stretch the back and the abdomen to a comfortable length.
4. Place the palms on the thighs.
5. If the ankle is uncomfortable, place a soft towel under the ankle.
6. Breathe deep to expand the chest and exhale contracting the abdomen.

Relax – Steps

- Lift the hip up and sit kneeling.
- Make space between the feet and gently sit down.
- Stretch legs forward and relax the knees.

Note from the Acharya

- This is a very meditative asana.
- If this asana is comfortable one can sit in this for a 5-minute meditation.
- It calms the mind and releases anxiety.
- If the knee begins to strain release the asana and massage the knees.

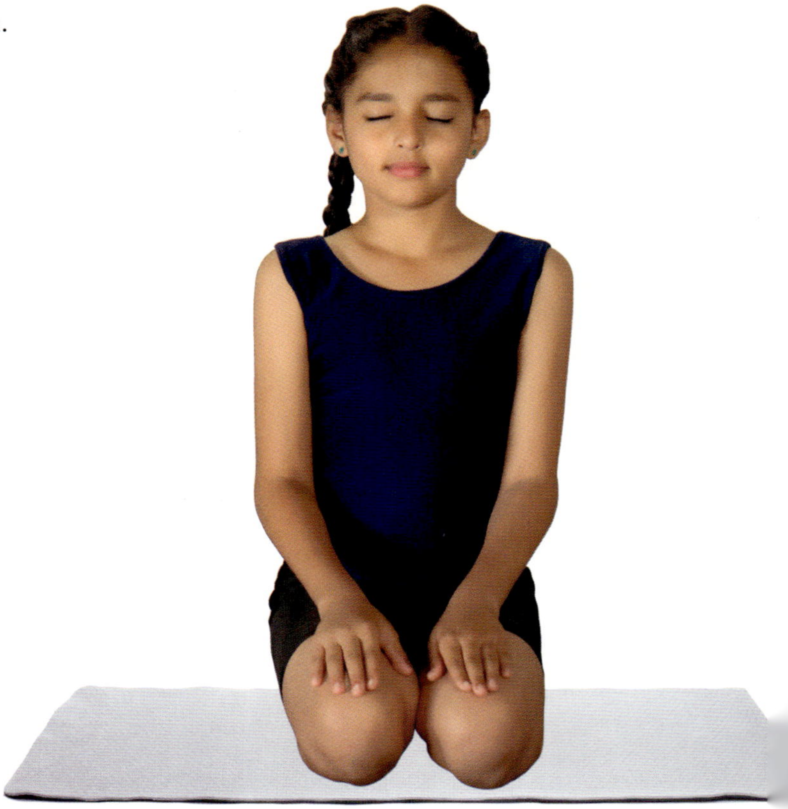

SHASHANKASANA (Rabbit Pose)

Facts

Yoga asanas were originally practised for healing physical problems.

PREPARE – Ready

- Sit in Vajrasana.
- Keep the back straight and head relaxed.

START – Steps

- Slowly raise hands up to lengthen the body completely.
- Stretch forward folding the body towards the thighs.
- Rest the chest on the thighs and relax feeling comfortable with deep breathing.
- Slide the chest forward away from the thigh until the chest reaches the ground.
- Stretch chin forward and gaze looking straight ahead (Samadrishti).

BENEFITS – WOW!

- Relaxes the back and shoulder muscles
- Relaxes the brain and calms agitation
- Makes the spine flexible and supple
- Increases blood circulation in the back
- A very beneficial asana for the kidneys

Note from the Acharya

- This is a very calming asana which can be used for relaxing the entire body.
- It keeps the back healthy and flexible.

Relax – Steps

- Slide back the body and place it on the thighs.
- Relax for a while.
- Place the hands on the floor for support and gently lift the body back to Vajrasana sitting position.

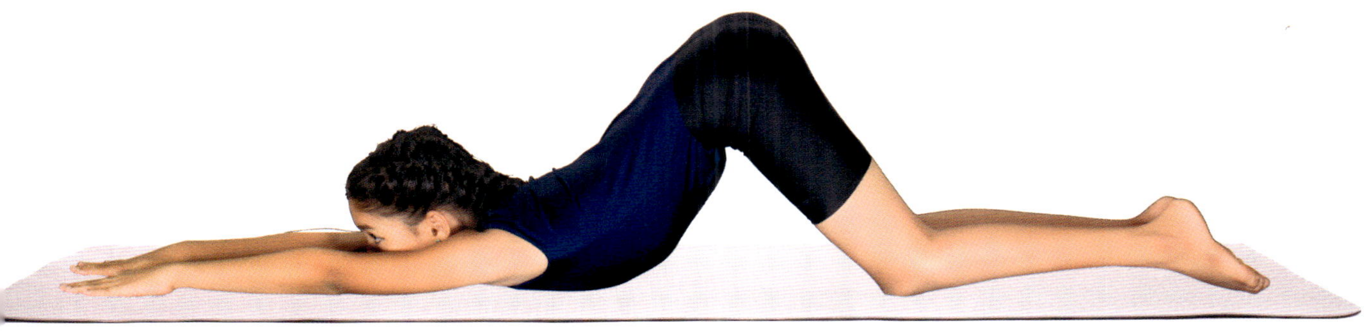

BALASANA (Child's Pose)

PREPARE – Ready!

- Sit in Vajrasana.
- Keep the back straight and head relaxed.
- Continue with normal and relaxed breathing.

START – Steps

- With extended spine fold the body forward.
- Let the abdominal length rest on the thighs first.
- Slowly drop the chin down to rest on the knees.
- Extend the back backwards so that the buttocks rest on the heels.
- Breathe deep 5 times.

BENEFITS – WOW!

- Rejuvenates the central nervous system
- Relaxes all the back muscles
- Gives a massage to the abdominal organs
- Encourages deep breathing.
- Relaxes tired leg muscles
- Helps blood flow towards the head

Relax – Steps

- Keep the head bent forward and tucked in the hollow of the throat.
- Lift the body up initiating the lift from the abdominal length.
- When the spine settles and becomes straight, then slowly lift the head up with eyes closed.
- Open eyes only when the neck is in line with the spine.

Note from the Acharya

- This asana is the best to release all tension from the entire body.
- After a hard day of work and play, just before you go to sleep do this asana for a relaxed sleep.

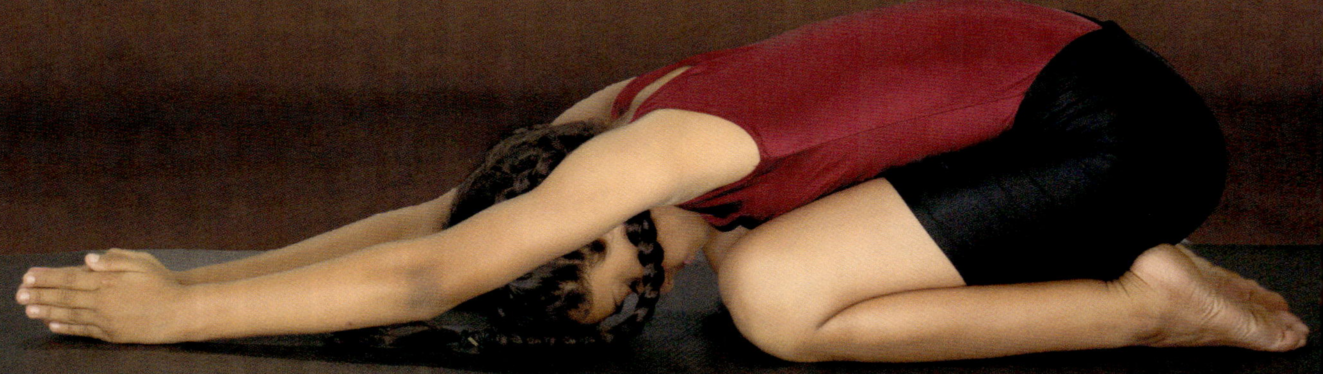

SUPTA VAJRASANA (Stretched Diamond Pose)

PREPARE – Ready

- Sit in Vajrasana.
- Keep back straight and head relaxed.
- Continue normal and relaxed breathing.

START – Steps

- Place the palms back with the body being supported by the arms.
- Gently fold from the elbows to the floor.
- Gently place the crown of the head to the floor (Pariyankasana.)
- Feel the neck stretch completely.
- Make sure that the hip is settled on the back of the knees and is stable.

Relax – Steps

- Slide back and neck to the floor and relax the body on the ground into a Supta Vajrasana.
- Relax for a while.
- Place the hands on the floor for support and gently lift the body back to Vajrasana sitting position.
- Relax.

BENEFITS – WOW!

- Relaxes the back and shoulder muscles
- Relaxes the brain and calms agitation
- Makes the legs flexible and supple
- Increases blood circulation along the length of the neck and throat
- Builds up respiratory strength and keep the lungs and heart healthy
- Improves postural defects
- Improves reflex action

Note from the Acharya

- Slowly raise hands up to lengthen the body completely to feel a complete stretch along the trunk.
- Relax the hands down and lean backwards taking support from the arms, keep stretching the back towards the ground.
- Place the elbows on the ground and stretch the neck backwards.
- Place the crown of the head firmly on the floor.
- If the head rests comfortably without neck strain, release the hand and raise it into a namaste upwards.

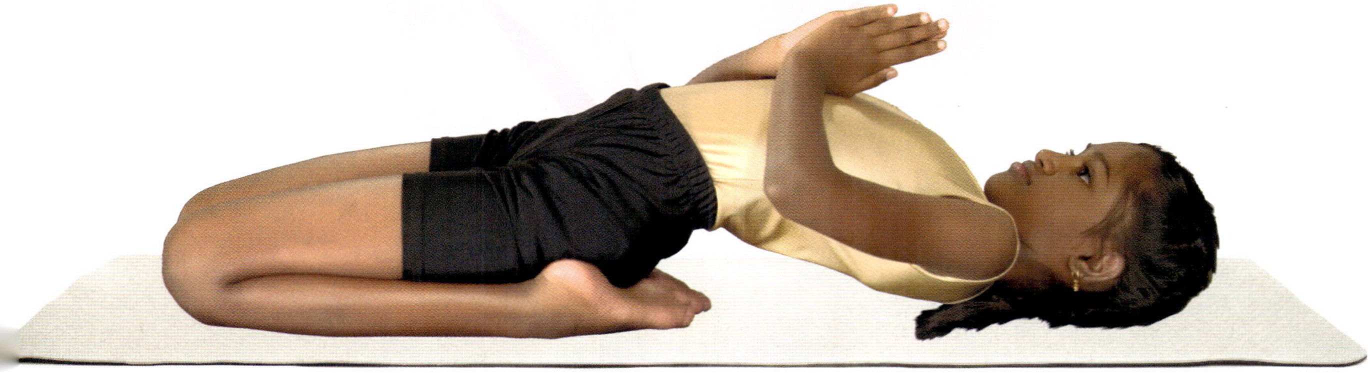

PARYANKASANA (Crown Pose)

PREPARE – Ready

- Sit in Vajrasana.
- Keep back straight and head relaxed.
- Continue normal and relaxed breathing.

START – Steps

1. Place the palms back with the body being supported by the arms.
2. Gently fold from the elbows to the floor.
3. Gently place the crown of the head to the floor.
4. Feel the neck stretch completely.
5. Make sure that the hip is settled on the back of the knees and is stable.

Note from the Acharya

- Slowly raise hands up to lengthen the body completely to feel a complete stretch along the trunk.
- Relax the hands down and lean backwards taking support from the arms, keep stretching the back towards the ground
- Place the elbows on the ground and stretch the neck backwards
- Place the crown of the head firmly on the floor.
- If the head rests comfortably without neck strain release the hand and raise it into a namaste upwards.

Relax – Steps

- Slide back and neck to the floor and relax the body on the ground.
- Relax for a while.
- Place the hands on the floor for support and gently lift the body back to Vajrasana sitting position.
- Relax.

BENEFITS – WOW!

- Relaxes the back and shoulder muscles
- Relaxes the brain and calms agitation
- Makes the legs flexible and supple
- Increases blood circulation along the length of the neck and throat
- Builds up respiratory strength and keep the lungs and heart healthy
- Improves postural defects
- Improves reflex action

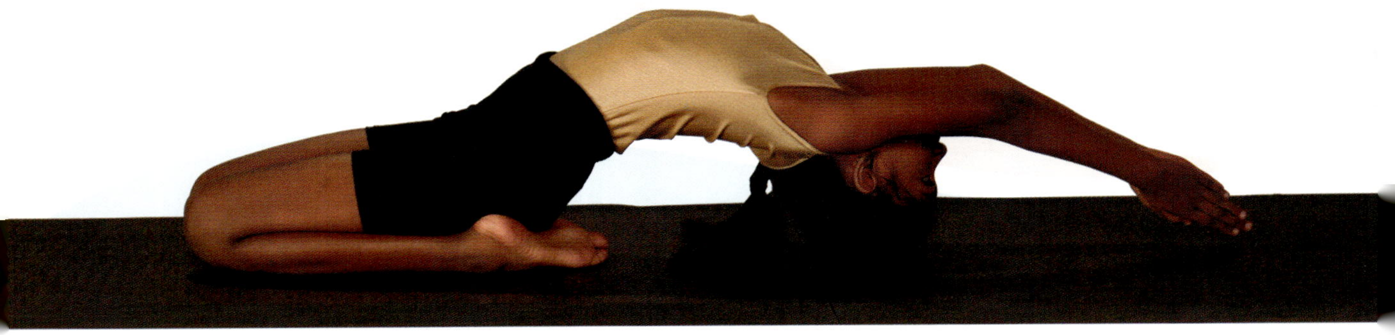

VYAGRASANA (A), VYAGRASANA (B), VYAGRASASANA (C) (Angry Lion Pose)

PREPARE – Ready!

- Sit with the leg folded backwards in Vajrasana.
- Place the hands firmly on the ground.
- Take a deep breath in and open eyes wide and big.
- Open the mouth as wide as possible and pull the tongue out with a strong outward breath.
- Breathe in and out in this position 3 times.
- Each time open the eyes wider and pull the tongue out.

BENEFITS – WOW!

- Releases fatigue and lethargy from the body
- Releases tension and anger from the body
- Cools the insides of the body
- Relaxes the brain
- Improves eyesight and works on the facial muscles
- Calms and relaxes the mind

Note from the Acharya

- Enjoy this asana and look as scary as possible!
- After completing this asana, don't forget to relax and smile.
- Enjoy.

Relax – Steps

- Relax the breathing.
- Relax the eyes and gently pull the tongue in.
- Keep the eyes closed.
- Relax and smile.

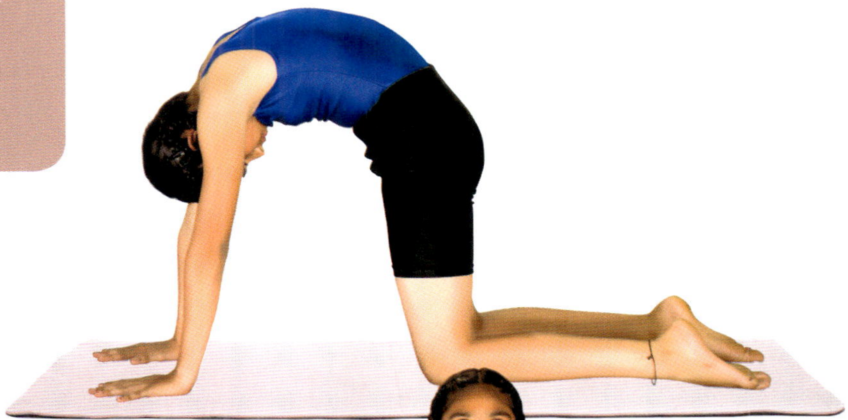

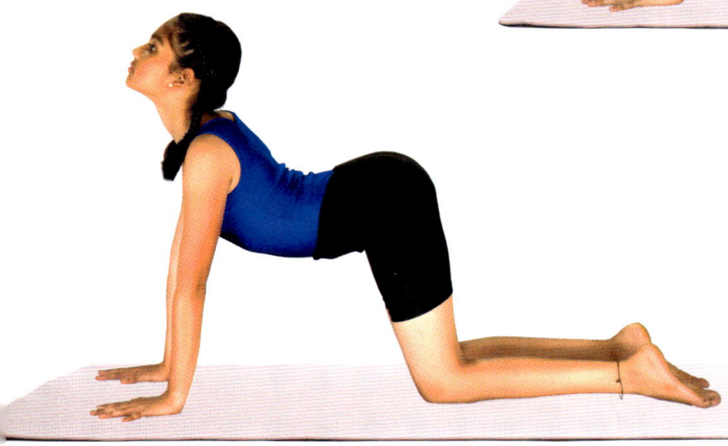

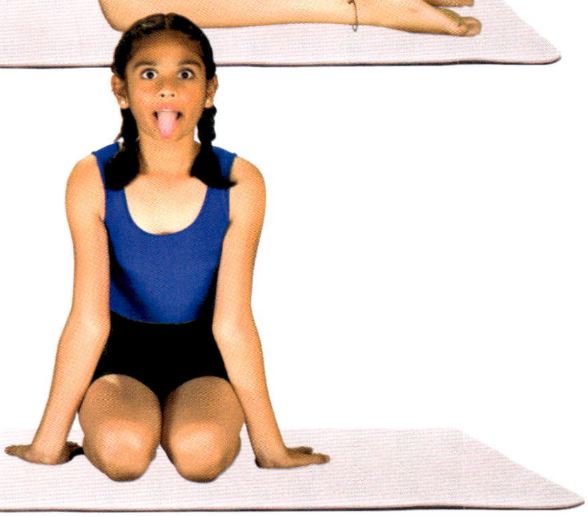

URDWA MUKHA SVANASNA (Upward Facing Dog Pose)

PREPARE – Ready!

- Lie down on stomach.
- Keep neck stretched forward with chin resting on the ground.
- Relax in that position with the hip bones firmly pressed to the ground.
- Keep the legs hip distance apart.

BENEFITS – WOW!

- Stretches the muscles of the entire back
- Shoulders, chest and abdomen benefit
- Opens up the chest and benefits deep breathing.
- Increases the flexibility in the spine and relaxes it
- Stimulates the organs of the abdomen and kidneys
- Relieves stress from the back and relaxes the tired body
- Elevates the mood
- Improves breathing and helps symptoms of asthma

START – Steps

1. Keep the palms by the side of the chest firmly against the floor.
2. Inhale and lift the chest up and keep it strong.
3. Lift the hips off the floor along with the thighs and legs.
4. Keep the muscles along the lower abdominals strong and hold for 3 to 5 deep breaths.

Note from the Acharya

- This asana is highly beneficial as it strengthens the back and helps the spine remain healthy.
- Try to keep the head relaxed to allow blood and oxygen circulation along the upper part of the body.
- Do not lift the shoulders.
- Stretch as far as possible as this asana progresses slowly.

Relax – Steps

- Slowly relax the hips and drop the chest down with an exhalation.
- Relax the head on the floor with chin tucked relaxing the forehead on the floor.
- Stay in position till the strain in the back settles down.

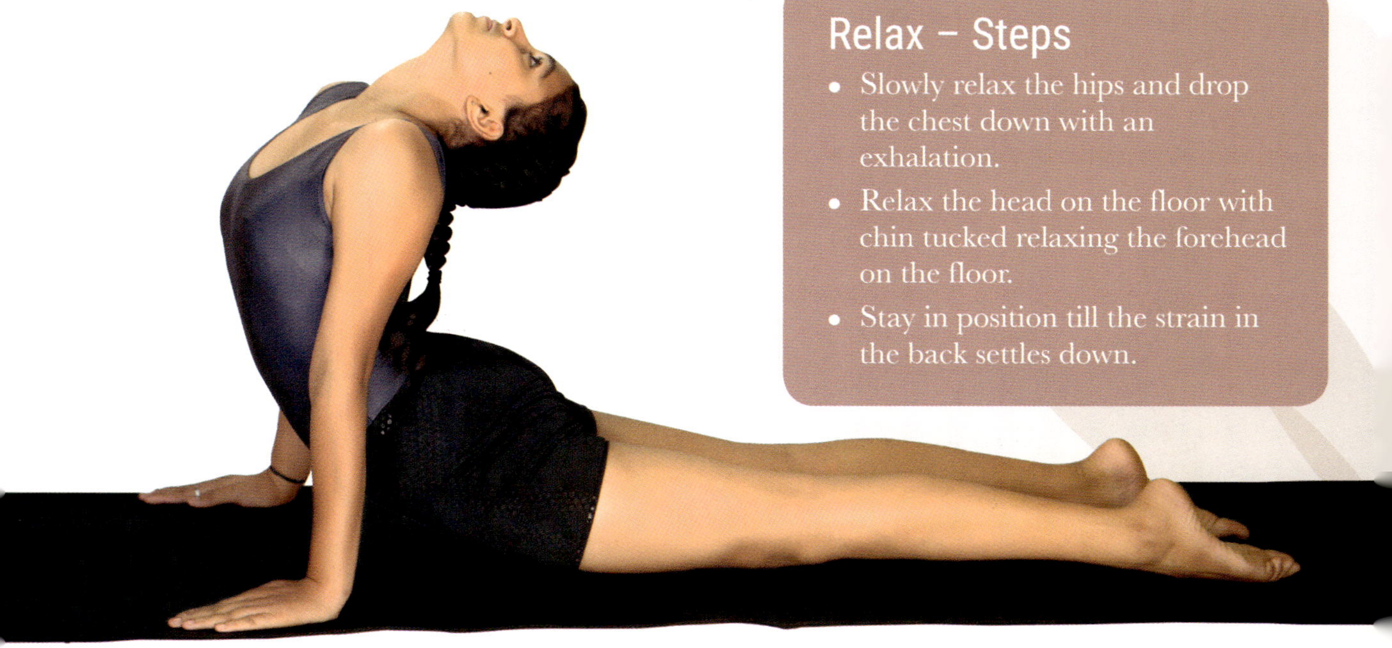

DWIPADA SHALABASANA (Locust Pose)

PREPARE – Ready!

- Lie down on the stomach.
- Keep the neck stretched inward with chin tucked in.
- Relax in that position with the hip bones pinned to the ground.
- Keep the legs hip distance apart.
- Keep the hands tucked under the thighs.

START – Steps

1. Keep the forehead pressed on to the floor with an exhalation.
2. With an inhalation, lift both the legs up as high as possible.
3. Let the palms support the thigh to keep the legs lifted from the ground.
4. Maintain the position for 30 seconds.
5. Breathe deep and strong.

BENEFITS – WOW!

- Stretches the muscles of the entire back
- Shoulder, chest and abdominal area
- Increases the flexibility of the spine and relaxes it
- Stimulates the organs of the abdomen and the kidneys
- Relieves stress from the back and relaxes a tired body
- Excellent asana to strengthen the legs
- Keeps the entire lower body strong
- Helps postural alignment for any defects in the hips and length of the legs

Note from the Acharya

- Rest after this asana with the palm placed like a pillow under the forehead.
- Stay relaxed until the breathing settles down.
- Do not hold your breath in this asana.

Relax – Steps

- Gently drop the legs down and relax.
- Turn the head, place the left ear on the ground, breathe for 10 seconds and then change direction for another 10 seconds of breathing.
- Relax.

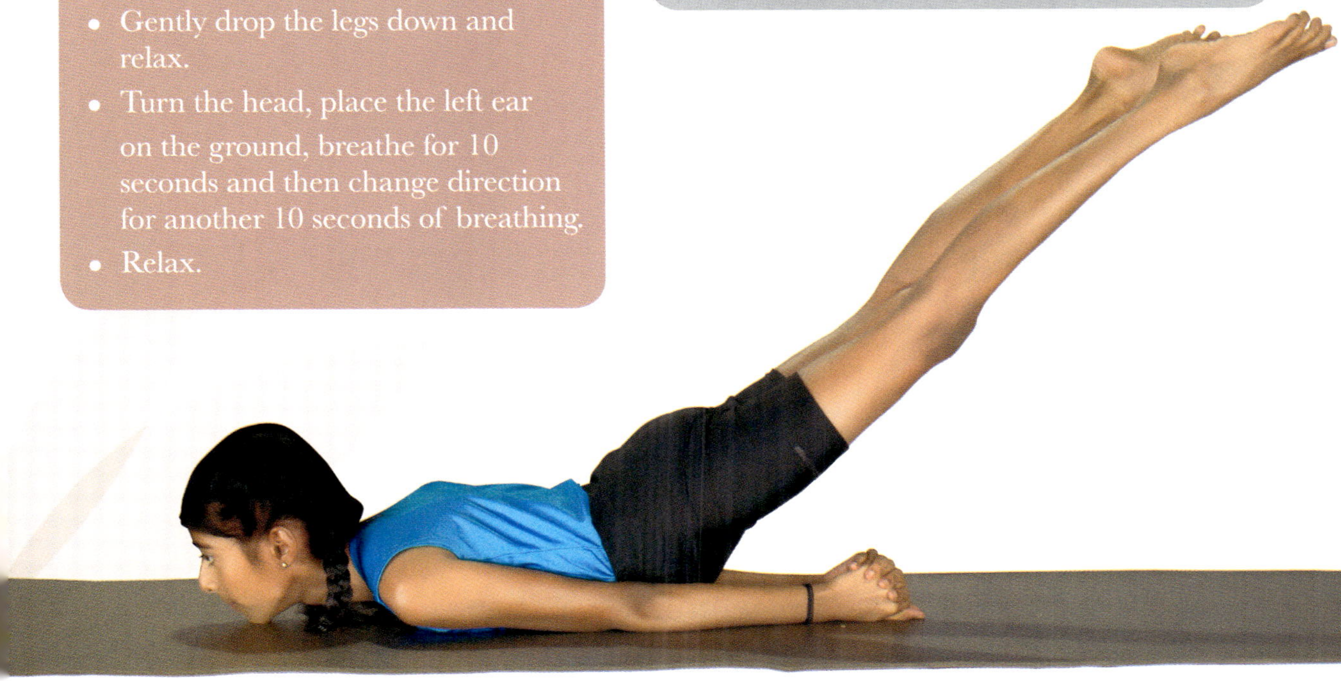

SAMPOORNA DHANURASNA (Circle Bow Pose)

PREPARE – Ready!

- Lie down on stomach.
- Keep neck stretched inward with chin tucked in.
- Relax in that position with the hip bones pinned to the ground.
- Keep the legs hip distance apart.

START – Steps

1. Fold the knees and firmly hold the ankles.
2. Lift the knees off the floor till it curves the lower back.
3. Lift the chest up and breathe deep.
4. Balance on the stomach and hold the position.
5. Slightly rotate the shoulders and hold the top part of the feet. Stay with deep breathing for 15 seconds.

BENEFITS – WOW!

- Strengthens the abdominal muscles and organs
- Opens up the back and increases the flexibility of the spine
- Improves blood circulation along the entire length of the body
- Strengthens the thighs, knees, legs and glutes.
- Expands the chest completely which benefits the organs of the chest
- Improves respiration
- Relieves stress from the body
- Improves posture
- Cures respiratory disorders like asthma

Note from the Acharya

- Deep breathe in this asana to reap the complete benefit of the stretch.
- Keep the shoulders relaxed and dropped away from the head position.
- Look straight with full focus on breathing.

Relax – Steps

- Relax the chest on the floor with an exhalation.
- Relax the thigh and knees on the floor.
- Gently let go of the grip of the ankles.
- Stretch the hands forward and rest till the heart rate comes down.

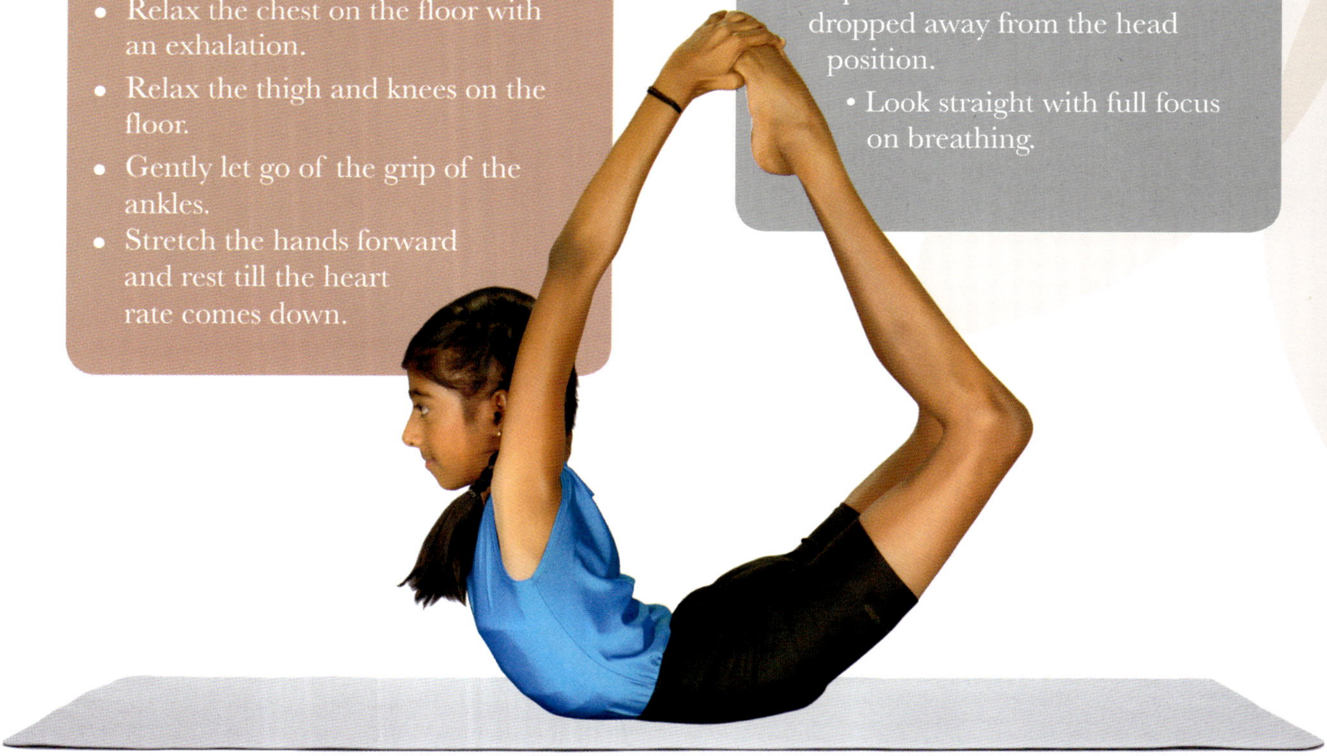

USHTRASANA (Camel Pose)

PREPARE – Ready!

- Sit in Vajrasana and relax.
- Kneel down with a namaste.
- Regulate breathing normally.

START – Steps

- From the position of kneeling down, lift the chest as high as possible. If required use the support of the hands to lift it from behind.
- Point the chest to the ceiling.
- Release the right hand downwards and grab hold of the right heel.
- Adjust the left shoulder to be in line with the right.
- Drop the left hand to grab the left heel.
- Lift the chest up and keep both shoulders stretched open.
- Drop the head backwards stretching the length of the neck.
- Hold the position for 5 deep breaths.

BENEFITS – WOW!

- Expands the chest completely and encourages deep breathing
- Correct posture and helps correct drooping shoulders
- Gently curves the spine increasing the spinal fluid secretion
- Alerts the brain and releases stress from the body
- Improves heart rate
- The lifting of the midriff releases tension and tiredness from the body
- Stretches the thighs and the knees
- Relaxes the lower back and glutes
- Stretches and improves blood circulation in the length of the thighs
- Reduces fat around the back of the abdomen, back of the shoulders and waist

Relax – Steps

- Release the position from the neck by gently lifting the chin up and point it towards the chest.
- Relax the shoulders and pectorals and release the hands from the heels.
- Straighten the spine and release the hands to place it at the side.

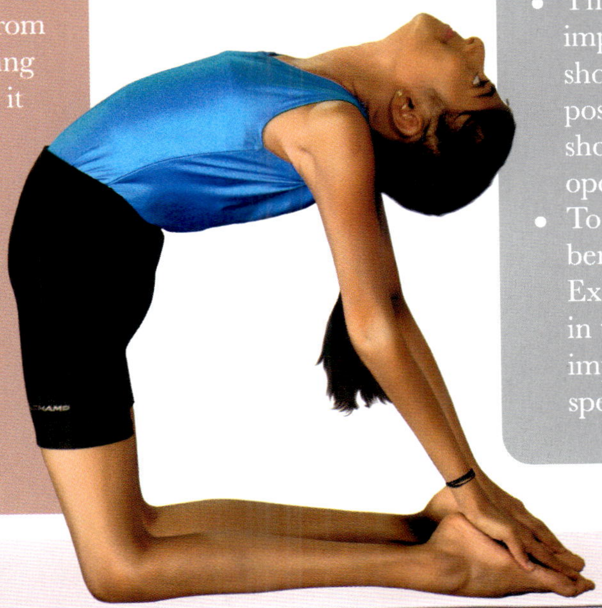

Note from the Acharya

- Try to keep the hips open and lifted.
- This asana helps improve drooping shoulders and correct posture. So keep the shoulders strong and open.
- To reap the best benefits breathe deep. Exhalation is difficult in this asana so it is important to pay special attention to it.

URDWA DHANURASANA (Upside Bow Pose)

PREPARE – Ready!

- Lie down on stomach.
- Keep neck stretched inward with chin tucked in.
- Relax in that position with the hip bones pinned to the ground.
- Keep the legs hip distance apart.

START – Steps

1. Bend hand from the elbows and place the palms by the sides of the upper part of the shoulders.
2. Elbows to remain perpendicular to the ground with fingers pointing towards shoulders.
3. Pressing the feet to the floor lift the hip up towards the ceiling.
4. Keep the thighs parallel to the ground.
5. Feel the weight of the body on the palms and keep the chest fully expanded.
6. Stay in position to deep breathe.

BENEFITS – WOW!

- This asana keeps the spine flexible
- It opens up the chest and increases the strength of breathing
- It also builds strength in the legs and tones the thighs
- It relaxes the mind and builds in courage and confidence
- Keeps the brain alert with increased blood and air circulation

Note from the Acharya

- Do not do this asana if there is a back injury.
- This asana should not be done while suffering from an upset stomach or just recovering from it.
- This asana is not to be done if there is a headache.

Relax – Steps

- With control slowly drop the hips to the ground and rest the spine on the floor.
- Relax the knees and thighs and pull it towards the chest to relax.
- Stay in position till the breathing becomes normal.

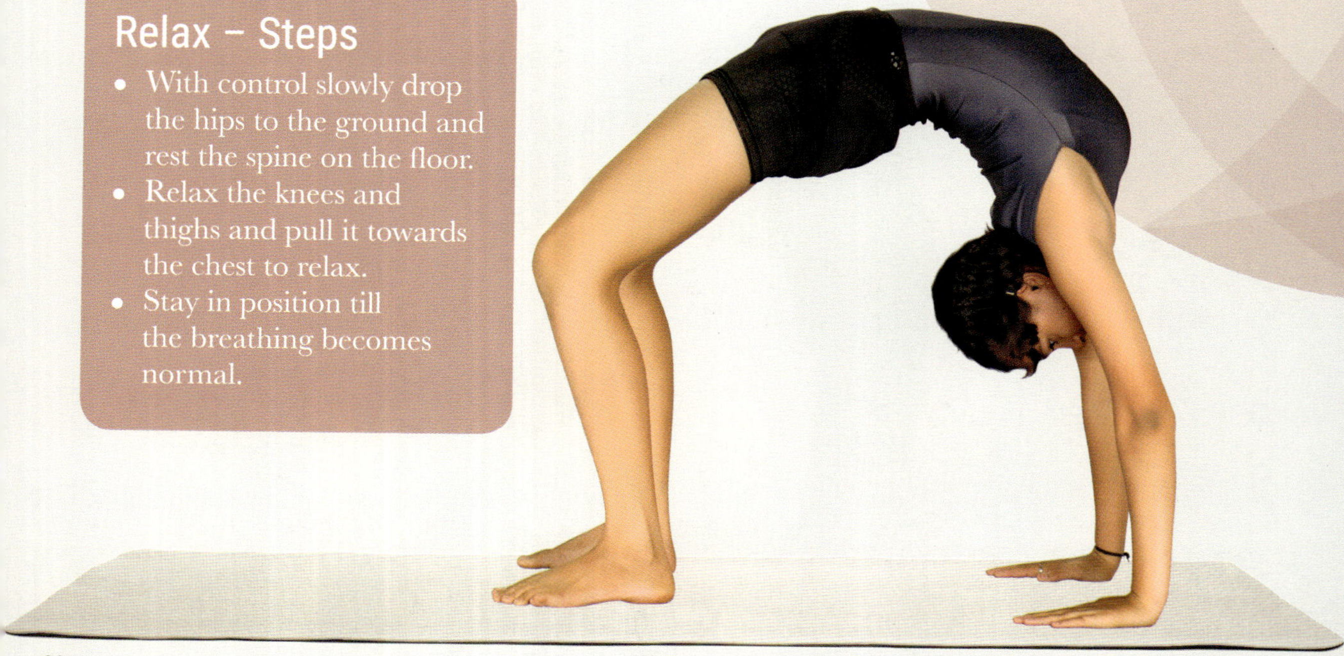

BHUJAPEEDASANA (Shoulder Balance Pose)

PREPARE – Ready!

- Take a squatting position with the thighs open with palms placed on the floor.
- Walk the legs forward in front of the palms as far as possible to go.
- Wrap the legs around the elbows and lock the feet one above the other.
- Relax in the position until a balance is established.

START – Steps

1. Keep the lock strong and lift it off the ground
2. Fix the knees comfortably on the upper region of arms and slightly hunch the back to create space for the feet to lift up.
3. Stay focused and look down at the floor.
4. Shift the weight of the body to settle on the arms.
5. Keep the feet lifted and locked closer to the chest.
6. Breathe calmly and focus on balance.

Relax – Steps

- Drop both feet down gently.
- Stay in the squat position and rest.

BENEFITS – WOW!

- Builds focus and concentration
- Strengthens the abdominal muscles
- Very helpful asana for children who are into sports
- Brings alertness to the mind
- Helps practise patience

Note from the Acharya

- A lot of patience is required while working on this asana.
- If the feel is that you are falling forward in the position, then you are not doing it right.
- The body has to stay strong and parallel to the ground before initiating the lift of the leg.
- It will take some time but once practised and achieved you will always enjoy doing this asana.

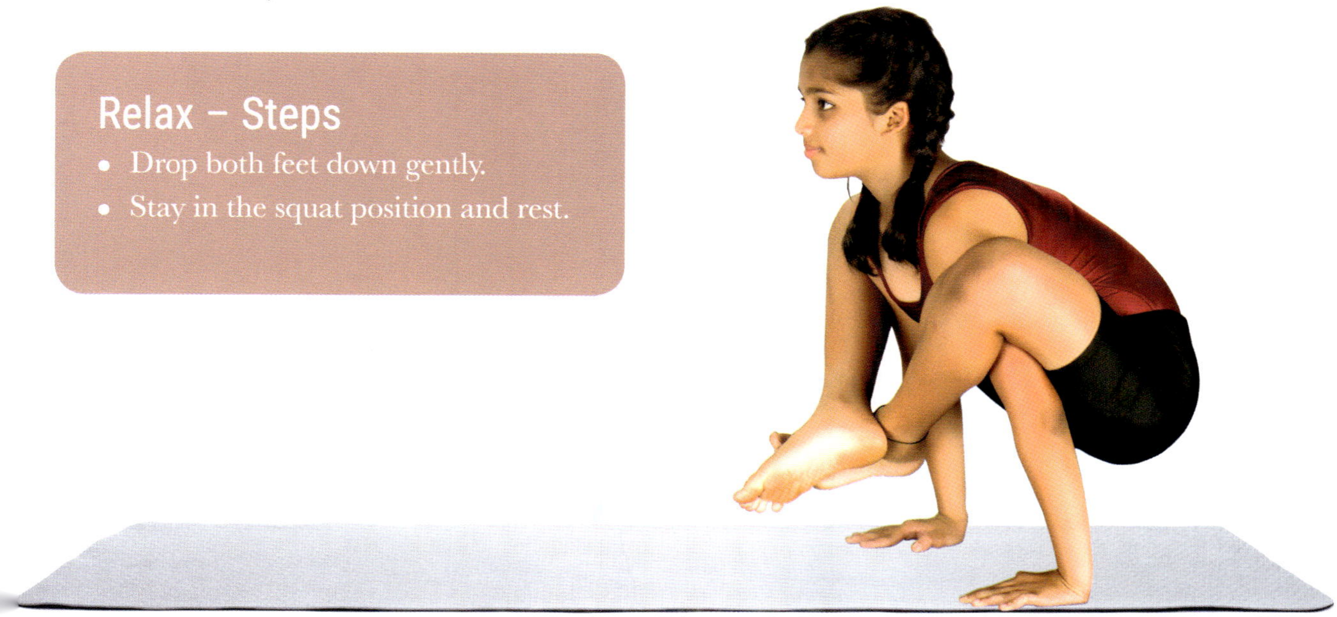

BAKASANA – (Big Bird Pose)

PREPARE – Ready!

- Take a squat position.
- Fix the knees comfortably on the upper region of arms above the elbows.
- Stay focused and look down at the floor.
- Relax and regularise breathing and focus on balance.

BENEFITS – WOW!

- Builds focus and concentration
- Makes the body feel light like a bird
- Strengthens the abdominal muscles
- Very helpful asana for children who are into sports
- Brings alertness to the mind
- Helps practise patience

START – Steps

1. Shift weight of the body to settle on the arms.
2. Practise by lifting one leg for some time.
3. Eventually lift up both the legs up and balance.

Relax – Steps

- Drop both the feet down gently.
- Stay in the squat position and rest.

Note from the Acharya

- A lot of patience is required while working on this asana.
- If the feel is that you are falling forward in the position, then you are not doing it right.
- The body has to stay strong and parallel to the ground before initiating the lift of the leg.
- It will take some time but once practised and achieved you will enjoy doing this asana all the time.

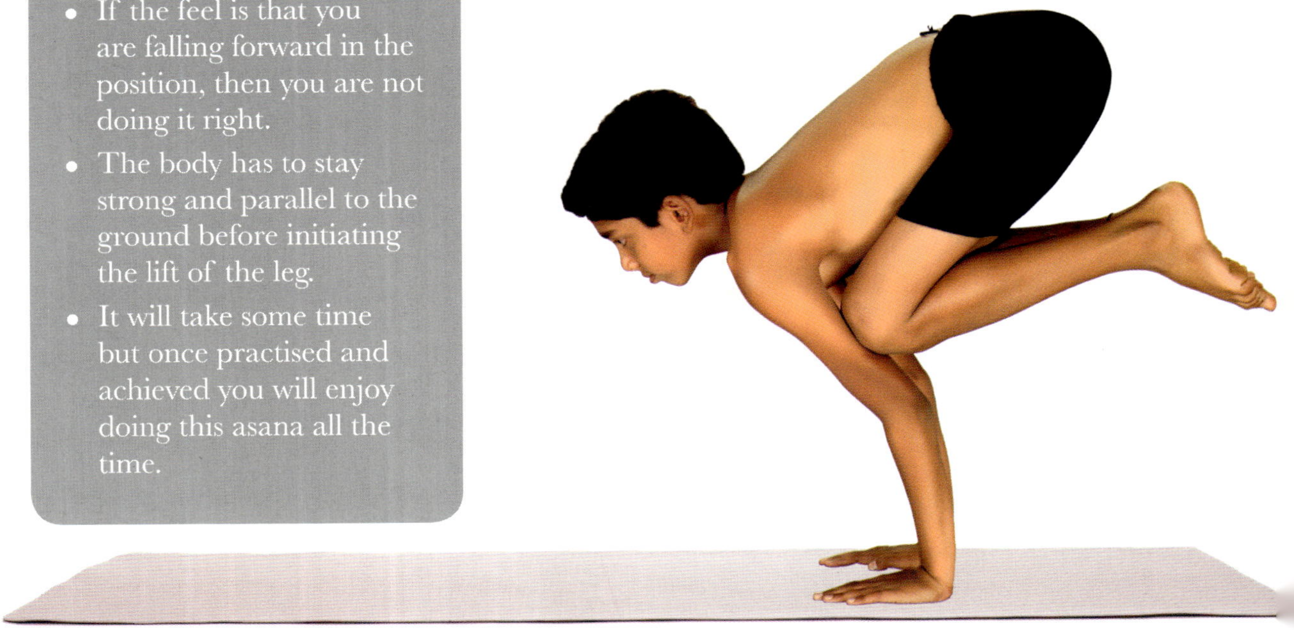

SHIRASASANA (Head Stand Pose)

PREPARE – Ready!

- Kneel down and sit comfortably.
- Make a triangle with the forearms and elbows and place closer to the wall.
- Keep the fingers firmly interlocked.
- Place the head on the floor and shift the weight of the body to the head.
- Keep the position and get used to the blood flow and the weight on your head.

START – Steps

1. The head should be now placed between the arms with the forearms pressing the ground.
2. Adjust the neck and keep it neutral.
3. Release all pressure from the neck and shift it to the forearm.
4. Keep the shoulders pulled away from the ears.
5. Gently lift one leg up and see how that feels.
6. Eventually lift the other leg up and steady.
7. Push all the weight to the forearm and balance it.
8. Hold the position for as long as possible with relaxed breathing.

Relax – Steps

- Gently drop the legs down and stay in the kneeling down position.
- Stay kneeled down with the head resting on the floor.
- Relax and breathe.
- Very gently roll up and stay with the eyes closed till breathing and heart rate settle down.

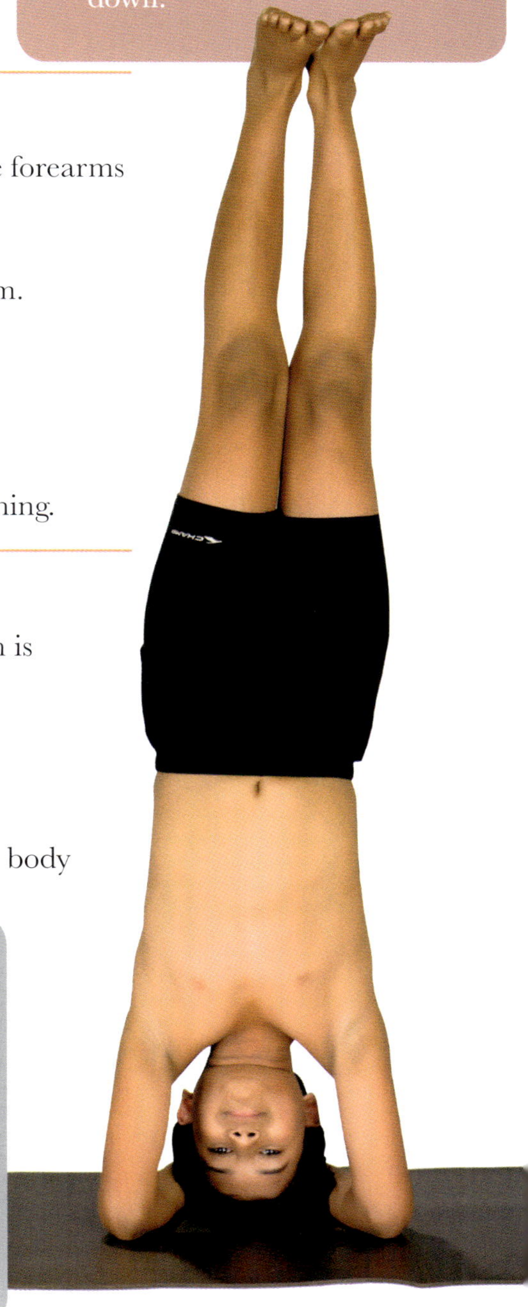

BENEFITS – WOW!

- The brain will get a rich supply of blood and oxygen which is highly beneficial
- This asana improves vision and keeps the brain alert
- Increases immunity
- Improves all the organ functions of the body
- Improves the quality of sleep and aids in the growth of the body

Note from the Acharya

- Practise the asana against the wall with the help of a guide.
- Try and keep all the muscles relaxed.
- Practice this asana only after completing practice of all other asanas.
- Do not practise this asana after intense physical exercise as vigorous workouts release toxins in the body.

GOMUKHASANA (Cow Face Pose)

PREPARE – Ready!

- Sit straight with legs stretched forward.
- Look straight and settle breathing.

START – Steps

1. Slide the left foot under the right knee to the outer side of the left hip.
2. Cross the right leg over the left.
3. Get the knees in line with each other.
4. The left foot must now slide in line with the right hip.
5. Make sure the both feet is arranged in a straight line on either side of the hips.
6. Lift both the arms and lengthen it.
7. Fold the left arm from up towards the shoulder.
8. First drop the right arm down towards the floor and the fold it upwards and hold.
9. Keep the neck straight and gaze straight.
10. Bend forward and press the abdomen along the length of the thighs.
11. Stay in position and deep breathe for 30 seconds.

BENEFITS – WOW!

- Improves flexibility of the back
- Relaxes the shoulders and stretches the arms
- A relaxing asana which helps release stress and anxiety in the mind and body
- Expands the chest and relaxes the diaphragm which benefits the respiratory organs

Relax – Steps

- Gently lift the body up with the hands still in place.
- Once the body is upright release the hand, lift it upwards to release arms and stretch the back of the shoulders.
- Release the hands to the floor.
- Slowly slide the legs back to Dandasana.
- Relax in the position for a while till the circulation settles down along the legs.
- Repeat on the other side.

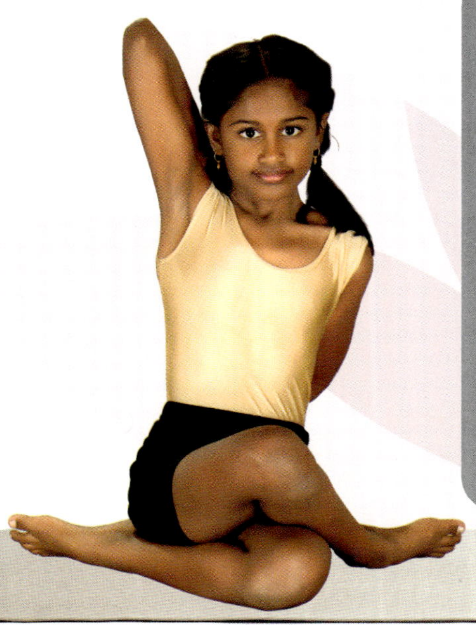

Note from the Acharya

- Make sure that the seat bones evenly rest on the floor.
- Keep the spine straight while tilting forward.
- This is a safe asana and extremely relaxing.
- If the seat is not settling, sit on a small pillow to avoid tilting of the hips.

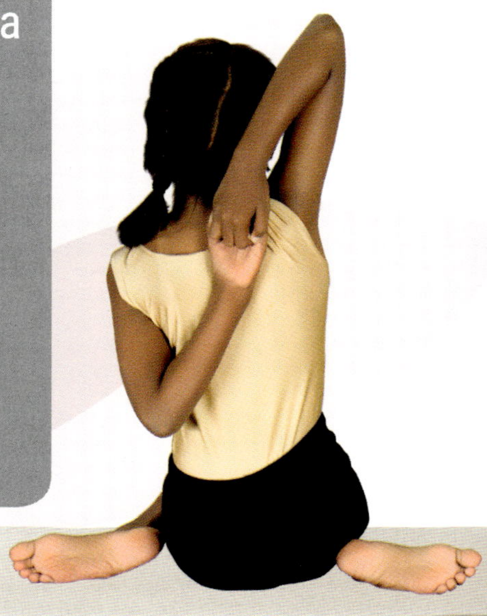

MARJARIASANA (Rabbit King Pose)

PREPARE – Ready!

- Sit with the legs folded backwards in Vajrasana.
- Keep the spine erect and eyes closed.
- Relax in the position for the knees to establish a stretch.

START – Steps

1. Keep the knees open to a hip distance apart.
2. Gently fold the body till the abdomen settles between the thighs.
3. Lift the hip up and push the chest towards the ground constantly adjusting the position.
4. Keep the lower back lifted up towards the ceiling.
5. Stretch arms forward as far as possible and hold the palm firmly on the floor.
6. Stay in position for 5 deep breaths with the body completely relaxed.

BENEFITS – WOW!

- Stretches the back, hips and thighs, knees and ankles
- Relaxes spine and shoulders
- Increases blood supply to the brain
- Improves vision and relaxes stress in the body
- Calms the mind
- Releases stress and fatigue from the body and mind

Note from the Acharya

- The asana should feel relaxed.
- Do normal breathing in the asana and rest.

Relax – Steps

- Release the length of the spine and the stretched arms.
- Keep the abdominal length pulled in and strong.
- Take the support of the arms and lift the body up gently to the sitting Vajrasana position.

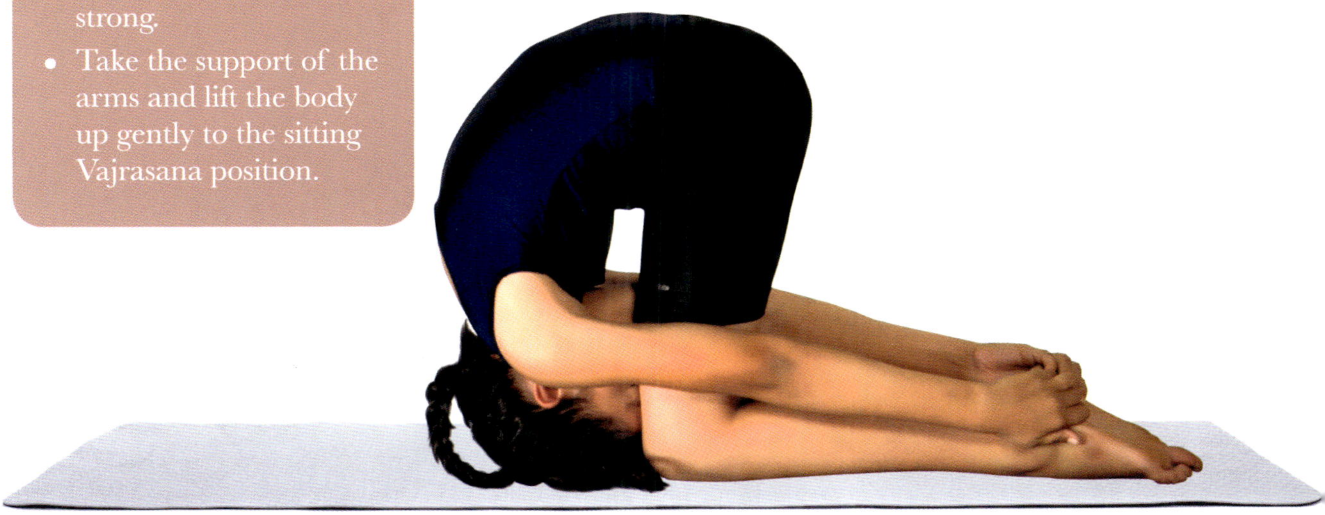

PASHASANA (Deep Squat Pose)

PREPARE – Ready!

- Squat down with thighs close together. If the heels are lifting off the ground, place a cushion under the heels.
- Keep the spine and back straight as possible.
- Keep shoulders open and chest relaxed.
- Head in line with the shoulders.
- Keep your *drishti* straight by fixing your eyes to a point in front of you.
- Smile calmly and maintain deep breathing.

CONSTRUCT – Steps

1. Keep feet pressed to the ground and together.
2. Keep the hips steady in a balance and open as wide as possible.
3. Keep the hands in a namaste, keeping the thighs as close to the abdominals as possible.
4. Keep the chest lifted up and each time you breathe, feel the chest expand.
5. Keep the eyes calm and focus on breathing as deep as possible.
6. Stay strong in the position.

Relax – Steps

- Relax the back and release the namaste. Let the arms rest on the floor.
- Gently press the hips down and sit.
- Slowly straighten the knees and relax by stretching the arms by the side of the hips or straighten the knees and relax in Dandasana.

BENEFITS – WOW!

- Improves flexibility of the hips and increases circulation around the area
- Releases tightness in the lower back area
- Strengthens knees and legs.
- Improves digestion and assimilation of food
- Builds focus and concentration
- Helps children sit for long hours comfortably

Note from the Acharya

- Keep the shoulders relaxed but chest open and lifted up.
- Can be done any time, especially when the back is feeling stiff after long hours of sitting or after sports.
- Girls can do this asana during menstruation.
- Do not do this asana while recovering from an upset stomach, indigestion or even constipation.

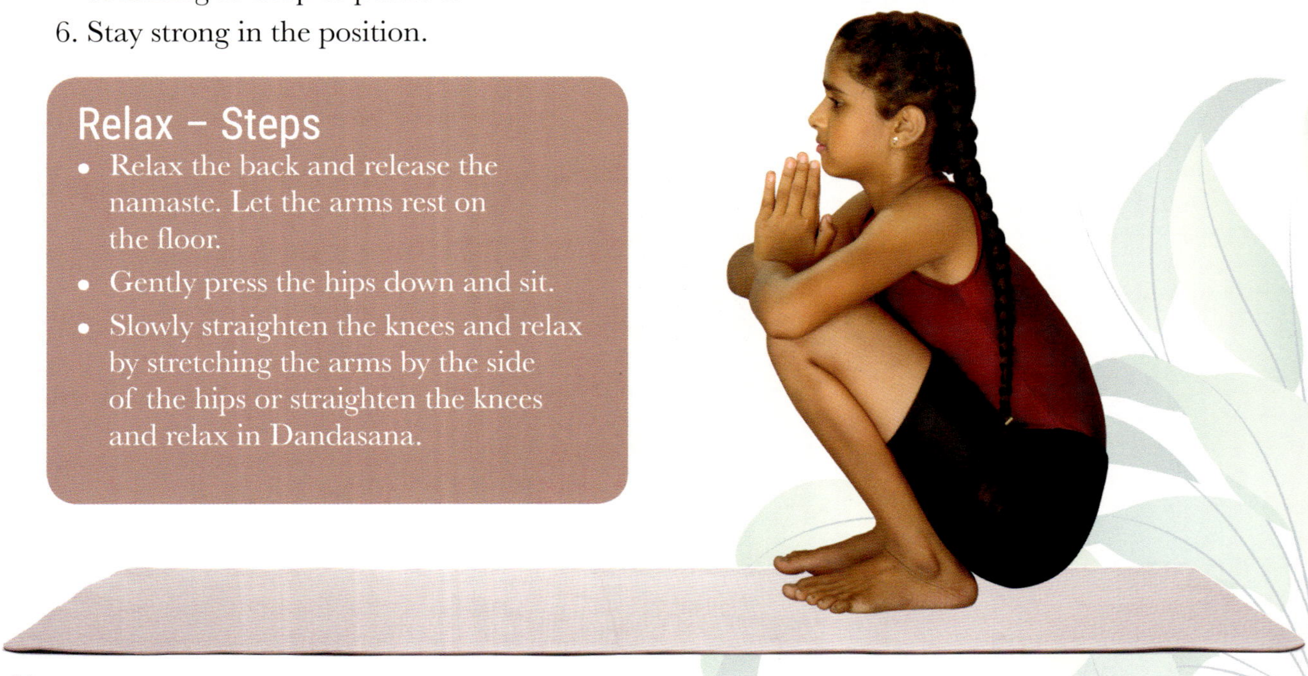

CHADURANGA DANDASANA (Plank Pose)

PREPARE – Ready!

- Sit on the floor with legs together and extended strong.
- Keep the seat bone pressed down and slightly forward to get a good grip.

START – Steps

1. Keep the abdomen pulled in and downwards.
2. The spine should be straight and pointing downwards.
3. Keep the ankles flexed with the feet pointing up and heels pressed downwards.
4. Keep the torso perpendicular to the floor.

Relax – Steps

- Release all muscular tension from the spine and legs and relax.

BENEFITS – WOW!

- Strengthens the back muscles
- Aligns posture and lengthens the spine
- Helps in the growth and length of the body
- Stretches and opens up shoulders and chest

Note from the Acharya

- It is important to keep the back straight in this asana. This is a preparatory asana for almost all sitting asanas as it sets the spine in a neutral position.
- A simple way to check alignment is to sit with the back against the wall. The lower back and the shoulder blades should be engaged to be pressed against the wall.
- This is a very beneficial asana to practise daily.

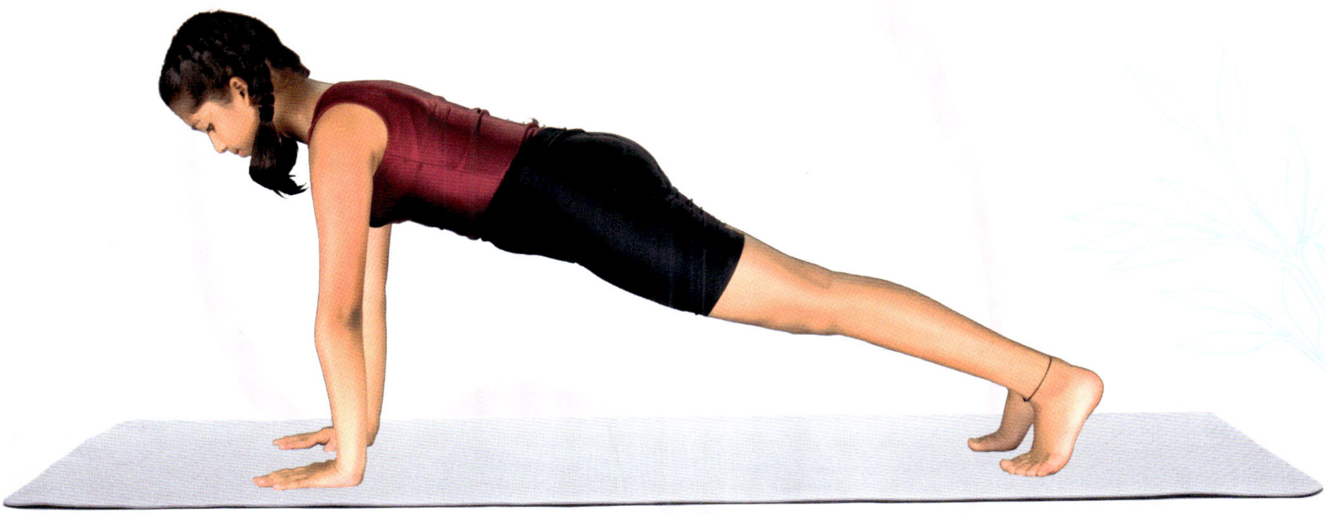

MARICHASANA (A) (Sage Pose)

PREPARE – Ready

- Sit straight with the legs stretched out and fix the seat bones firmly on the ground in Dandasana.

START – Steps

1. Fold the right leg and hold the knee close to the chest.
2. Breathe out completely before you start twisting the trunk towards the back (right shoulder pointing back).
3. Wrap the arms around the twist and hold the twist with strength, holding the arms tight.
4. Look back and stay in the position for 30 seconds.
5. Keep breathing and keep smiling.

BENEFITS – WOW!

- A cleansing and detoxing asana
- Stimulates the walls of the abdominal organs
- Clears the mind and regulates thoughts
- Reduces sugar levels from the body which helps body to calm down
- Trims the waist and melts abdominal fat
- Keeps the body strong

Note from the Acharya

- Do not hold your breath at any point of getting into the asana.
- Try not to jerk in the position of stretch.
- Do it as far as possible paying attention to your breathing.
- You can take help to get a grip on your hand.
- If you are recovering from an upset stomach/fever do not attempt this asana.

Relax – Steps

- Release the grip of the hand and relax the twisted shoulder.
- Rotate the shoulder front and stretch the folded leg forward and straight.
- Breathe out completely and relax before you start on the other side.

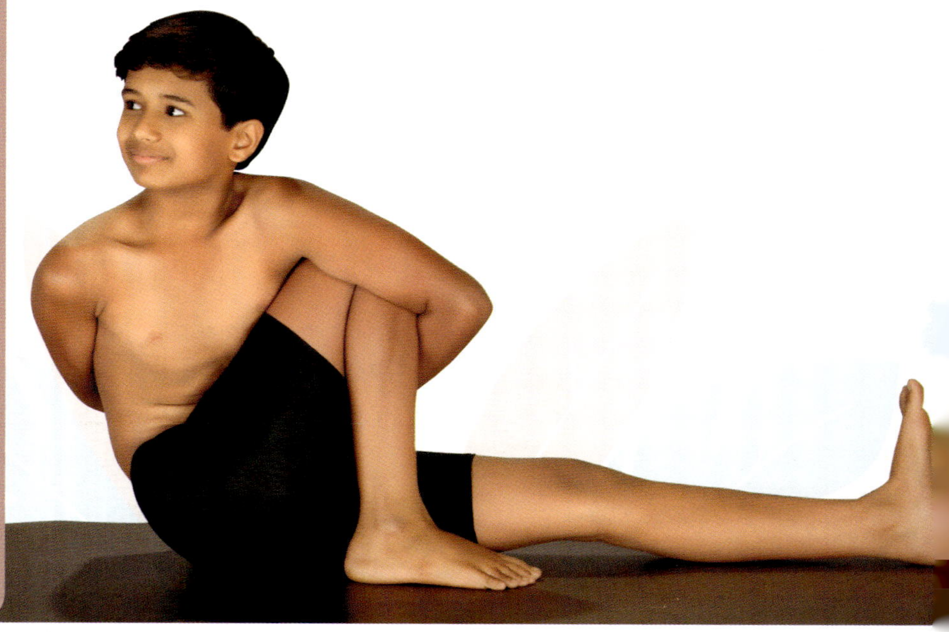

PASCHIMOTANASANA – (Forward Fold Pose)

PREPARE – Ready!

- Sit straight with legs stretched forward (Dandasana.)
- Look straight and settle breathing.
- While inhaling expand the chest and while exhaling deflate from the abdominal length.
- Practise deep breathing for 10 seconds.

START – Steps

1. Start folding the body forwards the thighs with the head reaching towards the knees.
2. The lower abdomen should touch the thighs first.
3. Keep breathing at every step while doing this asana.
4. Stay calm and focus on breathing and lengthening the spine.
5. Stay wherever comfortable and focus on breathing deep.
6. Don't force the stretch.
7. Stay calm and breathe for 30 seconds.

BENEFITS – WOW!

- Calms the brain
- Regular practice helps release depression in the body
- Releases anger and anxiety and keeps the mind calm and in control
- Reduces baby fat from around the lower belly
- Helps relieve discomfort during menstruation

Note from the Acharya

- If the back is feeling stiff due to sitting for a long time, this asana is the wrong asana to practise.
- If there is an injury in the back, this asana should be done carefully under supervision.

Relax – Steps

- Slowly lift the body up with an inhalation and sit straight and relax.
- Feel blood circulation in the back and observe the back, release and relax.

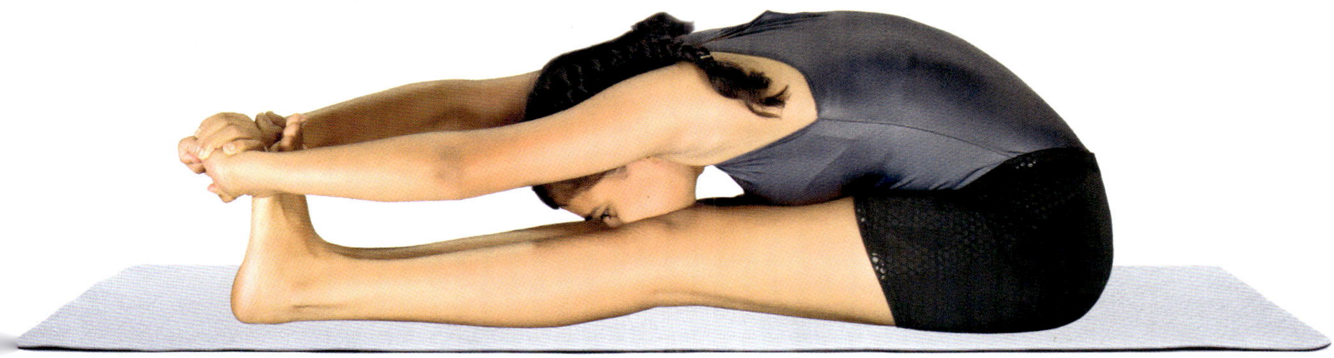

PURVOTTANASANA (Upward Plank Pose)

PREPARE – Ready!

- Sit straight with the legs stretched forward (Dandasana).
- Breathe in the position expanding chest and pulling the stomach in deep.

BENEFITS – WOW!

- Opens the chest and benefits the respiratory organs
- Benefits arms and shoulders and strengthens the wrists

START – Steps

1. Place the hands several inches behind the hips with the fingers pointing forward.
2. Bend knees and place the big toe on the floor by slightly tilting the legs.
3. Keep the arms firmly pressed to the ground and lift the hip up to be in line with the thighs.
4. Gently slide the feet forward keeping the buttocks strong so that the hip doesn't drop down.
5. Keep the torso and the thighs in the same height.
6. Keep the legs straight.
7. Keep the shoulder blades tucked in for better grip.
8. Without compressing the back of the neck slowly drop the head back.
9. Hold for 30 seconds and drop the hip down.

Note from the Acharya

- Do not do this if you have an injured wrist.
- Keep the chest strong so that the shoulders do not feel too much strain.
- Keep the shoulders pulled away from the ears before stretching the head back.

Relax – Steps

1. Gently lift head up to look into your chest.
2. Release the hip to the ground.
3. Get hand forward or to a namaste and relax your breathing.

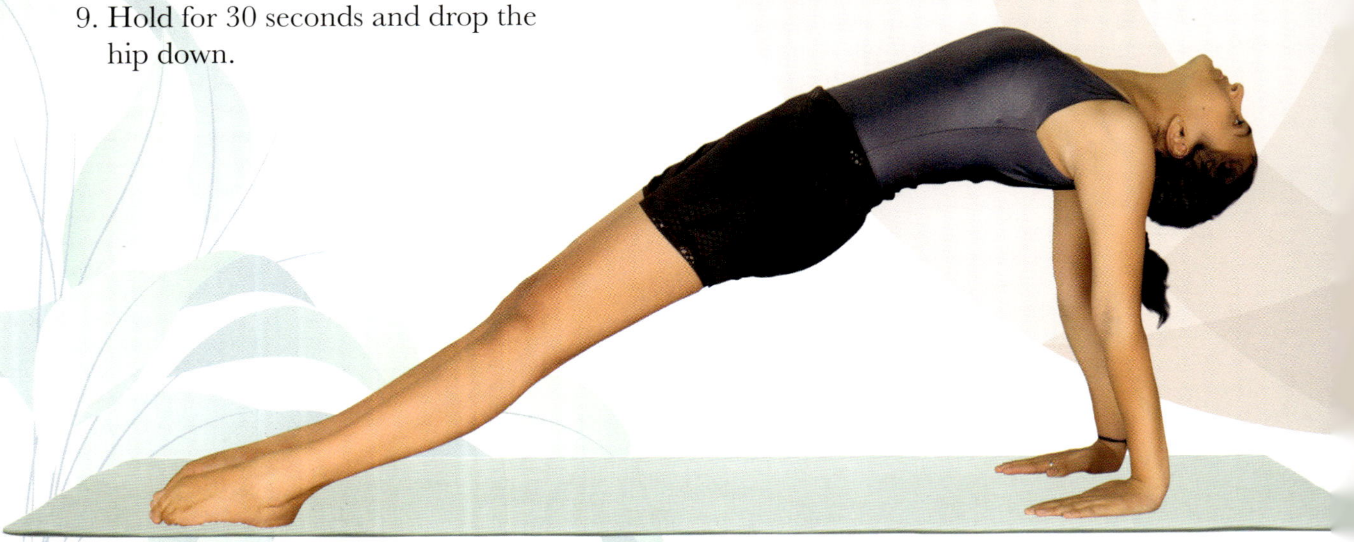

PADMASANA (Lotus Pose)

PREPARE – Ready!

- Sit in Dandasana keeping back straight and stomach pulled in.
- Regularise breathing and keep the seat bones pressed to the ground and spine erect.

START – Steps

1. Bend the right knee and place it on the left thigh.
2. Keep the soles of the feet turned upwards.
3. Now, bend the left knee and place in over the right thigh.
4. Keep both the heels close to the groin towards the abdomen.
5. Place the palm on the thighs and relax.
6. Keep breathing steadily for at least 30 seconds.

Relax – Steps

- Release the right knee and let it rest by stretching it forwards.
- Relax the left knee and keep the legs stretched.

BENEFITS – WOW!

- Relaxes the mind and makes the mind steady
- Benefits the digestive organs and improves digestion.
- Increases flexibility along the length of the legs and keeps them strong and supple

Note from the Acharya

- Do not do this asana if there is a knee injury.
- Make sure the legs are warmed up before doing this asana.

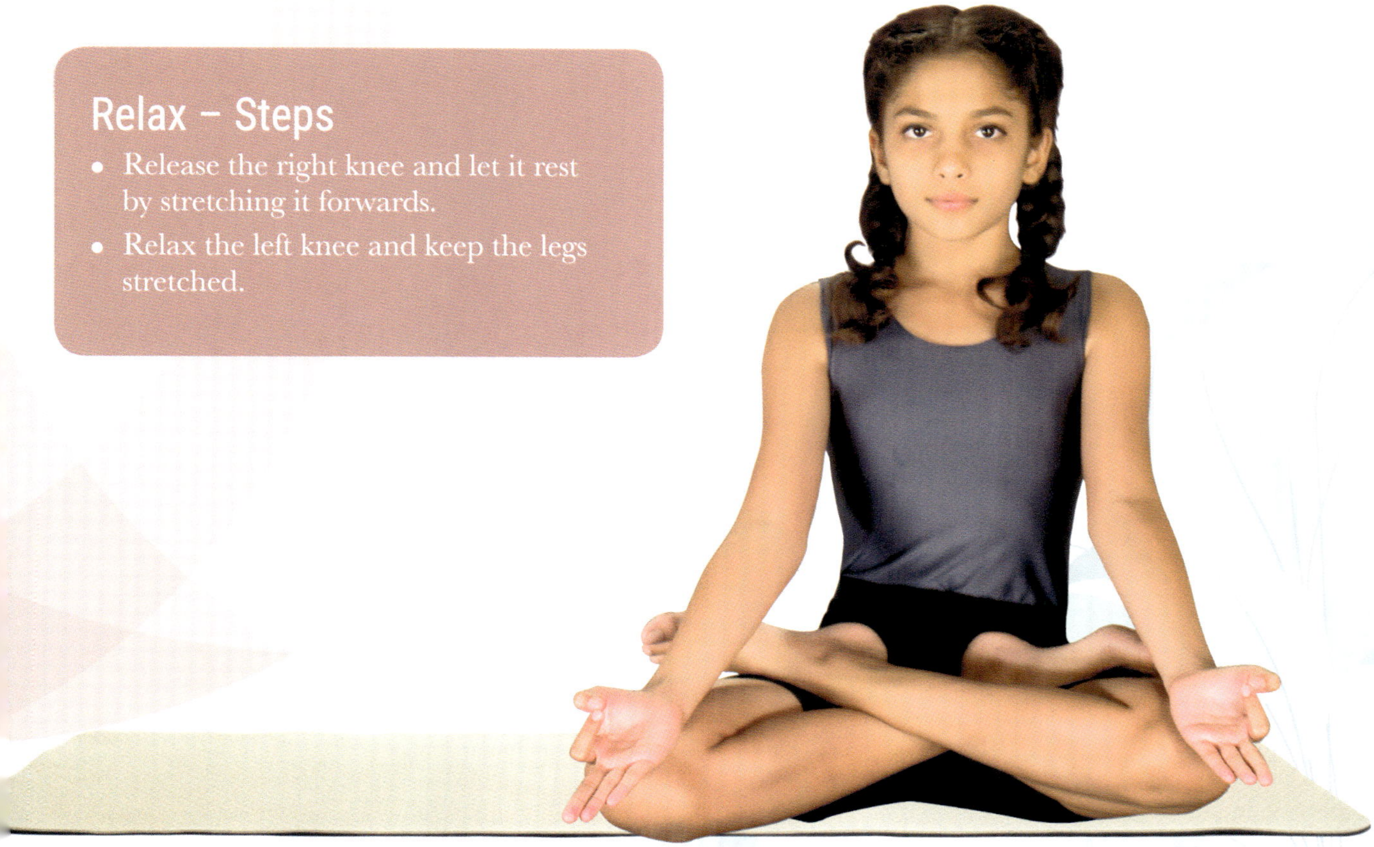

BADHAPADMASANA (Half-lotus Bind)

PREPARE – Ready!

- Sit in Dandasana keeping back straight and stomach pulled in.
- Regularise breathing and keep the seat bones pressed to the ground and spine erect.

START – Steps

1. Bend the right knee and place it on the left thigh.
2. Keep the soles of the feet turned upwards.
3. Take the right hand around the back and grab hold of your toe.
4. Lean forward without bending the knee and losing grip of the thumb which is holding the right toe.
5. Stay comfortable with deep breathing.
6. Hold in the bent-down position for 30 seconds.

Relax – Steps

- Release the right knee and let it rest by stretching it forwards.
- Relax the left knee and keep the legs stretched.

BENEFITS – WOW!

- This asana relaxes the mind and makes the mind steady
- Benefits the digestive organs and improves digestion
- Increases flexibility along the length of the legs and keeps them strong and supple

Note from the Acharya

- Do not do this asana if there is a knee injury.
- Make sure the legs are warmed up before doing this asana.

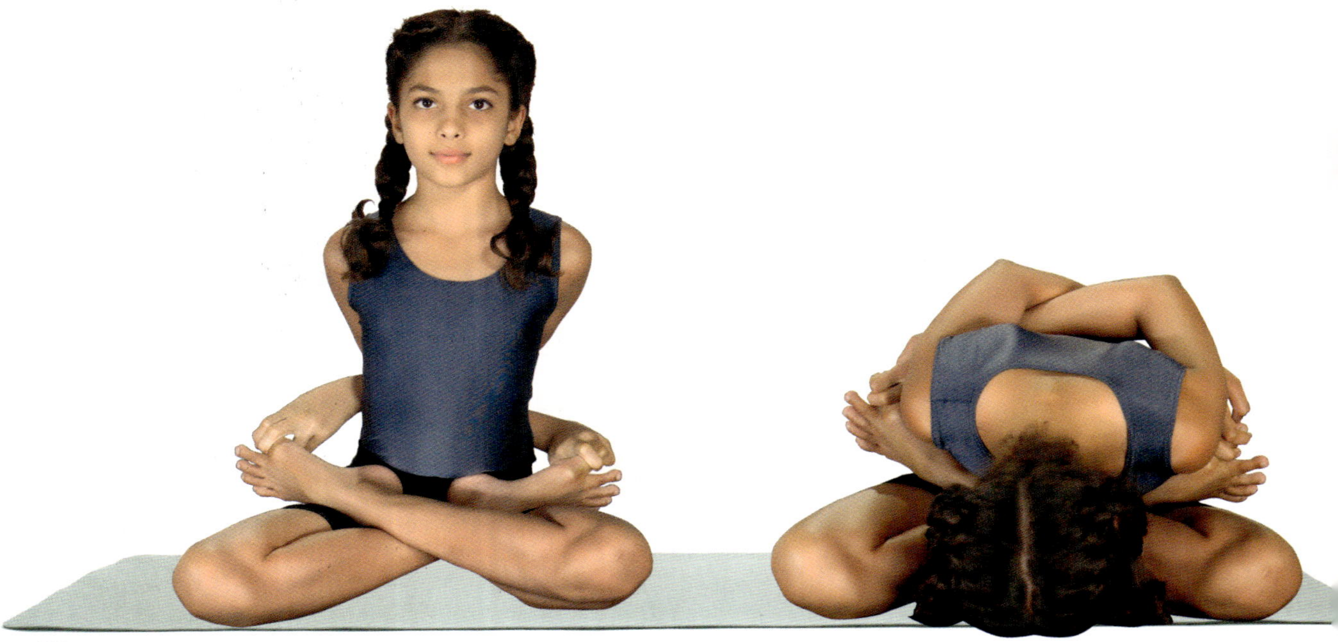

JANUSHIRASASANA (Head To Knee Pose)

PREPARE – Ready!

- Sit in Dandasana keeping back straight and stomach pulled in.
- Regularise breathing and keep the seat bones pressed to the ground and spine erect.

START – Steps

1. Bend the right knee and place the feet close to the groin.
2. Keep the soles of the feet turned upwards.
3. Lean forward without bending the knee and losing the grip of the thumb which is holding the right toe.
4. Stay comfortable with deep breathing.
5. Hold in the bent-down position for 30 seconds.
6. Repeat the asana on the other side.

BENEFITS – WOW!

- Relaxes the mind and makes the mind steady
- Benefits the digestive organs and improves digestion
- Increases flexibility along the length of the legs and keeps them strong and supple

Note from the Acharya

- Do not do this asana if there is a knee injury.
- Make sure the legs are warmed up before doing this asana.

Relax – Steps

- Release the right knee and let it rest by stretching it forwards
- Relax the left knee and keep the legs stretched

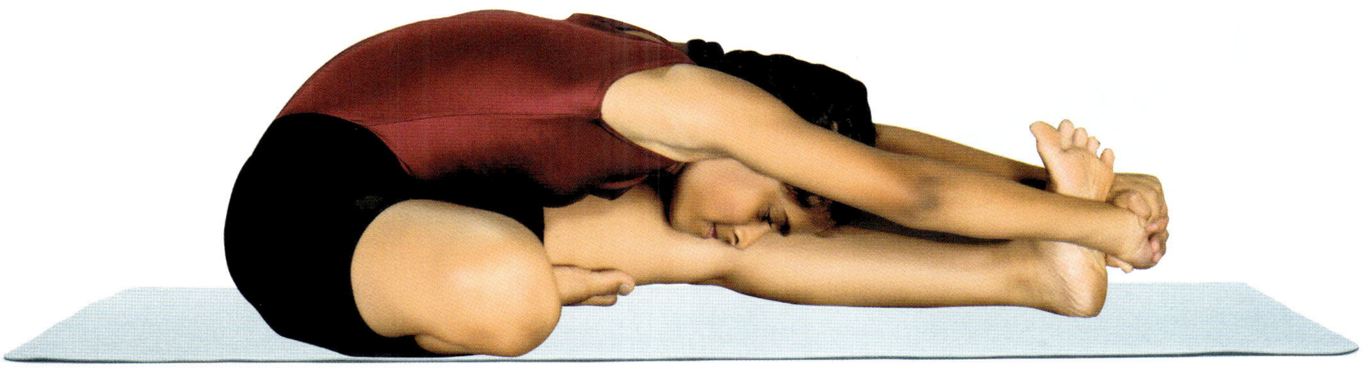

PARIVRITTA JANUSHIRASANA (Twisted Head To Knee Pose)

PREPARE – Ready!

- Sit in Dandasana with stretched legs, spine straight and gaze straight.
- Fold right knee and place the feet close to the groin.
- Stay in position breathing deep.

START – Steps

1. Exhale and lean to the right and press the back of the right shoulder to the inside of the right knee.
2. Drop the forearm on the floor close to the right knee.
3. Lengthen the right side of the torso along the inside of the thigh.
4. Reach the right palm to hold the edge of the right foot and reach the left hand over the head to reach the toe of the right foot.
5. Hold the position for 20 seconds and breathe comfortably.

Relax – Steps

- Exhale, release the hands and rotate the torso to face the floor.
- Gently, without straining the back, straighten the spine and stay still for a few seconds.
- Release the feet and keep in line with the left and relax.
- Repeat on the other side.

BENEFITS – WOW!

- A fabulous asana to relax a tired body
- Stretches the spine and shoulders and aids growth
- Stimulates the abdominal organs
- Releases fatigue and rejuvenates the body
- An excellent stretch for the back
- Relaxes neck and shoulder strain
- Improves digestion
- Relieves headaches
- A therapeutic asana for insomnia

Note from the Acharya

- Do not do this asana if recovering from diarrhoea.
- For girls, do not attempt this asana during menstruation.
- Progress into this asana slowly with consistent practice.

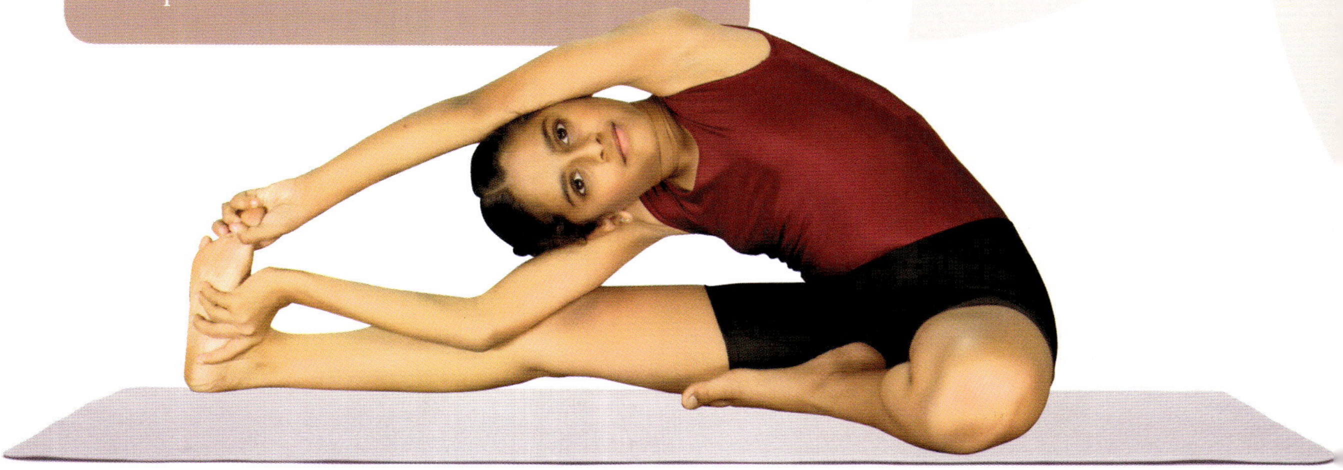

NAVASANA (Boat Pose)

PREPARE – Ready!

- Sit on the floor with legs stretched straight in front with the hands placed on the side in Dandasana.
- Inhale deeply, lift the sternum up and exhale completely, hollowing the stomach.
- Practise this breathing for a few seconds.

BENEFITS – WOW!

- Strengthens the abdomen, spine and hips
- Activates the digestive organs with rich supply of blood
- Relieves stress from the body
- Builds strength in the entire length of the body

START – Steps

1. Inhale and lift the chest up leaning back.
2. Exhale and bend the knees and lift the feet off the floor to an angle of 45 degrees.
3. Stay in position and balance.
4. Stretch the arms forward along the sides of the legs in line with the knees.
5. If possible, straighten the knees and balance in the position for 30 seconds.

Note from the Acharya

- Make sure the back is not rounded.
- The lower belly must be firm.
- Do not do this asana if there is a respiration problem.
- Girls do not do this asana during menstruation.
- Do not do this asana if recovering from diarrhoea.

Relax – Steps

- Exhale, fold the knees and drop the feet back to the floor.
- Straighten the back and release the hands to the floor.
- Relax in the position with normal breathing.

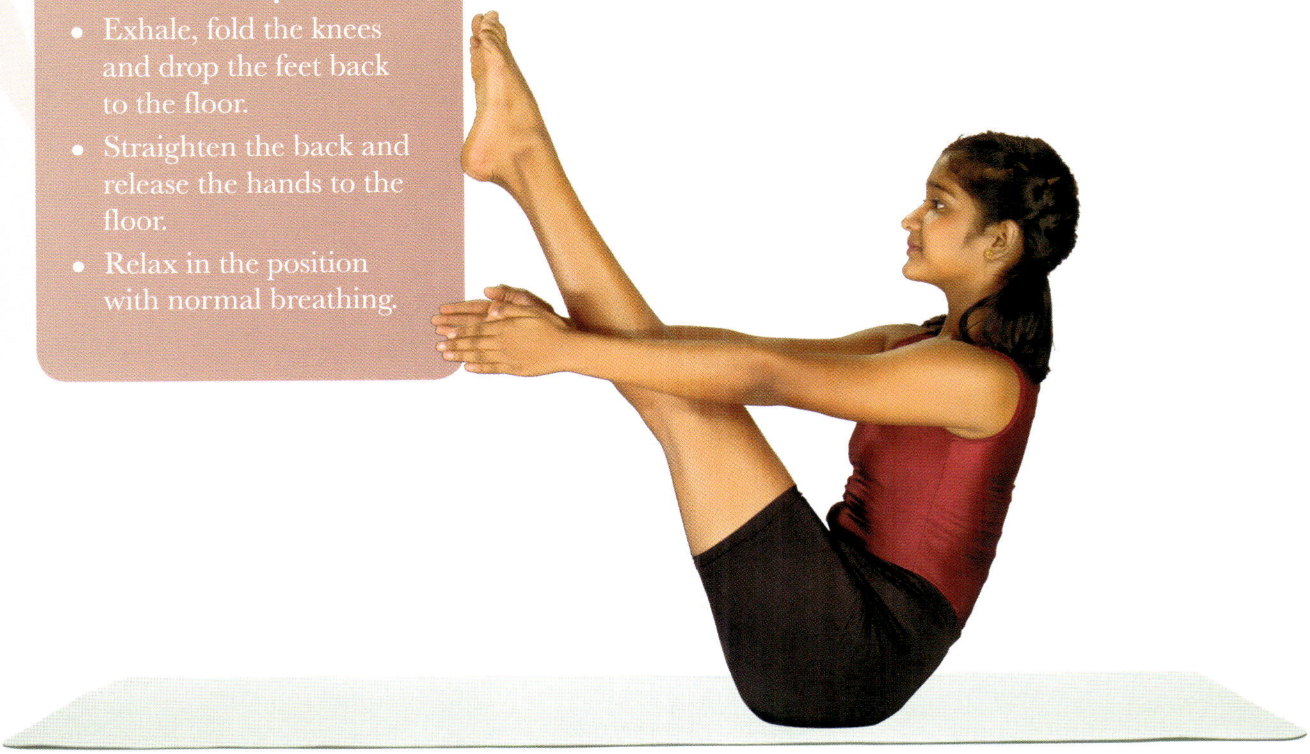

PINCHAMAYURASANA (Peacock Pose)

PREPARE – Ready!

- Sit down in Vajrasana.
- Lift hip up towards the ceiling and stay there until you are comfortable with the balance.
- Press the forearm to the floor firmly and lift the hip up and balance. Best to do it against a wall during initial stages.

CONSTRUCT – Steps

1. With the body's weight shifted on to the forearm, lift the hip up towards the ceiling with the feet still supporting and resting on the floor.
2. Let the hip be moved to be in line with the shoulders.
3. Keep the chest strong and stable.
4. Lift one leg off the floor with the knees straight.
5. Gauge for balance and lift the other leg also.
6. This requires practice to understand the point of balance.
7. Hold the balance in this position for 3 breaths.

Relax – Steps

- Bend the knees and release the hips gently towards the ground.
- The feet will automatically drop down.
- Drop the knees to the ground.
- Relax with the forehead touching the ground.
- Expand your chest and relax the shoulders.
- Gently lift the body up to kneeling down position.

BENEFITS – WOW!

- Helps develop strong arms and shoulders
- Builds a greater sense of balance of the mind and the body
- Makes the body feel light and supple
- Expands the chest and benefits the respiratory organs
- Calms the mind and helps maintain stability of the body

Note from the Acharya

- This is not a difficult asana.
- Good practice of a few preparatory asanas such as Adhomukha Svanasana, Uttanasana and Gomukasana will really help the practice.
- Practise this asana close to a wall and try pushing the legs against the wall.
  - Patience and constant practice will help you achieve this asana.

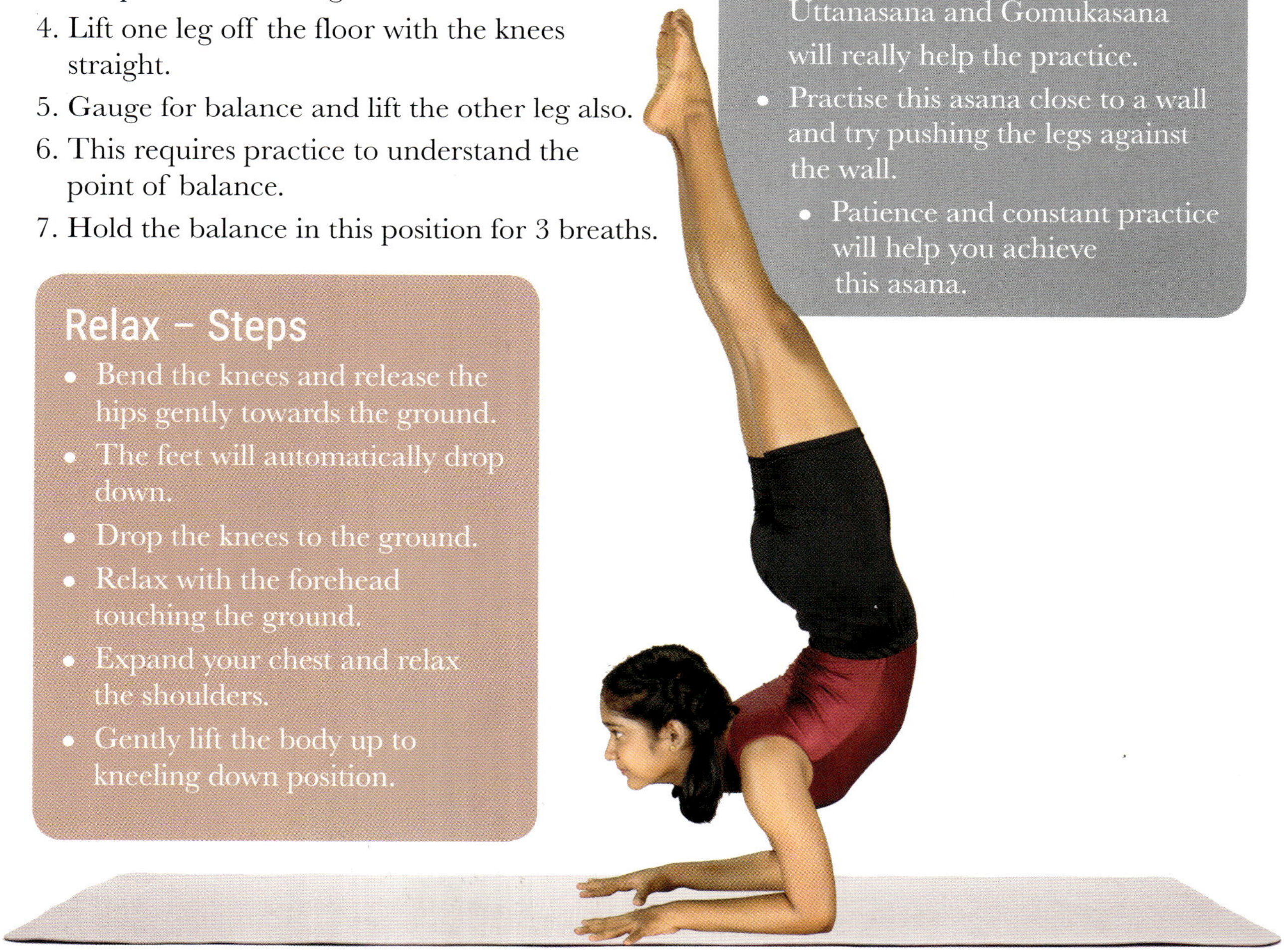

KOORMASANA – (Tortoise Pose)

PREPARE – Ready!

- Sit straight with the legs stretched out in Dandasana.
- Open legs a little more than hip distance apart and lean forward.
- Try to reach the ground and stay relaxed with deep breathing expanding the chest and contracting the abdominal muscles

START – Steps

1. Extend arms forward and lengthen the torso.
2. Bending the knees, slide the arms under the thighs and extend it.
3. Adjust the thighs and pull it towards the shoulders.
4. Stretch the arms to the sides completely.
5. Try to bring the chest and the head closer to the ground.
6. Hold the position for 30 seconds with deep and slow breathing.

Relax – Steps

- Relax and bend the knees again.
- Hunch the back a little and withdraw the hands from under the thighs.
- Get the feet together and straighten the back.
- Relax and breathe till the breathing is normal.

BENEFITS – WOW!

- Stretches the back completely
- Benefits the functioning of the digestive organs
- Relaxes the neck and shoulders
- Expands the chest and improves breathing
- This asana lengthens the spine and aids growth of the body
- A very good asana for the nerves
- Makes the mind quiet and calm
- Helps improve posture

Note from the Acharya

- A challenging asana. Consistent progress will help master this asana.
- If the knees or the arms pain, relax the shoulders and bend the knees.
- Do not push to do this asana. Keep practising and note the progress.

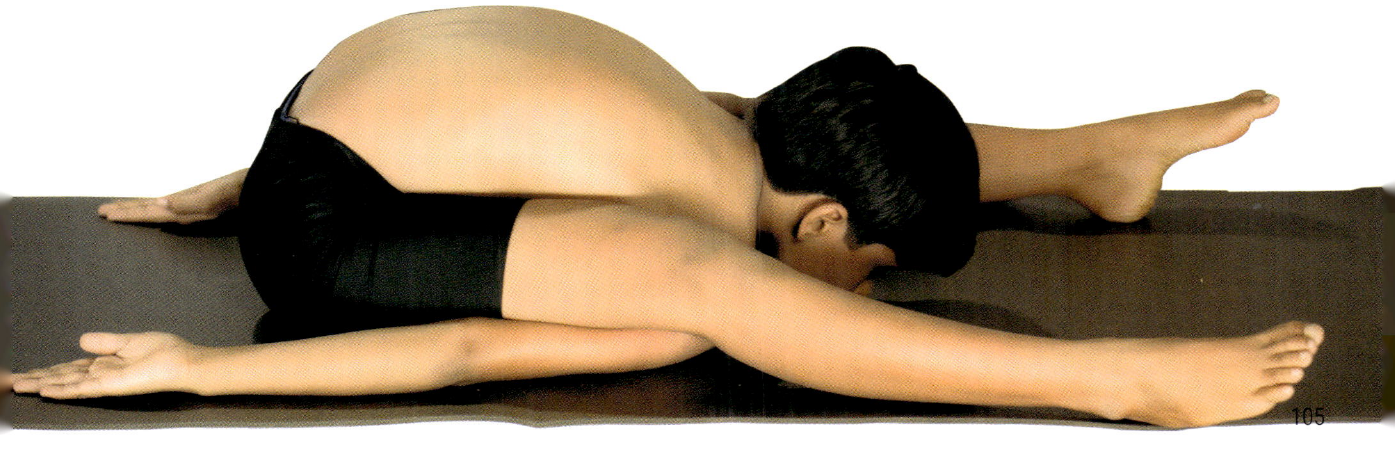

UPAVISTAKONASANA (Wide-angle Pose)

PREPARE – Ready!

- Sit in Dandasana with the legs stretched forward in a straight line and the spine straight.
- Open both the legs as wide as possible and stay in the position and feel the gentle stretch of the groin and legs.

BENEFITS – WOW!

- Stretches the insides of the legs and groin
- Lengthens and strengthens the spine
- Relaxes the back and releases strain from the body
- Calms the brain
- Stimulates abdominal organs

START – Steps

1. Inhale and lean the torso forward as far as possible.
2. Rotate the thighs outwards and pin the thighs against the floor.
3. Reach out to the heels as far as possible.
4. Exhale and stretch forward and lean towards the floor. Stop when it is not possible to go further.
5. Stay comfortable and do not impose this stretch.

Note from the Acharya

- Do not impose this stretch.
- It is a difficult asana which will progress slowly with consistent practice.
- While challenging yourself into this stretch, keep the knees bent slightly to avoid injury.

Relax – Steps

- Get the spine up straight.
- Slide the legs together back to Dandasana.

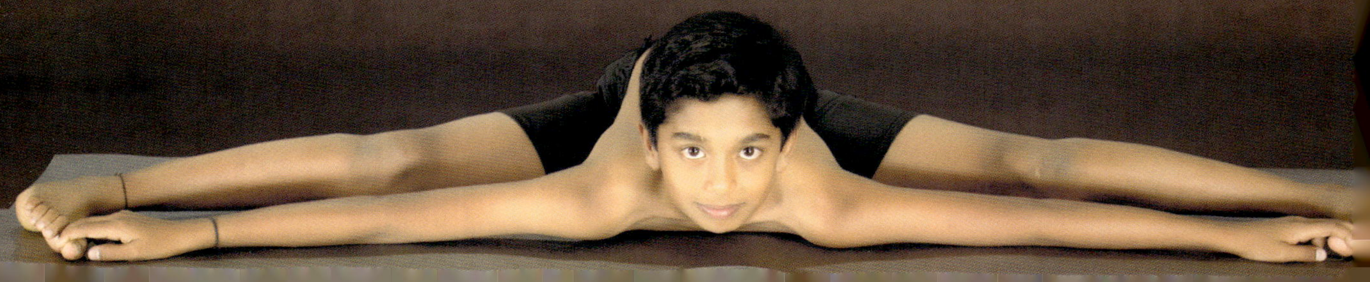

HANUMANASANA (Lord Monkey Pose)

PREPARE – Ready!

- Sit in Vajrasana.
- Put the right foot forward, bend forward to stretch and prepare the hamstrings
- Repeat with the left leg and feel the stretch.

BENEFITS – WOW!

- Increases flexibility of the thighs, hamstrings and groin
- Lengthens the legs
- Stimulates abdominal organs
- Increases flexibility of the hips

START – Steps

1. Exhale and lean torso forward, pressing the palms to the floor.
2. Slide the left knee back straightening the knees as far as possible carefully.
3. Gently push the right heel forward and try to straighten the legs forward.
4. Stay still once the stretch is complete.
5. Hold for 15–20 seconds breathing calmly.

Note from the Acharya

- Progress into this asana cautiously and with patience.
- Work on stretching and getting comfortable on one leg first and then work on the other leg.
- Monitor the intensity of the stretch with the pain which the stretch induces.

Relax – Steps

- Release tension from the length of the legs.
- Fold the right leg and place it comfortably.
- Keep the palm on the floor and slightly lift the hip up.
- Pull the left leg which is stretched back forward.
- Get back to Vajrasana and relax.
- Stretch the other leg forward and repeat.

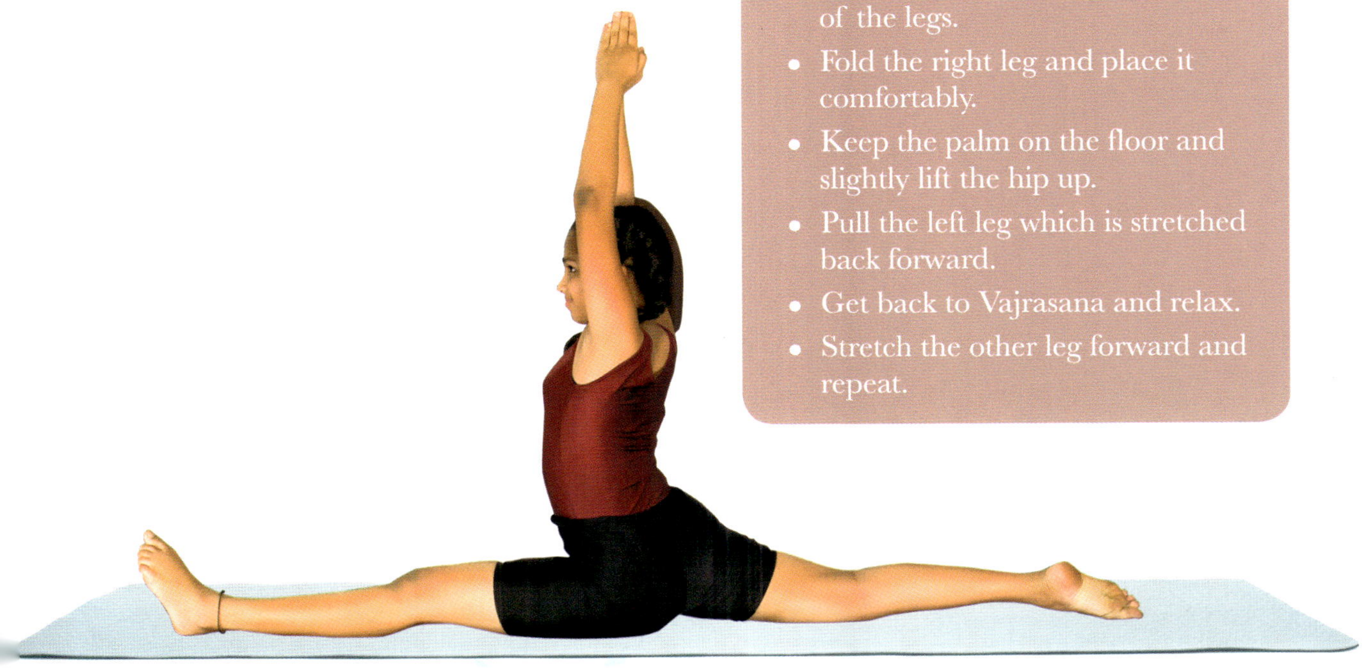

DHANURASANA (Bow Pose)

PREPARE – Ready!

- Lie on the belly with legs stretched straight and relax the back muscles.
- Keep the palms facing upwards.
- Relax and regulate breathing.

START – Steps

1. Exhale and bend the knees close to the buttocks.
2. Reach the hands back and hold the ankles.
3. Keep the shoulders dropped away from the ears and arms fully stretched.
4. Keep the knees hip distance apart.
5. Get a good grip of the ankles.
6. Inhale and strongly lift the knees with a good grip of the ankles.
7. Lift chest off the floor and the knees off the floor.
8. Stay in balance for 30 seconds.

BENEFITS – WOW!

- Stretches the entire body
- Increases circulation along the back
- Improves posture and keeps the back strong
- Expands the chest completely, benefiting the respiratory organs
- Improves breathing by increasing diaphragm strength
- Stimulates abdominal organs
- Keeps the spine healthy
- Releases fatigue from the body

Note from the Acharya

- It is sometimes difficult to lift the thighs up from the floor.
- Consistent practice will help understand the technique.
- Do not strain the neck, instead keep the chest lifted up.

Relax – Steps

- Exhale and release the tension in the arms which will relax the shoulders and chest.
- Relax the tension in the length of the thighs and drop it towards the ground.
- Stretch the arms forward and the legs backwards and stay in position for a few seconds allowing the spine to stretch back into length.

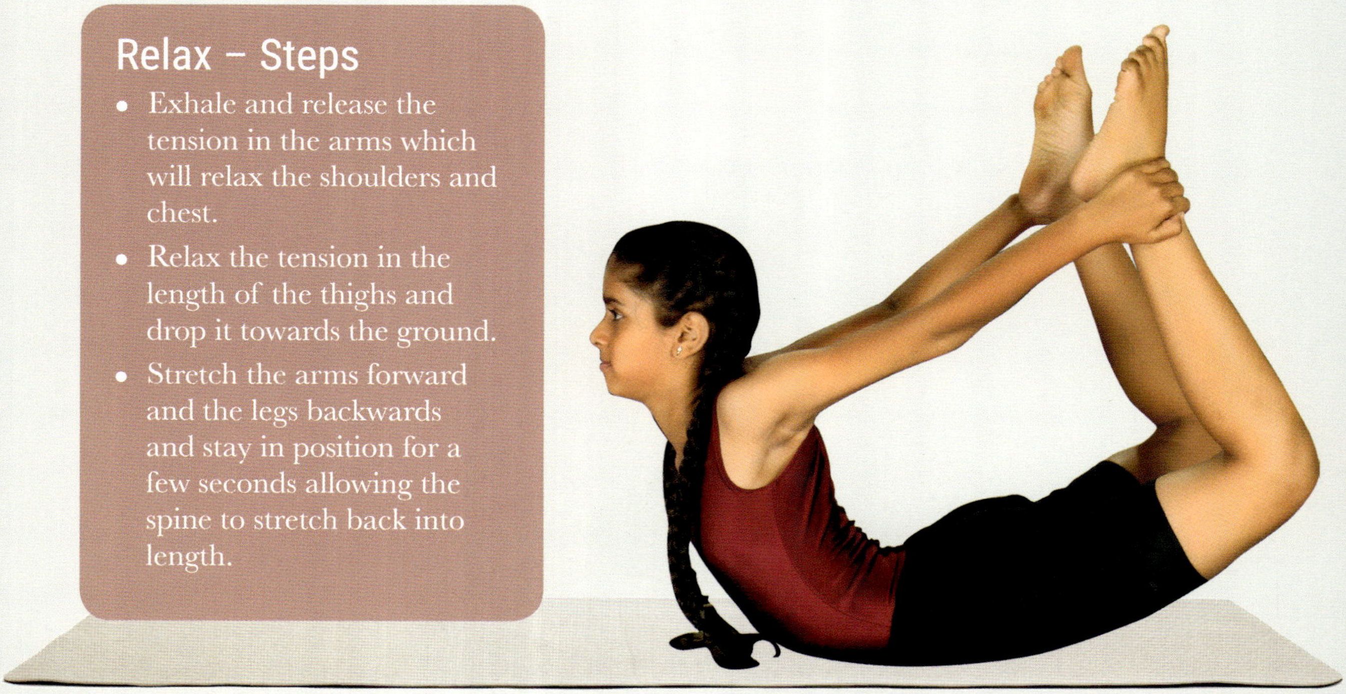

SARVANGASANA (Shoulder Stand)

PREPARE – Ready!

- Lie down on the floor with the head resting and the legs stretched forward.
- Keep the arms by the side of the hips and rest the spine with restful breathing.

START – Steps

1. Exhale and draw the knees (bent) towards the chest curling up the body.
2. Lift the hip up and then torso.
3. Immediately support the back with both the palms with elbows firmly placed on the ground.
4. Keep the elbows drawn closer together.
5. Keep raising the pelvis until it reaches in line with the shoulders.
6. Straighten the bent knees up towards the ceiling.
7. Tuck chin into the hollow of the throat.
8. Breathe comfortably and stay for 30 seconds.

BENEFITS – WOW!

- Benefits the entire body
- Benefits all the functions of the body by supplying a rich supply of blood and oxygen
- Rectifies disorders of the ears, nose and throat
- Helps maintain perfect weight
- Benefits menstrual disorders
- Purifies blood and increases immunity
- Refreshes the skin

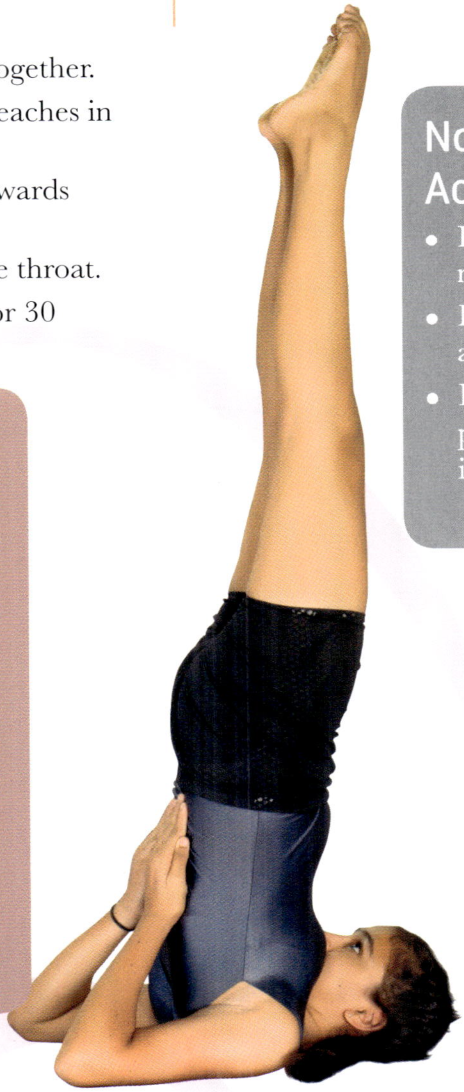

Note from the Acharya

- Keep the jaws and mouth relaxed.
- Keep the face calm and focus on breathing.
- Keep the abdomen pulled in to stay in balance.

Relax – Steps

- Exhale and bend the knees.
- Relax the hips and rest on the palms. This will naturally relax the chin which is tucked into the collar bone.
- Gently release the spine towards the floor carefully with control.
- Keep the arms balancing the back as the back drops to the floor.
- Gently stretch the legs to the floor and rest.

KARNAPEEDASANA (Knee To Ear)

PREPARE – Ready!

Sarvangasana

START – Steps

1. Fold the knees and take it towards the ears.
2. Press the knees towards the floor and drop the feet to the floor.
3. Keep the chin tucked into the hollow of the throat.
4. Breathe comfortably and stay for 10 seconds.

BENEFITS – WOW!

- Rectifies problems in the throat
- Deepens breathing
- Benefits the upper spine
- Rectifies thyroid disorders
- Strengthens the diaphragm
- Helps increase stamina

Note from the Acharya

- Keep the eyes closed and jaws relaxed.
- Pay attention to your breathing.

Relax – Steps

- Inhale and straighten the knees along the floor (Halasana).
- Relax and breathe.

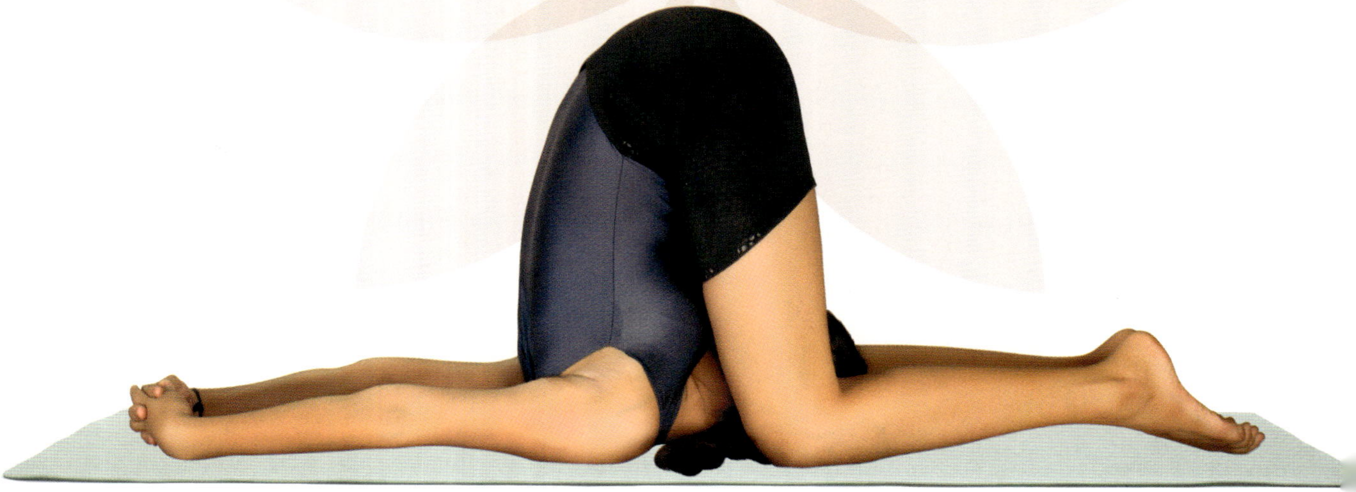

SARVANGASANA (Shoulder Stand)

START – Steps

1. Fold the right knee and take it close to the left side.
2. Keep the feet facing the chest.
3. Fold the left knee around the right and fix the feet under the right leg.
4. The toe to reach is to be placed on the left side of the groin.
5. Stay in position for 15 seconds.

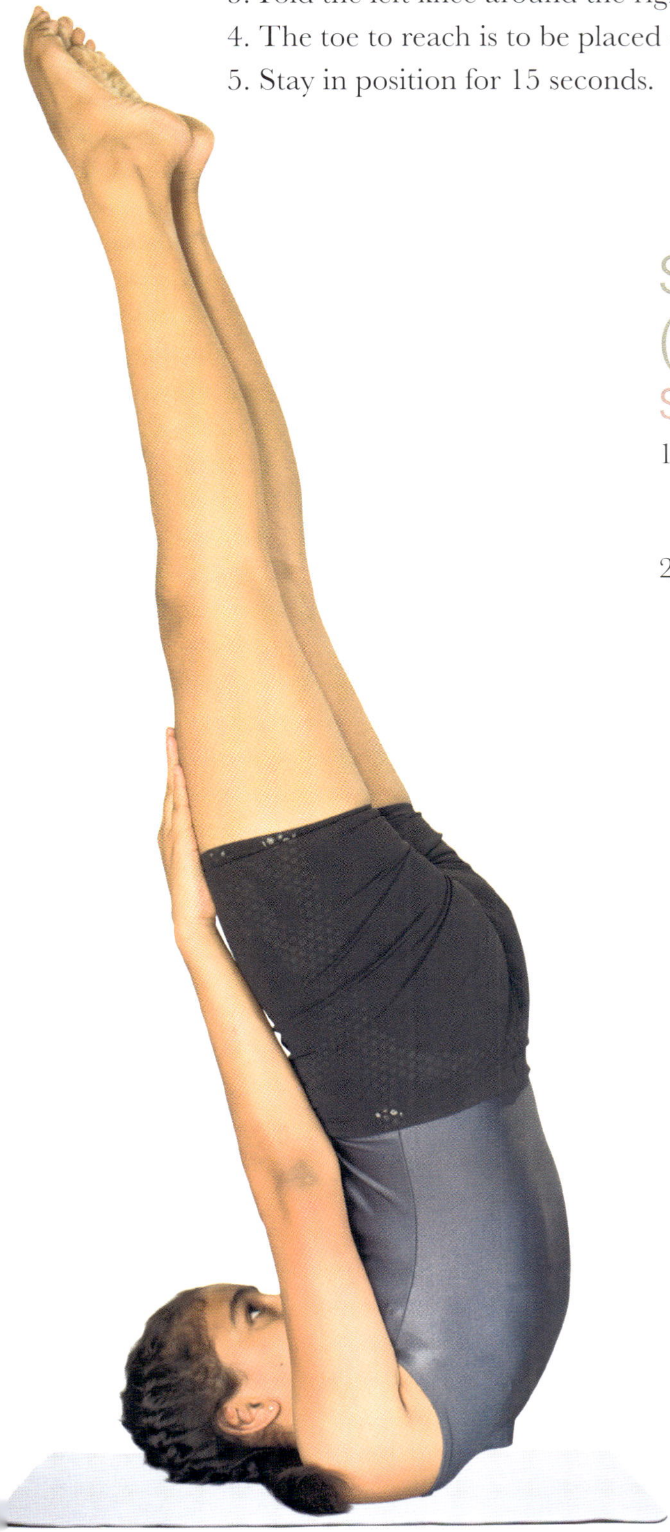

SARVANGAPADMASANA (Shoulder Stand – Lotus)

START – Steps

1. When the Sarvangasana feels stable, challenge the position without supporting the back.
2. Hold the balance of this position from the abdomen.

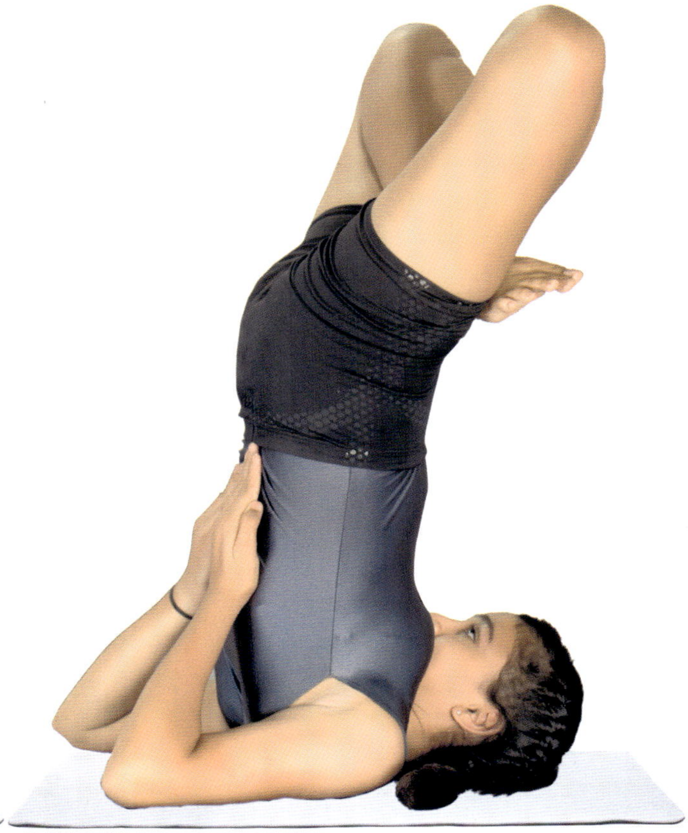

GARBA PINDASANA

PREPARE – Ready!

- Do not come out of Padma Sarvangasana position.
- Keep the chin tucked into the hollow of the throat and in balance on the shoulders.
- Get your breathing to be calm and even.

START – Steps

1. Gently and mindfully get the Padmasana to drop towards your forehead.
2. Make sure your hands are giving you enough support.
3. Keep your stomach pulled in and hip lifted away from gravity.
4. Make sure that there is no strain in your neck and shoulders.
5. The top part of your shoulder and the centre of your head should feel like a tripod giving you balance and support.
6. Stay in the position for 5 breaths.

Note from the Acharya

- This is a highly beneficial asana.
- Breathing is very challenging, but this challenge will help strengthen the lungs and the diaphragm.
- A good balance on the shoulder and head should be established.
- The chin to be positioned in the hollow of the throat comfortably.
- This asana has great benefits for all the organs and glands of the body.

BENEFITS – WOW!

- Strengthens the back and shoulder muscles and allows a rich supply of blood and oxygen along the neck and shoulder regions
- Relaxes the brain and calms agitation
- Makes the spine flexible and supple
- The squeeze and release of the throat region benefits the thyroid gland
- Builds up respiratory strength and keeps the lungs and heart healthy
- Improves reflex action

Relax – Steps

- Gently lift the Padmasana back to Sarvanga Padmasana.
- Release your legs up in the air towards the ceiling and release the breath.
- Slowly get back to Halasana.
- Mindfully drop the hip down towards the floor and relax.

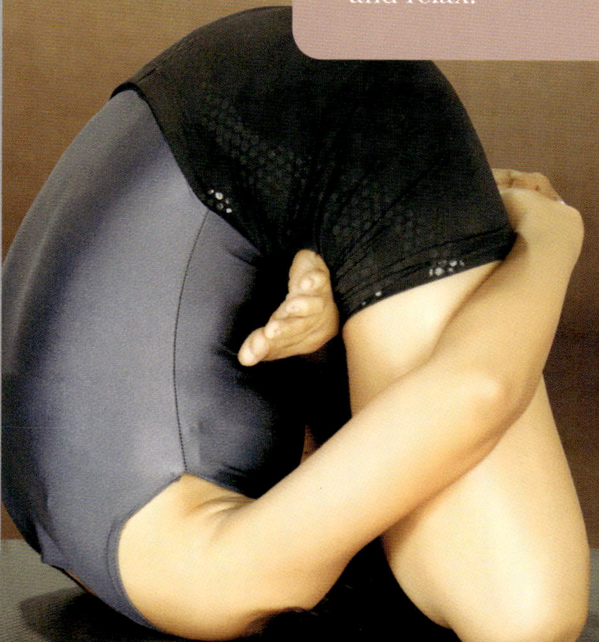

HALASANA (Plough Pose)

PREPARE – Ready!

- Sarvangasana

START – Steps

1. Exhale and slowly get both the legs to drop on the ground above the head.
2. Keep the knees straight and back curved upwards.
3. Keep the chin tucked and breathe deep.
4. Hold the position for 20 seconds.

BENEFITS – WOW!

- Relieves stress from the tired body
- Cools down the body
- Relaxes the spine and increases circulation along the nerves and veins
- Relaxes the back muscles
- Improves digestion
- Aids weight loss

Note from the Acharya

- Focus on your breathing.
- If the back is tired it will be difficult to reach the feet to the floor.
- Do not impose the stretch.
- Stay comfortable focusing on breathing.

Relax – Steps

- Inhale and lift both the legs of the ground straighten it towards the ceiling.
- Keep the chin tucked and body in balance.
- Keep the gaze fixed to the centre of the chest.
- Slowly relax the spine and drop towards the ground.
- Keep the knees pulled to the chest for a few seconds before releasing it along the floor.

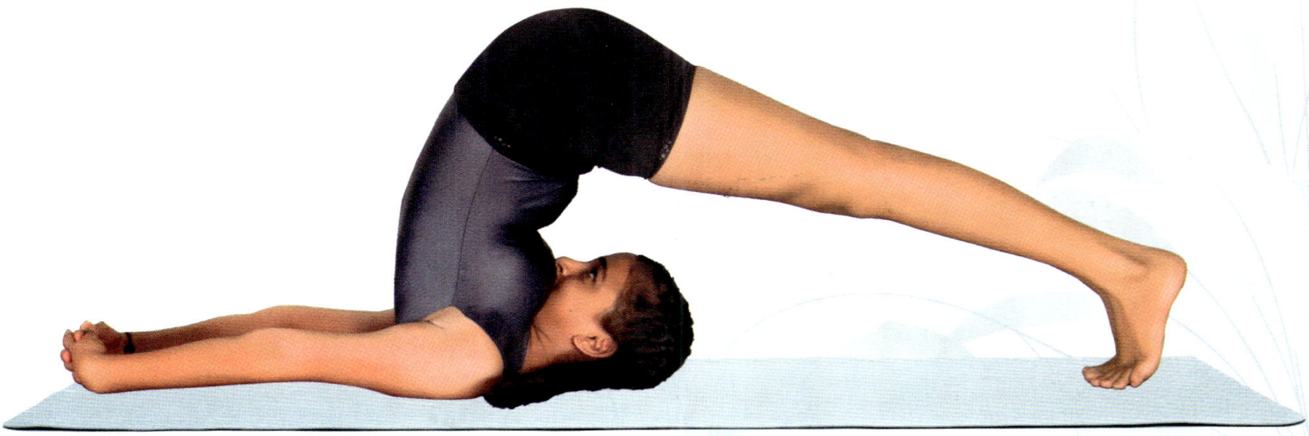

MATSYASANA (Fish Pose)

PREPARE – Ready!

- Lie down on the ground.
- Lift both the legs up and wrap the legs to do a Padmasana.

START – Steps

- Press the elbows on the ground and lift the chest up with the support of the elbows.
- Stretch the neck backwards and reach the crown of the head to the ground.
- Release the hand from the back and grab hold of the toes.
- With that grip, further lift the chest up and form a curve in the spine.
- Stay in position and deep breathe 5 times.

Relax – Steps

- Release the grip on the toes first.
- Take support of the elbows to relax the back, and gently slide the head to the floor.
- Relax.

BENEFITS – WOW!

- Strengthens the respiratory system
- Is helpful for kids with menstrual pain
- Relaxes the brain and calms anxiety
- Mild backaches will be relieved from doing this asana
- Improves posture

Note from the Acharya

- Do not do this asana if you have a headache.
- Do not do this asana if you have had a long day in the sun.
- If the body is tired, a combination of Sarvangasna and immediately Matsyasana, relaxes the body completely.

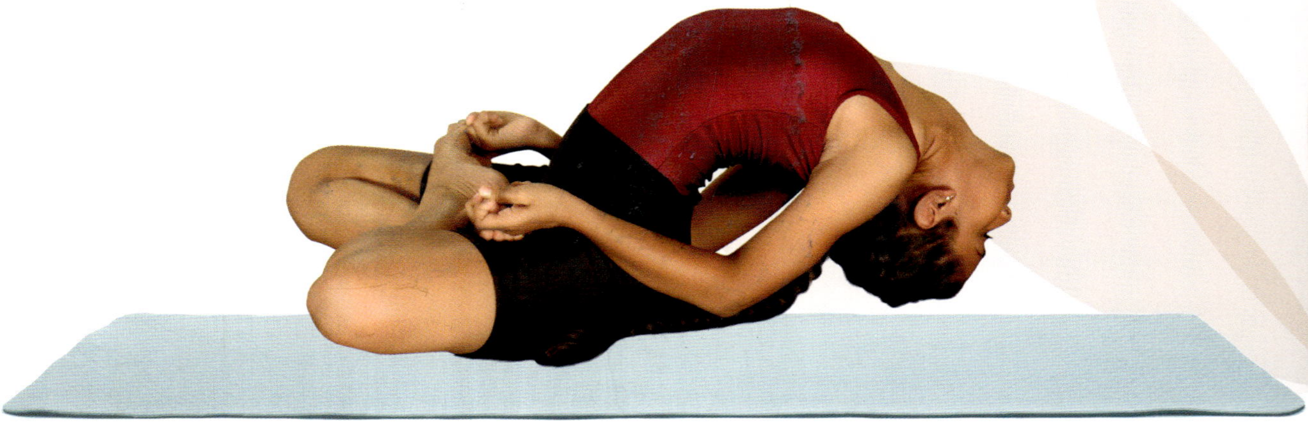

CHAKRASANA (Wheel Pose)

PREPARE – Ready!

- Stand with the legs apart
- Bend backwards as far as possible in the beginning (stand close to a wall if you need support.)

START – Steps

1. Bend backwards pushing the hips slightly forward.
2. Keep the arms stretched above the head lifting the chest up.
3. Press the feet to the floor push the tailbone up towards the ceiling expanding the hips.
4. Keep the inner thighs strong and parallel to each other.
5. Press the palm firmly to the floor, expand the chest and push it towards the arm length.
6. Maintain the curve and breathe for 30 seconds.

BENEFITS – WOW!

- Benefits the spine and the back muscles
- Stretches the chest and benefits the diaphragm and lungs
- Benefits the thyroid and related glands
- Strengthens the arms, wrist, legs, buttocks, abdomen and spine

Note from the Acharya

- If there is a back strain open up the feet outwards which will relax the lower back.
- Keep the neck relaxed to ease the breathing.

Relax – Steps

- Exhale and relax the back.
- Tuck the chin and rest the back of the head on the floor.
- Slowly release the length of the spine down and the hips.
- Relax the thighs and keep them pulled towards the chest to reverse the curve of the back.
- Stretch the knees and rest the leg on the floor.

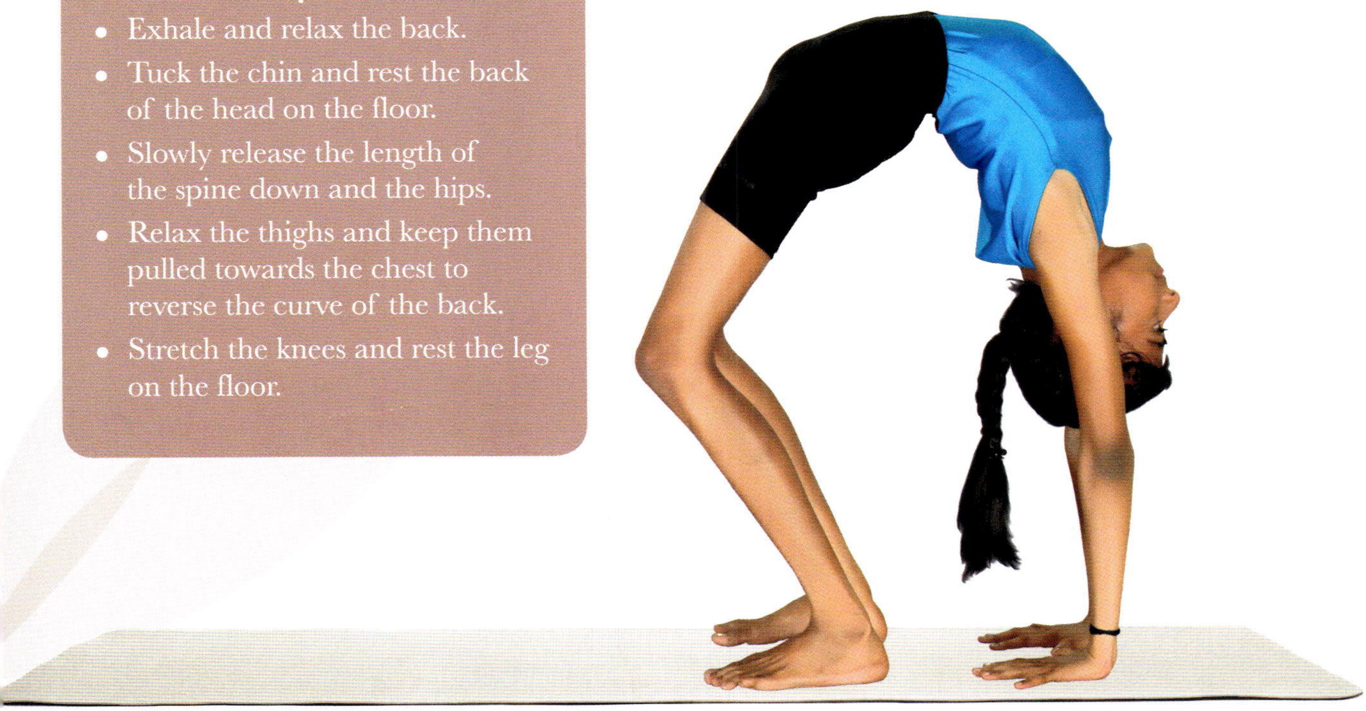

SHAVASANA (Total Relaxation Pose)

PREPARE – Ready!

- Lie down comfortably on the floor with the back flat and head relaxed.
- Inhale expanding the chest and exhale hollowing the abdominal length. Deep breathe for 30 seconds.

START – Steps

1. Close your eyes. Place legs comfortably apart.
3. Keep your arms one and a half feet away from the hips facing upwards towards the ceiling.
4. Slowly start drawing attention to every part of the body without leaving any part.
5. Relax the body step by step.
6. Starting from the toes and raise it upwards.
7. Keep the breathing relaxed.
8. Stay in the position for 5–10 minutes.

BENEFITS – WOW!

- Completely rests the body
- Brings the body to a meditative and relaxed state
- Helps to focus and concentrate
- Releases stress and calms the body
- Reduces anxiety and tension
- Heals the body from stain and stress
- Increases energy levels

Relax – Steps

- Start relaxing by paying attention to the head and neck region.
- Pay attention to every bit of the body as attention travels down towards the toes.
- Keep the breathing normal.
- Each time attention goes to a part of the body, gently move it.
- Once the attention reaches the toes fold the knees and take them close to the chest.
- Relax in this position for a few seconds and settle down.

Note from the Acharya

- This is one of the important asanas of a practice.
- Don't fall asleep.
- Keep your attention shifting from one part of the body to the next instructing that part of the body to relax.
- Pay attention to the breathing to become totally relaxed.
- It is best to lie down on a hard surface.

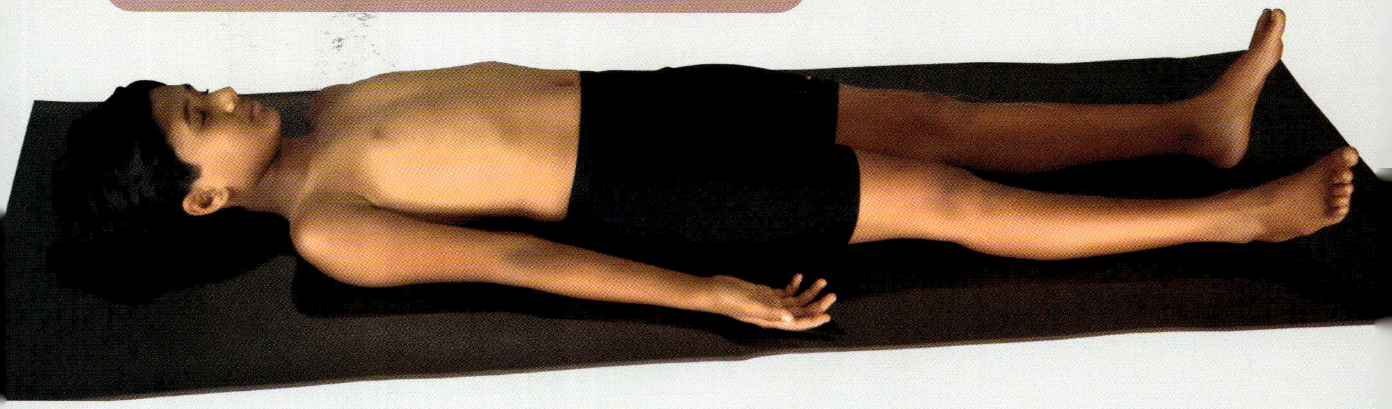

PRANAYAMA
THE ART OF BREATHING
Chapter 4

In the tradition of Yoga, *prana* (air) is considered the main and important life force for all living things. How do we get air to be our life force? It is through breathing. Now, there is a major difference between Pranayama and just breathing. Breathing happens naturally, without which life will end. So when it comes to Pranayama it is about breathing consciously with complete awareness. *Ayama* means control. When you do Pranayama, breathing is energised or charged with the flow of energy. It is difficult to experience this if you do not feel the air flow into the nostrils and out of the nostrils. Observing the breath is not as easy as it sounds. It requires immense focus and concentration. With consistent practice the benefits of Pranayama can be observed.

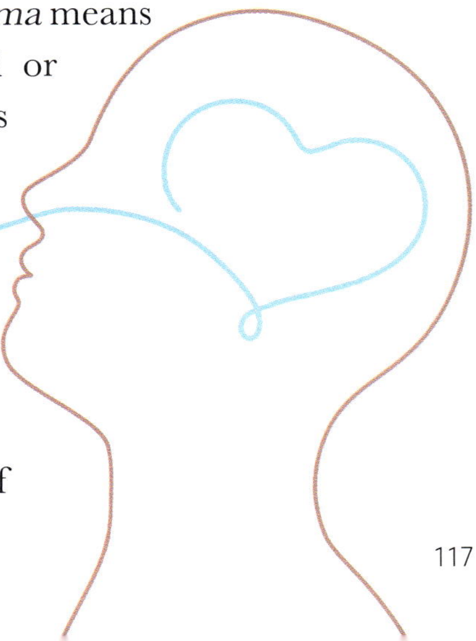

The practice of Pranayama charges the entire body with valuable energy. All the body's energy systems are vitalised to perform their functions better. There are different types of

Pranayama, each with specific benefits.

In this chapter, we look at breathing techniques to understand more about Pranayama. Pranayama is a very powerful tool. Conscious breathing requires intelligence and is the fuel that makes the body work. In this chapter, we are going to try and understand a little more about breathing and how important it is to pay attention to our breathing techniques to live a healthy and peaceful life.

You might have many questions. Why does breathing require conscious attention? Doesn't it happen naturally? Does yoga practice instruct us to learn to breathe in different ways? The answer to this lies in the knowledge of the powerful role breathing has in generating energy in the body which increases our concentration and helps us do whatever we want to do very efficiently.

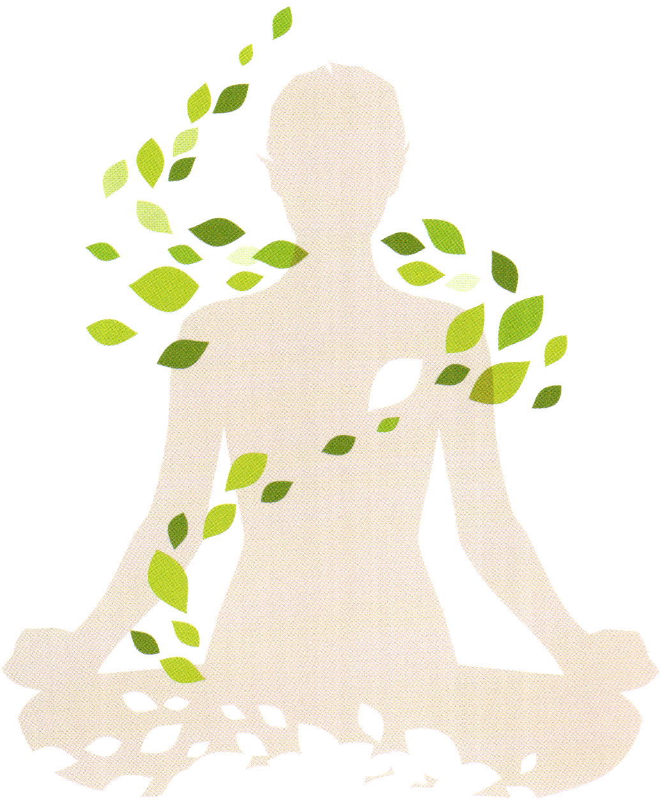

Pranayama is the art of breathing and breath control. Pranayama is practised to build awareness on breathing. When breathing is mastered, you will naturally become alert. When you breathe consciously, the organs of the body, which are like machines, start to work efficiently, resulting in good health and lots of power to do more things tirelessly.

As the practice of Pranayama progresses, the body learns to relax, muscle tension softens, emotions settle down, concentration improves, nerves calm down and awareness deepens.

Now let us try a few exercises to understand the technique of breathing. As it happens naturally we sometimes fail to notice our own breath. But before that it is important to make note of a few points.

POINTS TO REMEMBER FOR PRANAYAMA

- Do not practice this immediately after eating food as the lungs are constricted when the stomach is full.
- A correct posture has to be maintained. Whether you are standing, sitting, kneeling, lying down you should make sure the spine is straight. I would suggest that while doing Pranayama, being in an asana is the best. Try Padmasana or Vajrasana. You can also sit on a chair. Keeping the spine straight is very important.
- The midriff or the breastbone has to be kept lifted during breathing in and also while breathing out. The diaphragm

can then move freely, allowing a lot of air intake and this produces a lot of energy.

- Breathe in and out of the nostrils only as it filters and protects the lungs from pollution and infections. If you feel that you are not breathing out completely and your nose is making a sound, then use mouth for breathing out only.
- Develop a habit of watching your breathing and play with your breath. Keep count of how long you can breathe in and how long you can breathe out.
- Slowing down your breathing helps monitor breathing and also let you take control of any emotions which disturb the mind. Slow breathing helps gain conscious control over the nervous system.
- Do not do practice continuously but take breaks with natural breathing in between deep breathing practice to monitor how you feel in the body.
- In the process of breathing if the mind gets distracted it is important to calm it down and then continue.
- Choose a quiet, clean and airy place for practice.
- Ideally, you need to do Pranayama only after a good 30 minutes of yoga asana practice or just after sports to calm down.

A Few Exercises for Pranayama

OBSERVATION EXERCISE 1

- Close your eyes.
- Breathe normally without imposing

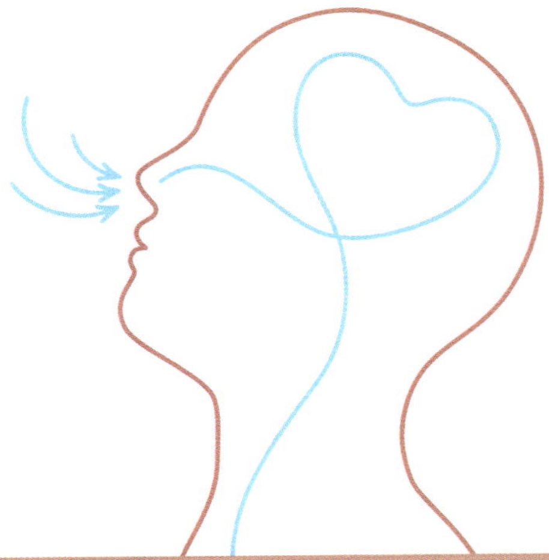

A NOTE ON THE PROCESS OF RESPIRATION

The lungs are not muscles. They cannot expand and contract when you are breathing. The lungs need assistance to stretch and expand during inhalation and deflate during exhalation. This work is done by a large muscle called the diaphragm, which lies below the lungs. It is dome-shaped and tucked under the ribcage. Both the lungs and the heart rest on the dome of the diaphragm, which is spread to the front and behind the chest. The lower part of the diaphragm arches over the liver, the stomach and other abdominal organs. If you notice the movement of the diaphragm while breathing, it benefits both the upper part also known as the thoracic cavity and the lower part which is the abdominal cavity.

deep breathing.

- Observe the air flow in through your nostrils as you breathe in and observe air flow out as you breathe out.
- Now observe the coolness of the air as you breathe in and the warmth of the air as you breathe out.
- Observe the gentle expansion of the lungs as you breathe in and gentle contraction of the lungs as you breathe out. The slower you breathe, the more you will be able to focus on your observation.

OBSERVATION EXERCISE 2

- Close your eyes and start observing your breathing.
- Visualise the dome of the diaphragm spread around the ribcage/midriff.
- The lungs expand as the air gets drawn in.
- Next, pay attention to the diaphragm gradually getting soft and releasing its hold on the lungs.
- The lungs start to contract and the diaphragm dome slowly moves up for the air to flow out.
- Do this exercise around 5 times.
- Slowly open the eyes and experience a feeling of freshness.

(When you are feeling tired and sleepy, try doing this exercise. You might fall asleep. But you will also wake up feeling refreshed.) With each inhalation, the walls of the diaphragm contract, drawing the dome of the diaphragm down. Now, in addition to the contraction, the diaphragm has another important effect–it presses down the abdominal organs. This gently massages the abdominal organs, increases circulation and helps the organs to function better.

TRAINING BREATH EXERCISE 3

- Sit in a comfortable position.
- Start by observing normal breathing up to 10 counts.
- Slowly increase the depth of the breath and make it go deep into the length of the chest so that you feel the lungs expand.
- Try to observe the contraction of the diaphragm.
- Do this 3 times.

- Now count as you breathe in and observe what the count is.
- Now count as you breathe out and observe the count.
- Make sure the breathing out count is at least 2 times more than the breathing in count. (eg. if your breathing in stops at count 4, your breathing out should be at least 8. It can be more, but not less.)
- Do this 10 times and rest with normal breathing.

PRANAYAMA BREATHING TECHNIQUES (2 VARIATIONS)

Ujjeyee (Deep Sound Breathing) is the fundamental breathing technique in Pranayama. It helps circulate fresh oxygen and pumps energy into the body. This Pranayama variation generates internal body heat which is vital in boosting energy for the entire body.

- Sit in a comfortable position or in any one of the recommended asanas.
- Back has to be comfortable and straight.
- Keep gaze straight for 10 seconds without fluttering your lashes.
- Now close eyes and calm down the breathing.
- Bring awareness to normal and existing breathing.
- Allow the breathing to go deeper and slow.
- Draw awareness to the throat. Feel air entering the hollow of the throat.
- As you keep practising the above breathing for a while you will start noticing a sound like that on the seashore. This sound only happens when the breathing is strong and deep and when the throat hollows and squeezes the supply of air.
- Consistent practice will help master this powerful breathing.

  (Note: If you find it difficult to get the sound of the breathing practice, inhale deep and exhale with the whispering sound of 'ha...' This sound should come from the back of the throat.)

Benefits of Ujjeyee

- Brings fresh energy, which in turn awakens the senses
- Promotes clarity in the mind and improves focus
- Slows the breath and relaxes the body and mind
- Improves the immune system
- Helps the body feel light and energised

Anulom Vilom (Alternate Nostril Breathing)

Best breathing exercise to calm the nerves down, eg. during exams.

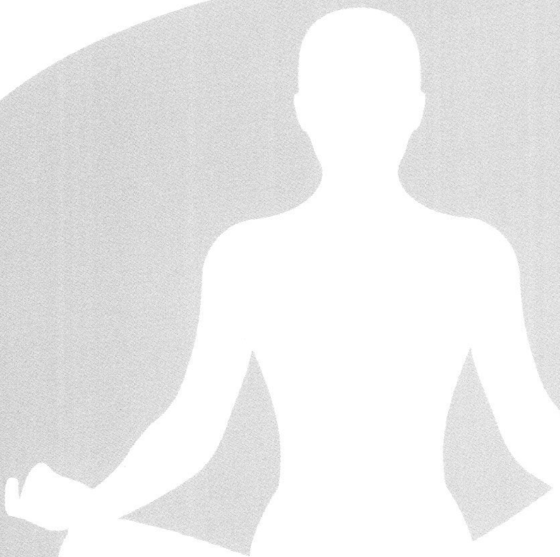

Steps

- Sit erect with your left hand on the knee and the right hand in a mudra.
- Now, your thumb has to close the right nostril, while your index finger and middle finger are closed inwards and placed on the mound of the thumb.
- Keep the ring finger close to the left nostril.
- Keep your eyes closed gently and without movement.
- Close the right nostril and breathe in through the left and close the left nostril and breathe out of the right. (This is the first round.)
- Keep repeating this breathing for at least 5 rounds.
- Rest and repeat again if you feel like it.

Benefits of Anulom Vilom

- Relaxation: Practising this Pranayama immediately relaxes the brain and relieves all tension from the body. This Pranayama has the power to heal many serious health conditions. This is a popular Pranayama which balances the nervous system. The mind feels calm and centred even when done for 5 rounds.
- Therapy: This Pranayama is therapeutic for children suffering from heart conditions, asthma, headaches, common colds, fever and other day-to-day stress-related conditions. It also helps improve any conditions of the eyes and helps maintain healthy skin even when there is hormone disruption during puberty. The immune system is strengthened.
- Balance: Practising this Pranayama balances the temperature in the body. It also helps to change habits that are deeply ingrained and need changing. Pranayama is especially useful for girls when they face emotional imbalances during PMS.

PRATYAAHARA, DHARANA, DHYANA, SAMADHI: THE ART OF CLEARING THE MIND

Chapter 5

Just as a healthy body can fight toxins and pathogens, practising Pratyaahara, Dharana, Dhyana and Samadhi can help the child reject negative influences from external sources and stay free from the turmoil around.

This chapter covers child-friendly ways to:

- Declutter thoughts
- Clear, calm and refresh the mind
- Eat the right kind of food to nourish the physical body

Children are generally open-minded and you might be surprised when they get excited to know more about this chapter. I have prescribed a few simple techniques as experiments which both you and your child can try. These are some of the deeper aspects of yoga which are important to understand in order to get the complete benefit of the practice.

- Dharana (one-pointed focus)
- Dhyana (meditation)
- Samadhi (peace and harmony)

These concepts are not elaborated in detail as they are too advanced for a child's practice. However, awareness of the philosophical aspects of the practice is important. The child must understand the core aspects of the practice and not think of yoga as just a physical exercise routine. Yoga is to be understood as a philosophy.

PRATYAAHARA (SELF-ANALYSIS)

Sutra I.30

| | Vyadhistyannasamsyapramadalasyavirati –
Bhrantidarsanalabdhabhumikatvanavasthitatvani
Cittaviksepastentaryah | |

This sutra says the mind is always challenged by interruptions which create disturbances and stop us from seeing our issues clearly. If we don't see the issue clearly that will distract us. When we start valuing these distractions then it will start showing symptoms like disease; mental imbalance; doubt; carelessness; laziness; inability to withdraw, compose, and rest; hallucination; inability to reach, grasp, or comprehend the goal; and inability to remain grounded.

In the yoga texts, our ancient masters emphasise that the mind is the best tool nature has given to humans. By using this tool, limitless knowledge that lies in the world becomes accessible. However, the mind always finds it difficult to recognise this. Why? Because the mind is habitually distracted and the brain gets easily confused. Only an intelligent mind stops running after distractions. To understand this and overcome confusion, some preparation, understanding and practice are required. Pratyaahara teaches you how to recognise and evaluate what is important at that particular moment and teaches you to focus only on what is useful and healthy.

Pratyaahara means to pull away from all distractions. It is a practice by which you feed the mind with good thoughts and keep the body clean with good food. Pratyaahara is like a formula to realise your own desires easily. Before you walk that path, you may have to answer a few questions for yourself. These are your secret questions. You don't have to show the answers to anyone.

Exercise 1

1. Start by writing your name on a piece of paper.
2. Think of all the things you want to do.
3. Think of all the ways in which you can do those things.
4. If you think it is not possible to get it, then, write down the reason why.
5. If you think it is possible, then do you have a plan?

Answer these questions. You must try to answer these questions once a week.

But before you sit down to answer these questions, spend a few minutes sitting quietly with your eyes closed. Let the mind settle with the image of something pleasant like a sunrise, garden, sea, hills, anything of your choice, but it should be nature. Slowly listen to the thoughts that float in the mind. When that happens, pay attention to the air flowing in and out of your nostrils. Slowly open your eyes. Read the questions and try to answer them in not more than 2 sentences. You might find the questions difficult to answer, but if you keep answering them every week you will start finding the right answers yourself. Eventually you will also know what to do.

Now, Try Exercise 2

Nidra is an important exercise which will also help the practice of Pratyaahara. It can be done once in two weeks. *Nidra* means sleep but this sleep is all about systematically relaxing the mind and body and gaining clarity. Though this is called sleep you are still aware and really awake! You are just instructing the body to sleep and observing the body sleep. It is a beautiful experience when the body and mind relaxes with your instructions.

Next, Try This

1. Lie on your back with arms and legs in natural position.
2. Adjust the shoulder blades to rest comfortably tucked underneath the body.
3. Let the palms be turned upwards and fingers point upwards towards the sky.
4. Relax the chest and see if the breathing is comfortable.
5. Pay attention to the hips and keep the buttocks pushed more towards the thighs.
6. Keep the thighs rotated outwards which will make the knees and the feet also relax and drop outwards.
7. Pay attention to the body and crosscheck if there are any tensions in the body.

Note to parents

- Parental guidance necessary
- To deal with issues like anxiety, depression and lack of self-esteem. These mindfulness exercises will help children get a grip on their feelings and help calm them down.

8. Pay attention to the head. The neck should feel completely relaxed with the chin pointing towards the chest.
9. Keep the mouth slightly open and tongue relaxed. Please do not breathe in and out of the mouth.
10. Stay still without moving for a couple of minutes.
11. Now, pay attention while breathing. The breath should be smooth and not jerky or noisy.
12. The breath should be deep and gentle.
13. Try not to hold your breath.

Now, observe the mind automatically feeling restful, centred and calm.

Nidra is to be held without movement for at least a minimum of 5 minutes. This is enough to feel the relaxation. It should be held for at least 10 minutes to feel the benefit and 20 minutes to feel completely rejuvenated.

After *Nidra*, Exercise No. 1 will be easy to answer. This is because the mind will reach a point of clarity.

One more important aspect of Pratyaahara includes regulating some important habits or disciplining thoughts so that the body and mind are healthy and not disturbed. The body can face disturbance due to undigested food and the mind can face disturbance owing to bad thoughts and bad company. The yoga texts outline 3 levels of *aahara* (food):

- The food we eat for physical nourishment.
- Sensations of sound, touch, feeling, smell and taste are considered food for the senses.
- The association we make with people and things is also considered as food for the mind.

These 3 levels influence the health of the body and the mind. Therefore, working on Pratyaahara helps us understand which food is unhealthy so that you withdraw from it. The wrong food releases toxic chemicals in the body creating discomfort and irritation. Foods that are too spicy, cold, oily and too much food are considered bad.

Similarly, wrong impressions are quite common in this age of the internet and unlimited information, observing the kind of information you consume gives clarity. For instance, viewing disturbing images is not advisable as it can result in muddled thoughts. This is not helpful in the long term.

Even the kind of company you keep influences your sensory impressions. Therefore, Pratyaahara built up as a practice helps to develop a disciplined all-round personality.

Dharana, Dhyana, and Samadhi

These 3 points (listed below) that form the Ashtanga limbs could seem a little complicated, but they have been simplified for your sake. Outlined are a few simple techniques as experiments, which can be tried. These are some of the deeper aspects of yoga.

1. Dharana involves exercises to develop concentration.

2. Dhyana is a state of mind free from the effects of distraction.

3. Samadhi is the blissful state when the mind is tranquil and totally free from all distraction.

These concepts are not elaborated in detail as they are too advanced for a child's practice. However, awareness of the philosophical aspects of the practice is important.

DHARANA

This limb of yoga helps the mind to concentrate. Regular practice of Dharana techniques enhances the practitioner to stay focused. It trains the mind to remain calm and increases mental strength.

The power of concentration is indispensable to success in all walks of life. Whether you wish to be a scientist, doctor, businessman or woman, chef, artist, political leader, parent or gardener, you require concentration. The sacred texts define concentration as one-pointed focus on a specific object or thought. Great things can be achieved with concentration. An archer must concentrate on hitting the target, a pianist on his/her keynote, a dancer on movement. All you need to excel is concentration and it will be easy to achieve anything in the world.

Let us try a small exercise to enhance concentration. In the initial stages, it is ok to not have complete focus. We will get there.

Note to parents

- These are higher techniques of concentration and focus which are not advised to be practised by children. However, the knowledge of yoga is incomplete without understanding these.

Exercise 1

Try this exercise to check your focus. Keep your mind focused for 12 seconds on any object of your choice. There should be no interruptions. Keep a timer if required to count to 12 seconds. See how that goes and if it goes fine without any problems then try it for another 12 seconds and see if that goes well too. If you can do it then you are ready to understand Dharana.

Dharana can enhance awareness and concentration and help you focus on the here and now. Why does concentration come at the end in the Ashtanga Yoga discussion? In order to focus and concentrate, it is important to be physically healthy and mentally strong. Pranayama or breathing practices enable the breath to be regulated properly in the body. *Prana* is an important energy, essential for the functioning of the body. When the breath is smooth and regulated, it becomes easy to focus.

When you concentrate inner focus comes alive. In this state of concentration, all your distracted mental faculties come together.

Exercise 2 (Focusing on a chant is an easy way to improve concentration)

a. Try to learn a chant/mantra

b. If learning a long mantra is difficult then just stick to the universal chant 'Aum'.
This chant has huge benefits.

c. Learn it well by repeating it with your parent or teacher.

d. Now find a comfortable quiet place.

e. Put your yoga mat on the floor and sit down in Padmasana or any comfortable seated posture.

f. Get comfortable. Pay attention to the entire body. Every part of your body should be relaxed and there should be no movement. Listen to the sounds around you. Even if the sounds are disturbing, try not to care. Just sit calmly.

g. Observe your breathing, which should feel easy and calm.

h. Once you are ready, take a lengthy breath and repeat 'A…U...M'. (Try doing this 11 times.)

i. If you can do it without losing focus you are good at Dharana.

j. But you might lose focus. The mind is clever and will do everything to distract. When thoughts creep in, learn to ignore them. Initially, it will be difficult. But eventually with some practice you will learn how to ignore your thoughts. Then, you will gain full concentration.

k. If you feel like you can repeat this again, try another session of 'A…U...M' 11 times.

If you succeed, you have almost mastered it.Next, you need to detach yourself from all thoughts that distract the mind. The disturbed energy will convert into a fresh new energy, which is very powerful.

Exercise 3 (Monitoring and Ignoring Thoughts)

a. The mind is very clever and will do everything to distract you. So thoughts will come creeping in.

b. Pay attention to all your thoughts. You will see them come one after the other.

c. As one thought comes you can ignore it. Then ignore the next as well.

d. After a while, the thoughts get tired of coming.

e. When this happens, you will start to observe the sound of your chanting.

f. This will be the next stage of Dharana.

g. These are difficult exercises. Even elders find it difficult and get even more thoughts because of all the responsibilities they have. That's why it is best to practise concentration when you are young so that by the time you grow up, you will be a master of concentration and enjoy success in life.

The third is most important as it awakens an inner quietness which will help the mind to fully focus on only one specific object, with no distractions at all.

Exercise 4 (Inner Quietness)

a. Once you start ignoring your thoughts, they will get tired of disturbing you.

b. This is when you start focusing on the sound of the mantra.

c. After chanting the mantra 11 times, don't say anything but stay still and be quiet.

d. Initially, the inner silence will last for a few seconds.

These exercises will not show you any immediate results but its benefits will manifest in different ways. Keep the practice going and enjoy the results of a joyous, clean and clear mind.

DHYANA

While you work on focus and concentration in Dharana, you automatically move towards the most important stage of yoga practice which is Dhyana or meditation. Meditation is deeper concentration. Concentration will prepare you with knowledge and focus. Once it becomes effortless and continuous, it becomes meditation. Dhyana or meditation takes you into an inner world of knowledge.

Here's an example of extreme focus. Even before Sir Isaac Newton discovered the law of gravity, people have been seeing apples fall from trees. Sir Newton's deep focus on the subject reflected an inner world of knowledge which led him to discover the law of gravity. While doing meditation, the meditator becomes one with the object of meditation. So concentration is the primary stage. Concentration involves seeking knowledge and building up conviction. Sometimes it is mingled with reasoning and sometimes rational thoughts can also arise.

Concentration can put an end to doubt but meditation can transform the thought into deeper knowledge. Sir Newton's concentration cleared his doubts, but as he concentrated deeper on the subject, he discovered something very valuable.

Sometimes meditation is linked to prayer. Some people find it easier to link meditation to a symbol or a personal deity. Focusing on an image or a symbol helps during the initial stages but eventually meditation goes beyond images and symbols, which are just stepping stones.

Meditation is about gaining mastery over the mind. The mind is a funny thing. It is our best friend when we control it and our worst enemy when we do not. Meditation is a technique to let the mind rest and rejuvenate. A disturbed and agitated mind can do nothing but repeat and imitate old thoughts and behaviours. Meditation rejuvenates the mind and helps to give rise to new and fresh thoughts, which will make life comfortable and enjoyable.

Dhyana requires lot of practice and knowledge. It takes preparation and time. This is the most difficult stage of yoga. Everybody, young or old, struggles to get to this stage. The people who have experienced and mastered the art of meditation with rigorous practice and study have experienced the benefits and bliss of the art of meditation.

Meditation makes life more joyful. Nothing in the world will bother you and you are free from all kinds of trouble the mind constantly gets into. The mind will become smarter and calmer. You will enjoy the world you live in better and you will find everything beautiful.

SAMADHI

Samadhi is an advanced state of meditation which has to be experienced and therefore explanation is very difficult. It is the final stage of meditation. Great sages and seers meditate for years, becoming one with whatever they are meditating upon. Samadhi is supposed to be a complete and joyous state of mind.

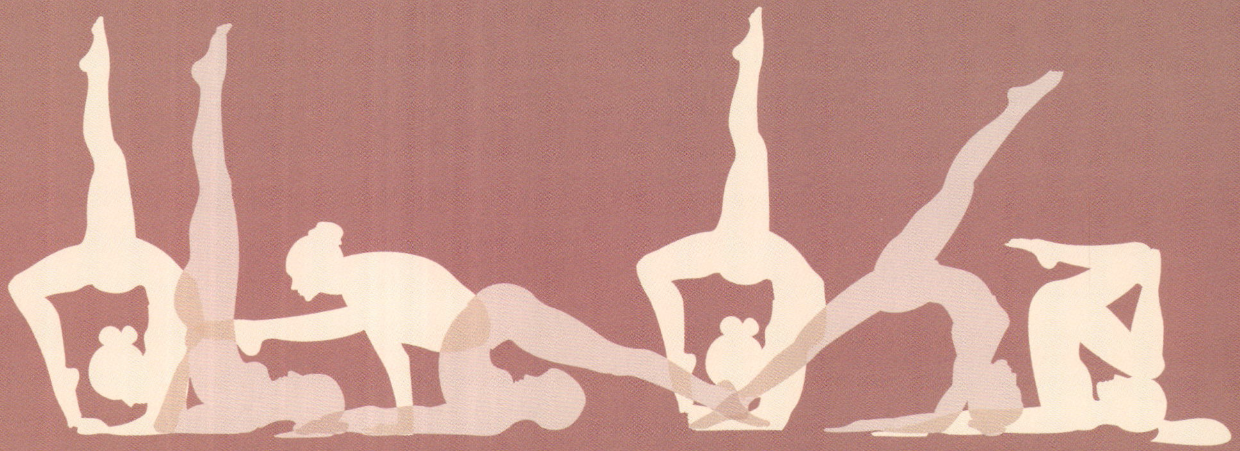

PRACTICE CHARTS

MONDAY

Asanas for good appetite and balance in body weight

Standing Asanas

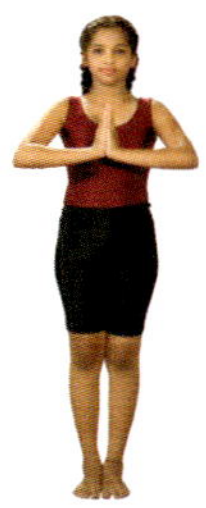

Tadasana/ Samasthithi – Tall Pillar Pose

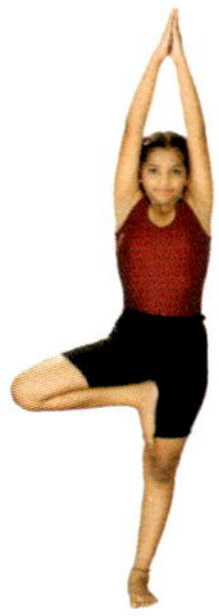

Vrikshasana – Tree Pose

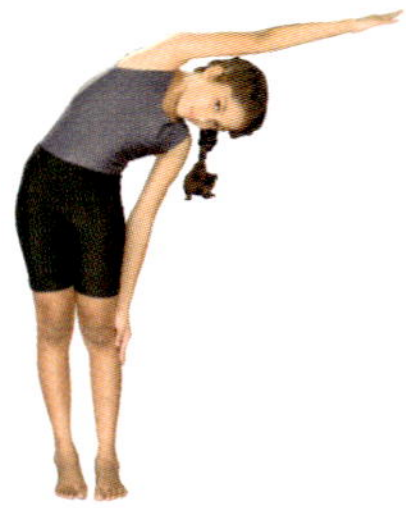

Ardha Kati Tadasana – Half Side Wheel

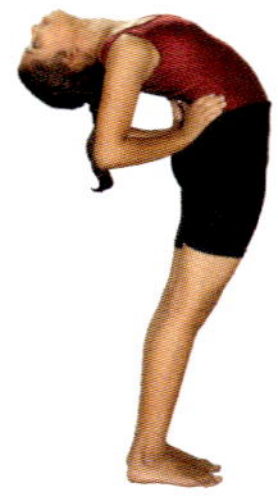

Ardha Chakra Tadasana– Half Back Wheel

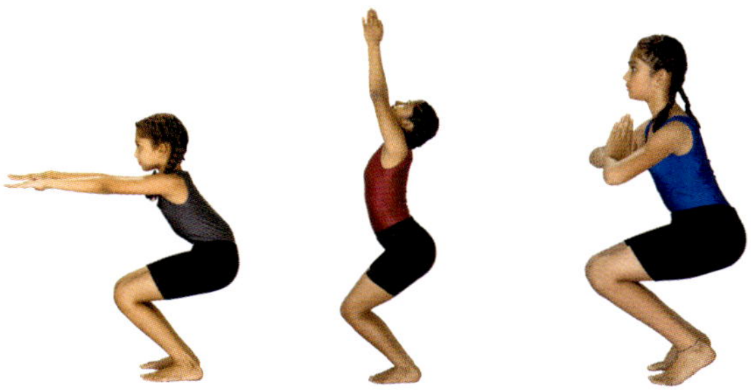

Utkattasana A. B. and C – Chair Pose

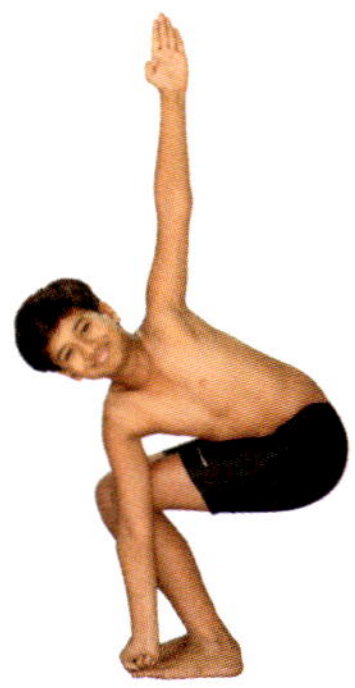

Parivritti Utkatasana – Twisted Chair Pose

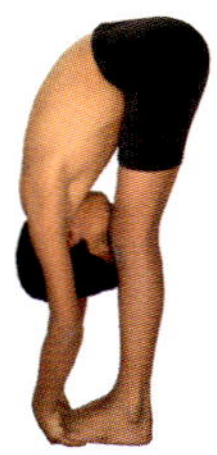

Pada Hastasana – Toe Hold Pose

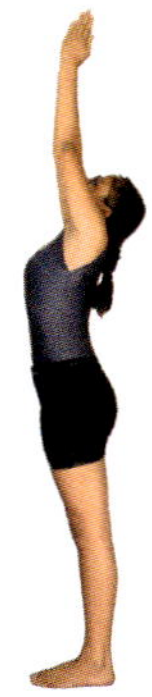

Surya Namaskara A & B (3 times)

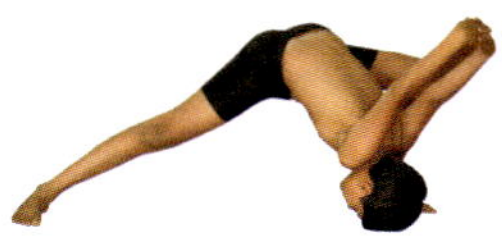

Shirasa Parsvakonasana – Head Downward Stretch

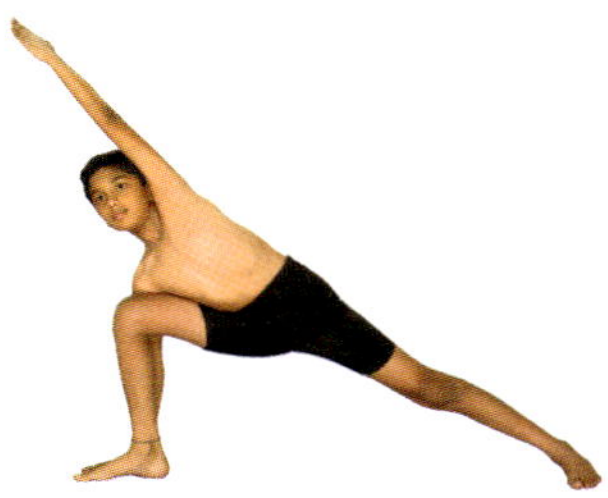

Parsvakonasana – Side Angle Stretch

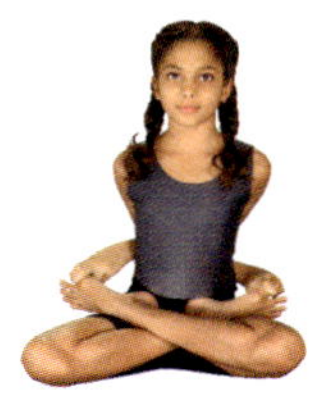

Badha Padmasana – Half Lotus Toe Hold

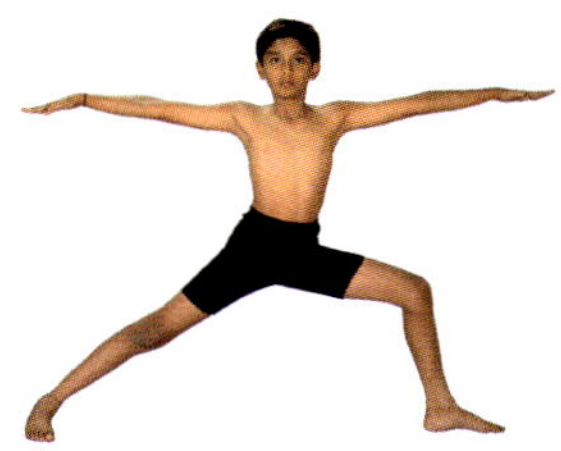

Veerabhadrasana D – Warrior Pose

Note to parents

- The asanas listed here help increase the peristaltic movement in the abdominal muscles, which is a wave-like movement in the oesophagus, stomach, and intestine. Practising these yoga asanas will instill a good appetite in the child and will balance the weight in the body adequately.
- It is important to observe the child's sudden loss or gain in appetite. Loss of appetite will result in weight loss and increase in appetite will result in weight gain. It is important to consult a doctor before starting any therapy for the child.
- The asanas listed here are good for children who are underweight and overweight. How it works is that yoga increases the child's mindfulness and the way the child relates to the body. With this kind of awareness, it is easy for the child to make some decisions and choices which are good for them.

Floor Asanas

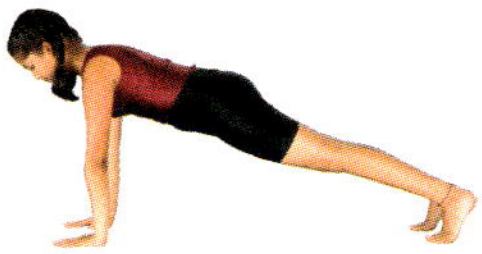

Chaduranga Dandasana – Plank Pose

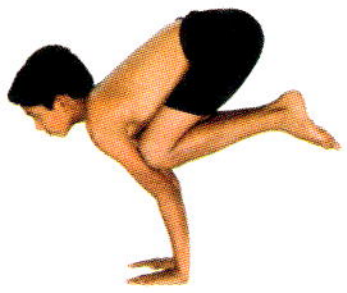

Bakasana – Bird Pose

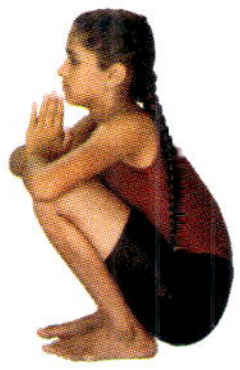

Pashasana – Deep Squat Pose

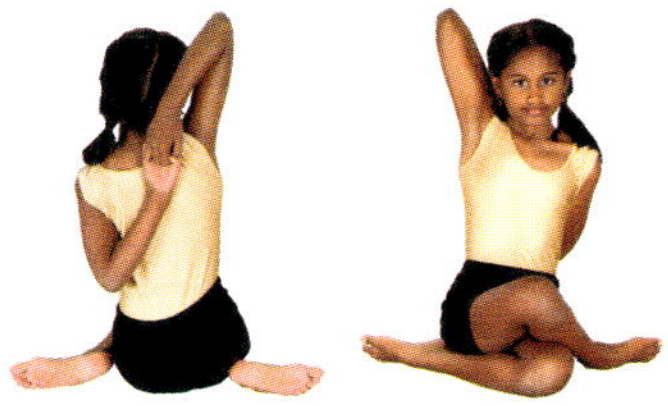

Gomukasana – Cow Face Pose

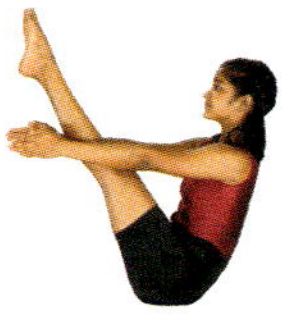

Navasana – Boat Pose

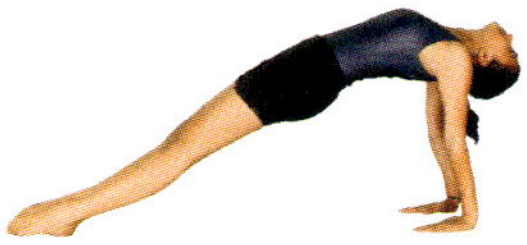

Purvottanasana – Backward Stretch Pose

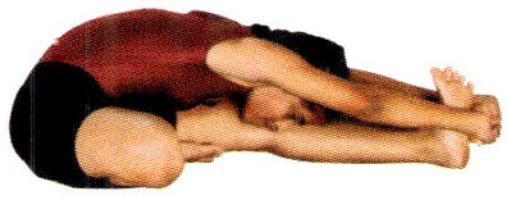

Janushirasana – Head On Knee Pose

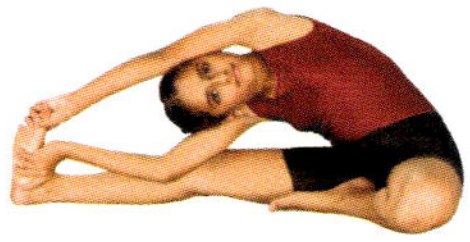

Parivritti Janushirasanana – Twisted Head on Knee Pose

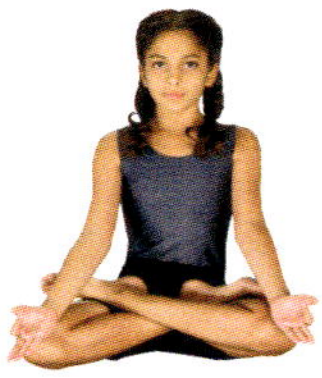

Padmasana – Lotus Pose

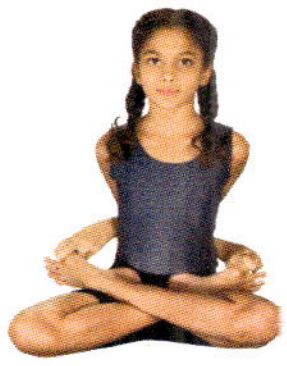

Badha Padmasana – Half Lotus Toe Hold Pose

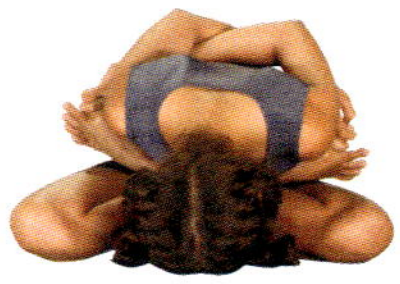

Badha Padmasana – Folded Half Lotus Toe Hold Pose

Cooling Down Sequence

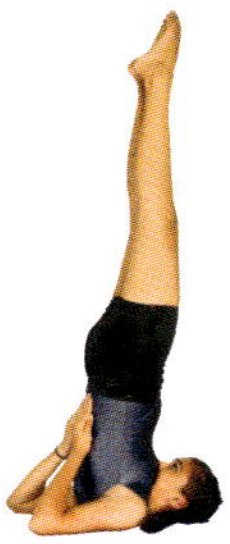

Sarvangasana – Shoulder Stand Pose

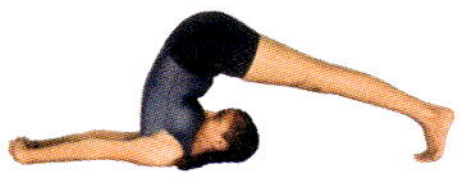

Halasana – Plough Pose

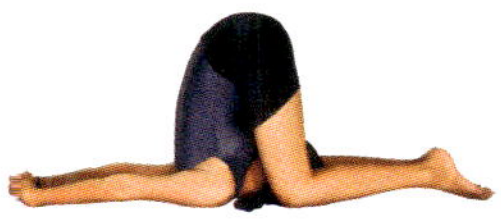

Karnapeedasana – Knee to Ear Pose

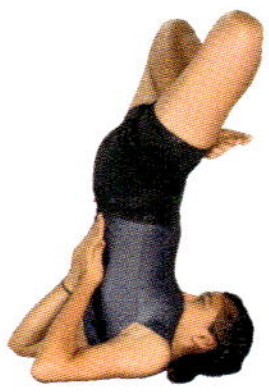

Sarvanga Padmasana – Upward Lotus Pose

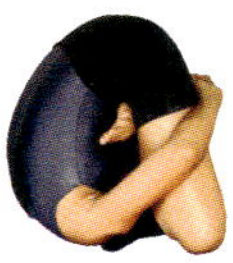

Garbha Pindasana – Baby Pose

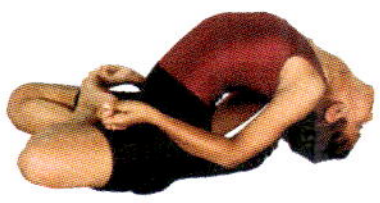

Matsyasana – Fish Pose

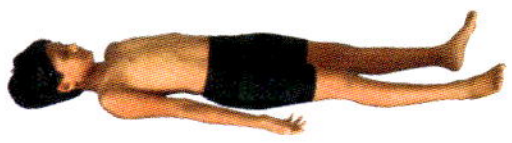

Shavasana – Total Relaxation Pose

Pranayama

As explained in **Anulom Vilom**

1. Please note that asanas have repeated across sequences as each have numerous benefits. In each of the sequencing patterns it is important to build an intention for the purpose of doing that particular asana. For eg. in the Concentration sequence Urdwa Tadasana is performed with an intent on of using concentration to balance the mind and focus on stability. The same asana in the Strengthening sequence is done with the intention of maintaining a strong and firm muscular length in the legs.
2. All the asanas which are therapeutic sequences from the author's experience as a teacher and practitioner of yoga for the past 30 years. These sequences cannot replace a doctor's treatment or diagnosis. Please consult a doctor if necessary and then introduce the asana practice.

TUESDAY

Asanas to deal with lethargy

Standing Asanas

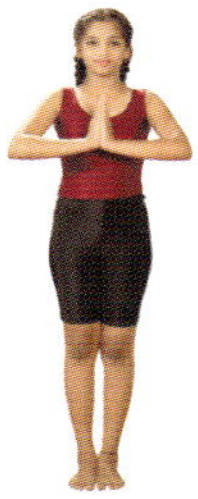

Tadasana – Pillar Pose

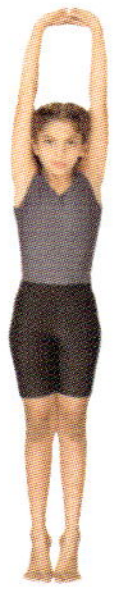

Urdwa Tadasana – Tall Pillar Pose

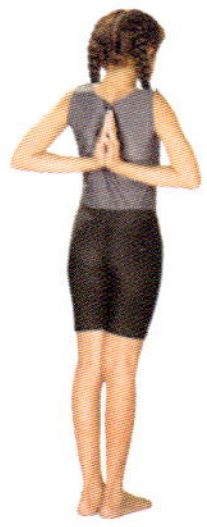

Parshwa Hasta Tadasana – Twisted Pillar Pose

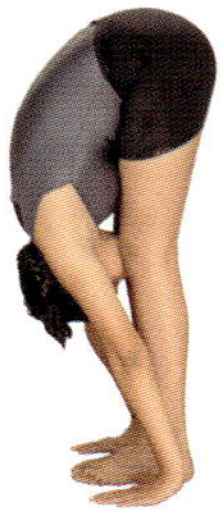

Pada Hastasana – Hand to Feet Pose

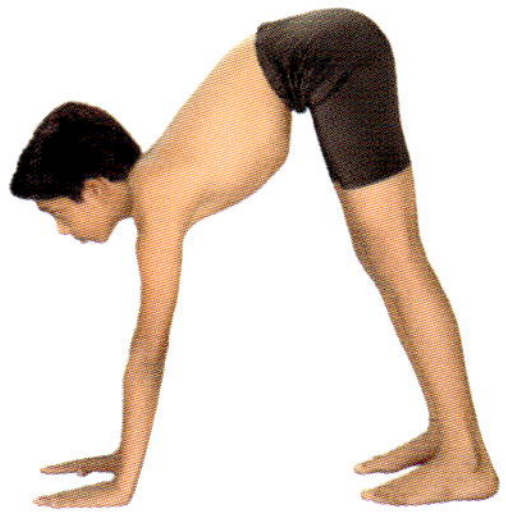

Chatuspadasna – Four-legged Pose

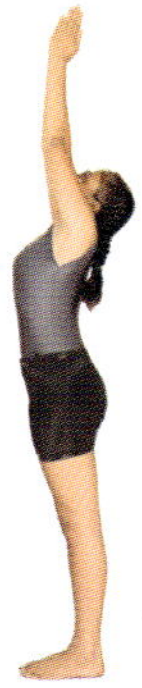

Surya Namaskara A & B (3 times)

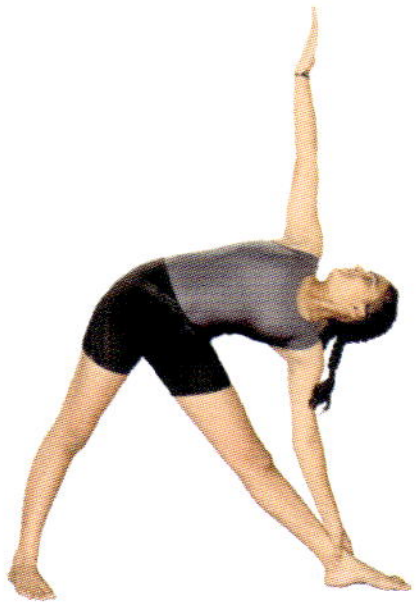

Trikonasana – Triangle Pose

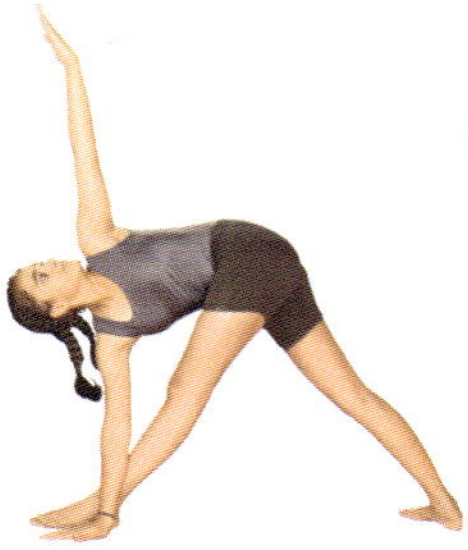

Parivritti Trikonasana – Twisted Triangle Pose

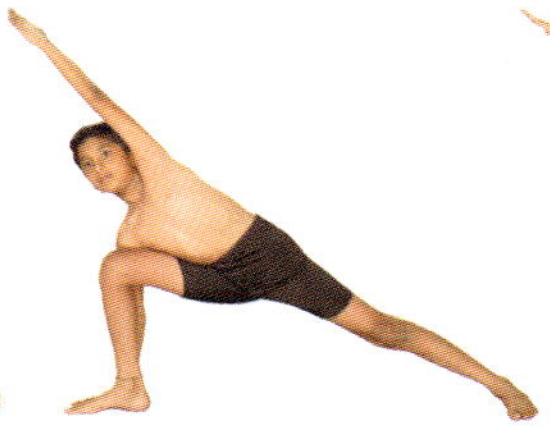

Parshvakonasana – Stretched Angle Pose

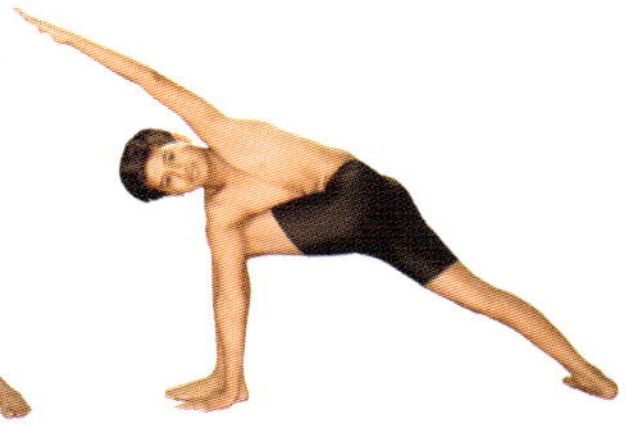

Parivriti Parshvakonasana – Twisted Stretched Angle Pose

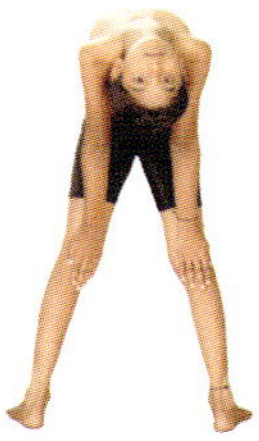

Triranga Mukothasana – Tabletop Pose

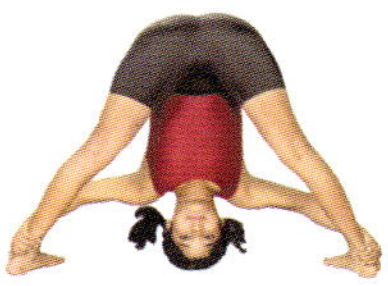

Prasaritha Padottanasana – Pyramid Pose

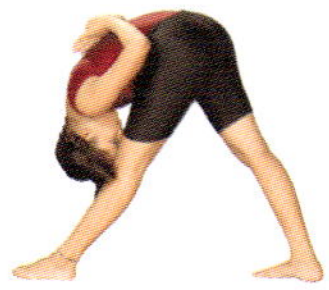

Parsvattanasna – Forward Fold Pose

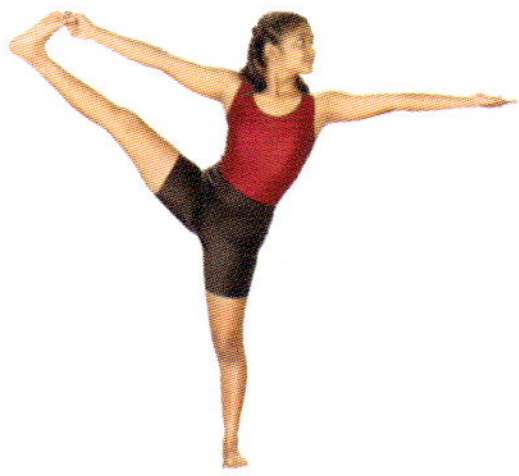

Uttita Hasta Padangustasana – Lifted Toe Hold Pose

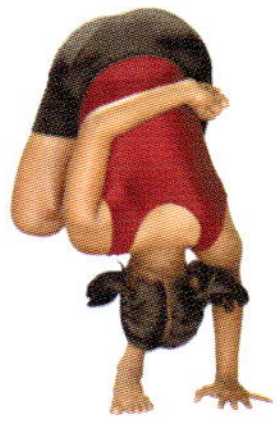

Ardha Baddha Padmottanasana – Half Lotus Toe Hold Pose

Note to parents

- Lethargy in a child could be due to medical reasons like exhaustion, stress, allergies, postural defects and infections. It is important to consult a doctor and treat it. Lifestyle-related causes can be easily dealt with by doing the asanas mentioned below.
- The asanas listed below mainly deal with lifestyle-related causes like poor posture, wrong eating habits, lack of sleep, too much of screen and internet time, etc. The asanas aim to invigorate the body and stretch the tired and lazy muscles. These asanas will wake up the body's intelligence and bring in a balance into the lives of the practitioners.

Floor Asanas

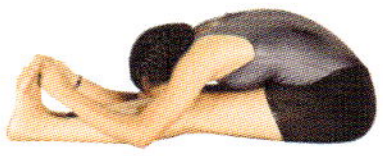

Paschimottanasana – Forward Bend Pose

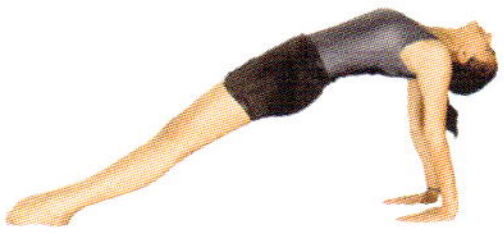

Purvottanasana – Backward Stretch Pose

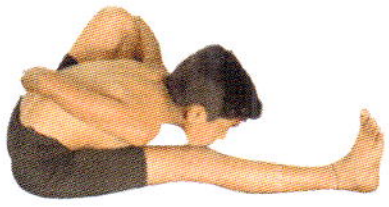

Marichasana A – Sage Pose

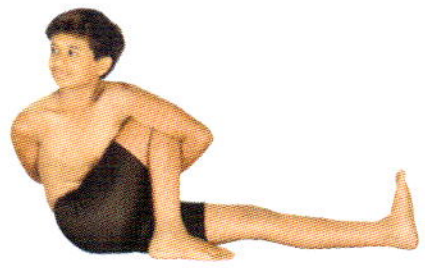

Marichasana B – Sage Pose

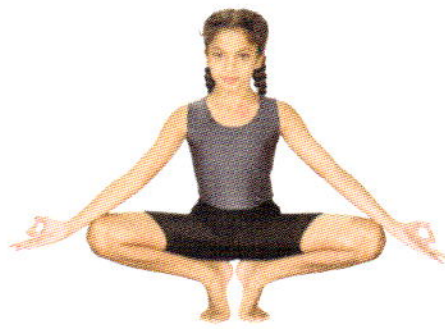

Bhadrasana – Lifted Cobler Pose

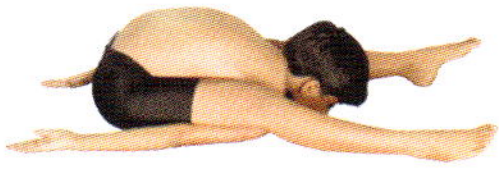

Kurmasana – Tortoise Pose

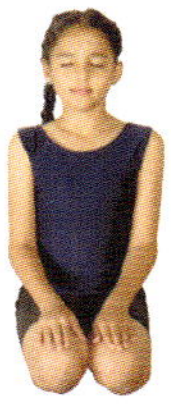

Vajrasana – Diamond Pose

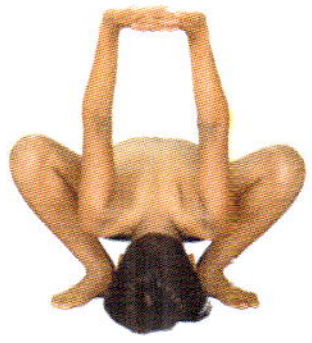

Malasana – Garland Pose

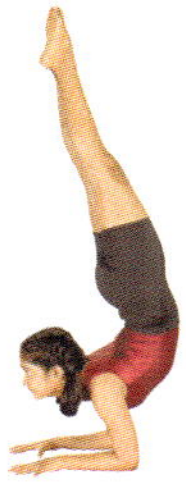

Pinchamayurasana – Peacock Pose

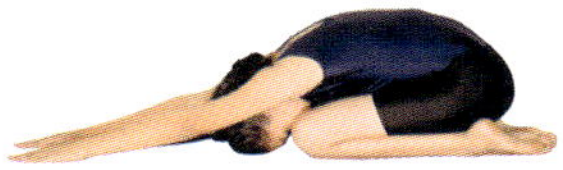

Balasana – Child Pose

Cooling Down Sequence

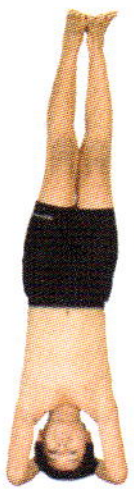

Shirasasana – Headstand Pose

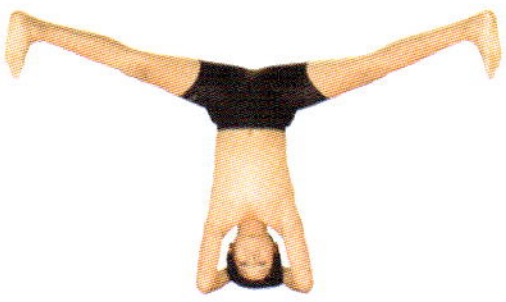

Shirasa Upavishtakonasana – Wide-angle Headstand

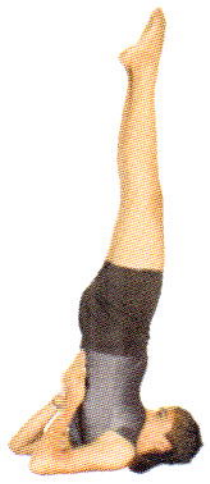

Sarvangasana – Shoulder Stand

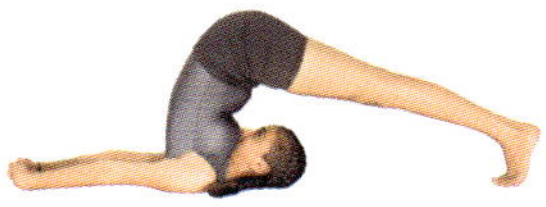

Halasana – Plough Pose

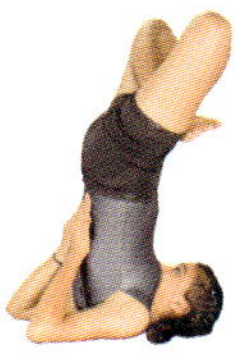

Sarvanga Padmasana – Upward Lotus Pose

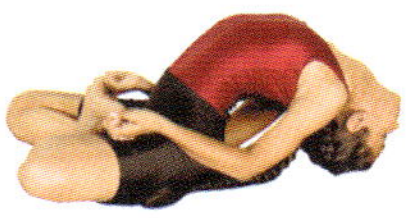

Matsyasana – Fish Pose

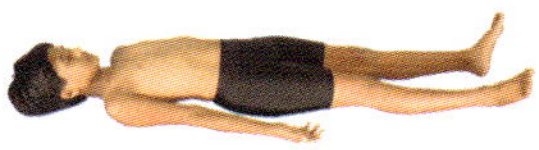

Shavasana – Total Relaxation Pose

Pranayama

As explained in **Anulom Vilom**

1. Please note that asanas have repeated across sequences as each have numerous benefits. In each of the sequencing patterns it is important to build an intention for the purpose of doing that particular asana. For eg. in the Concentration sequence Urdwa Tadasana is performed with an intention of using concentration to balance the mind and focus on stability. The same asana in the Strengthening sequence is done with the intention of maintaining a strong and firm muscular length in the legs.
2. All the asanas which are therapeutic sequences from the author's experience as a teacher and practitioner of yoga for the past 30 years. These sequences cannot replace a doctor's treatment or diagnosis. Please consult a doctor if necessary and then introduce the asana practice.

WEDNESDAY

Asanas for concentration

Standing Asanas

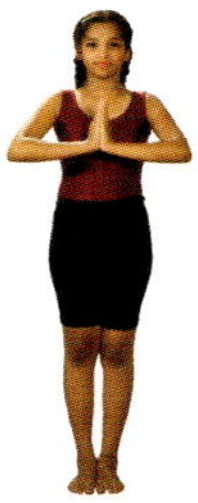

Tadasana – Pillar Pose

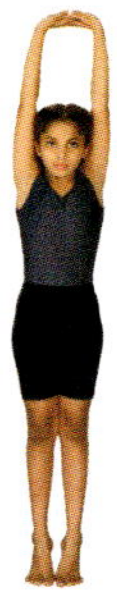

Urdwa Tadasana – Tall Pillar Pose

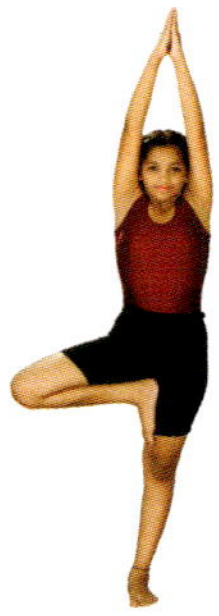

Vrikshasana – Tree Pose

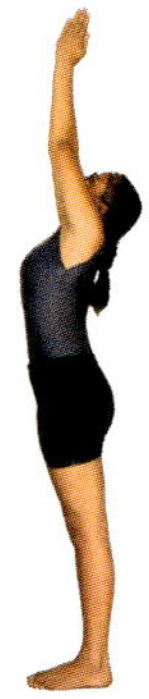

Surya Namaskara A & B (3 times)

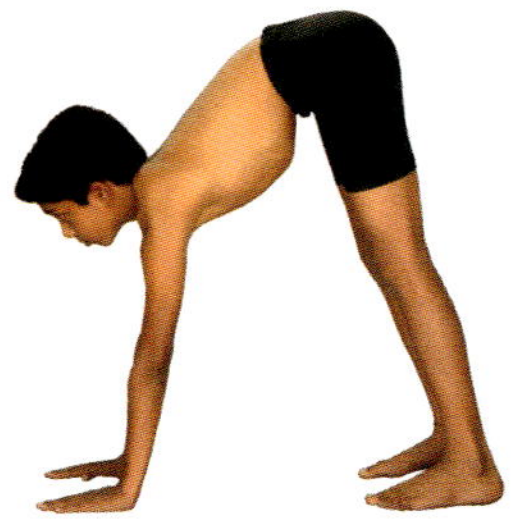

Chatuspadasna – Four-legged Pose

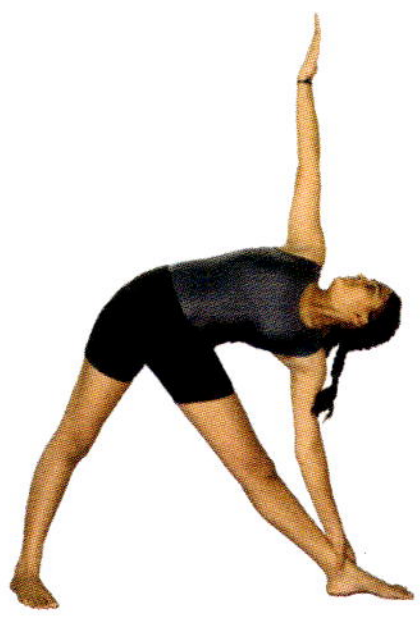

Trikonasana – Triangle Pose

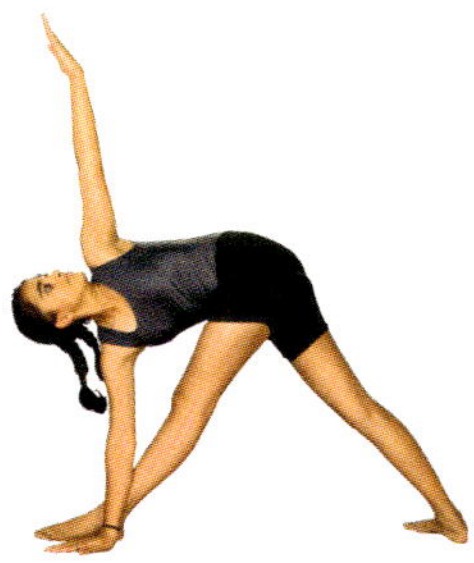

Parivritti Trikonasana – Twisted Triangle Pose

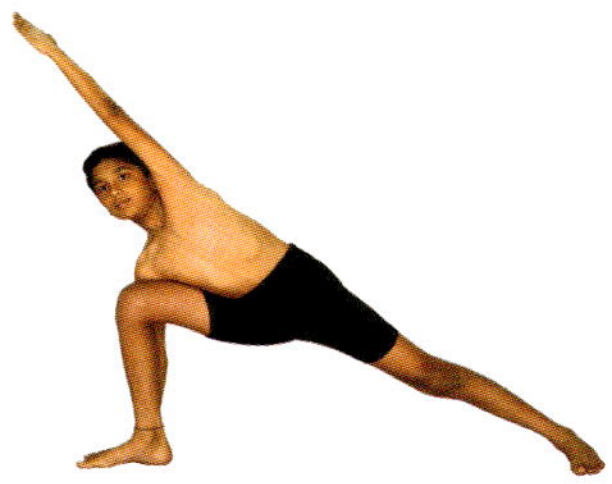

Parsvakonasana – Side Angle Stretch

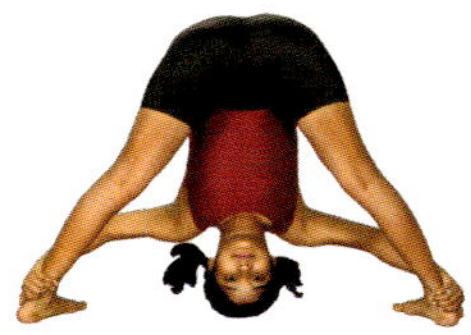

Parsaritapadottanasana – Pyramid Pose

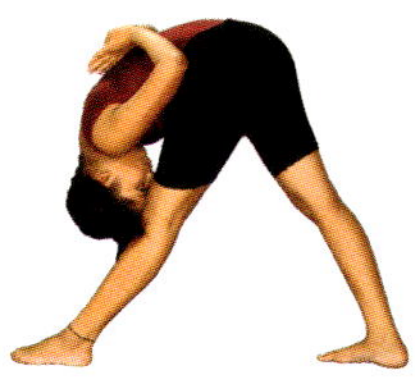

Parsvattanasna – Forward Fold Pose

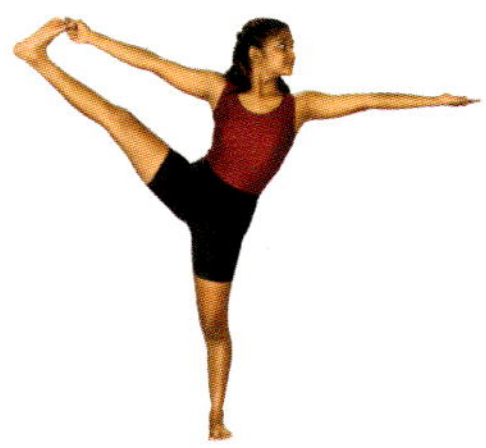

Uttita Hasta Padangustasana – Lifted Toe Hold Pose

Note to parents

- A common complaint with all parents is that it is extremely difficult to get their children to focus when it comes to studies. They get distracted very fast and very often. However, it is nothing to get worried about. Something certainly can be done to bring in balance.
- Setting up a routine is key and ensuring the child sticks to it is very important. It helps the child focus better. The parents should make it a point not to compromise with a set timetable. This will help overall development and enhance child performance. It will also help them become well-rounded and focused individuals in the long run.
- Paying attention to what they eat is also key. Focus and concentration will improve manifold if the child is given food rich in vitamins like A, C, D, E, important for their cognitive functions. Food rich in minerals like zinc, iron, copper and selenium also enhances their power to concentrate.
- The series of asanas sequenced here will quieten the mind and will challenge them to focus. They will learn to increase mental strength along with physical strength. It will also tone their muscles and build up core strength which will keep the child strong and focused.

Floor Asanas

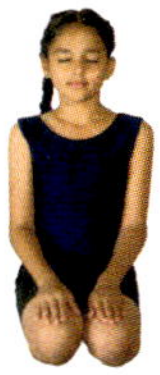

Vajrasana – Diamond Pose

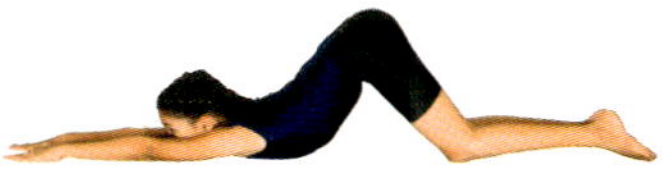

Shashankasana – Rabbit Pose

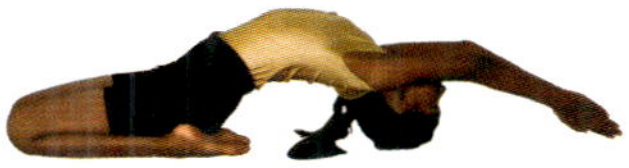

Paryankasana – Backward Fold

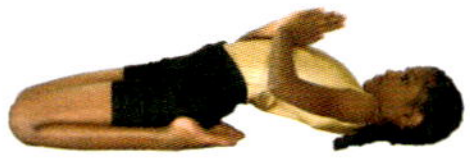

Supta Vajrasnana – Stretched Diamond Pose

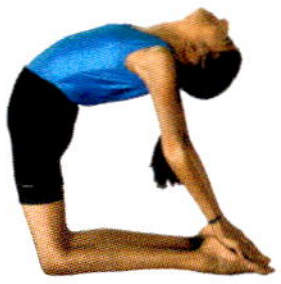

Ushtrasana – Camel Pose

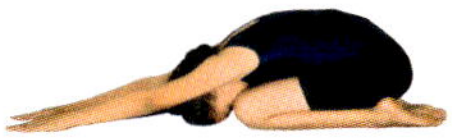

Balasana – Child Pose

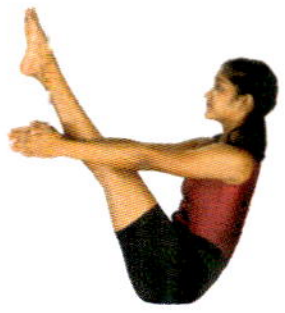

Navasana – Boat Pose

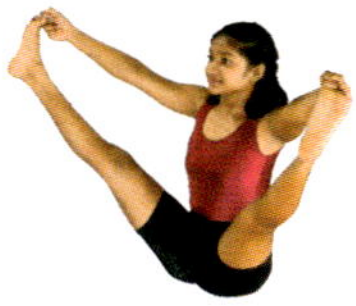

Upavishta Navasana – Wide-angle Boat Pose

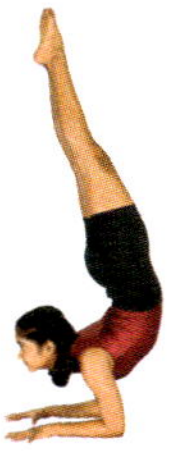

Pinchamayurasana – Peacock Pose

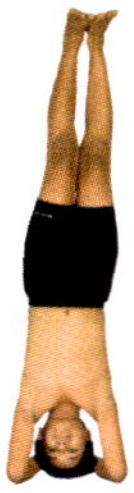

Shirasasana – Headstand Pose

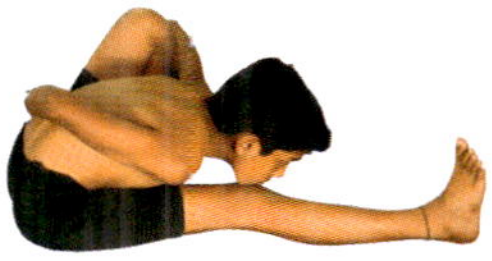

Marichasana A – Sage Position

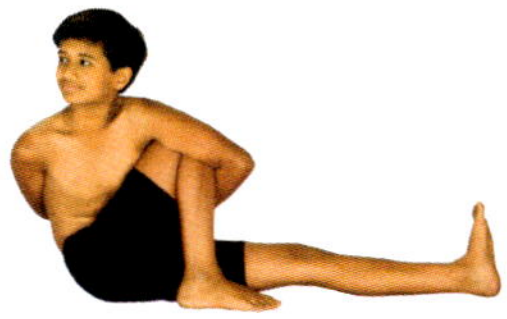

Marichasana B – Forward Bend Sage Pose

Cooling Down Sequence

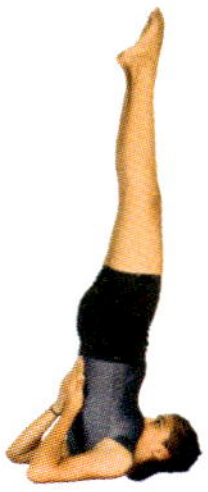

Sarvangasana – Shoulder Stand

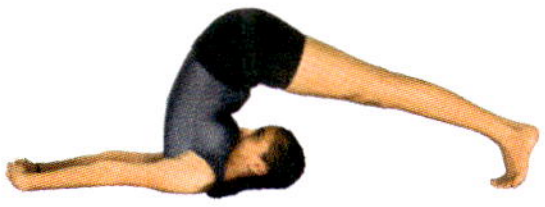

Halasana – Plough Pose

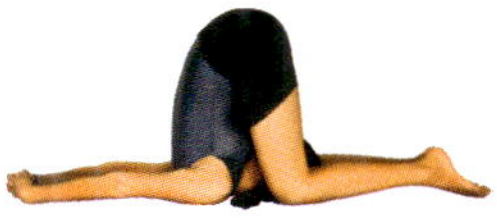

Karnapeedasana – Knee to Ear Pose

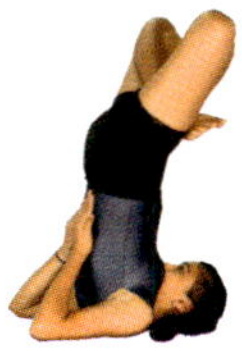

Sarvangapadmasana – Upward Lotus Pose

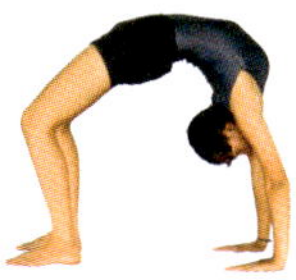

Urdhva Dhanurasana – Lifted Bow Pose

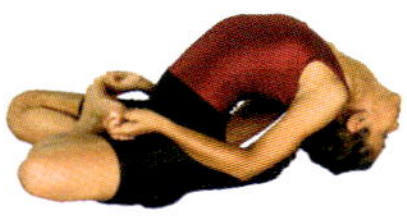

Matsyasana – Fish Pose

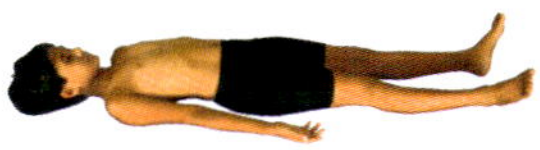

Shavasana – Total Relaxation Pose

Pranayama

As explained in **Anulom Vilom**

THURSDAY

Asanas to strengthen immunity to fight allergies

Standing Asanas

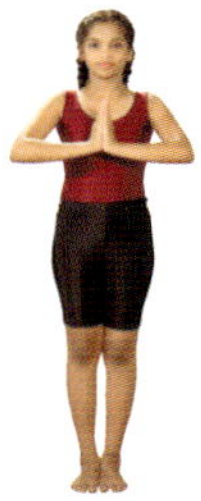

Tadasana – Pillar Pose

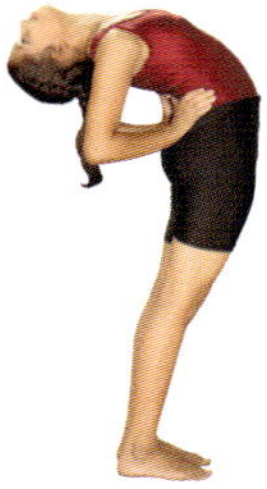

Ardha Chandra Tadasana – Half Side Wheel

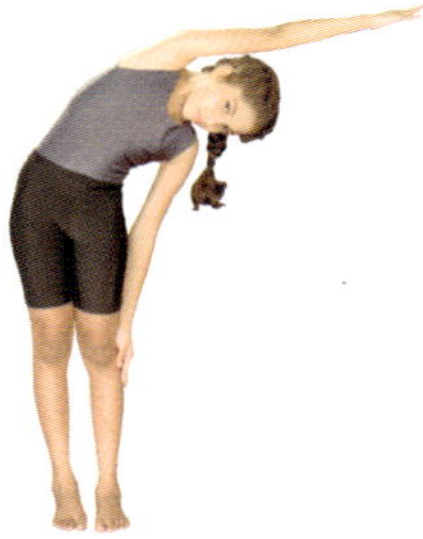

Ardha Katti Tadasana – Half Wheel Pose

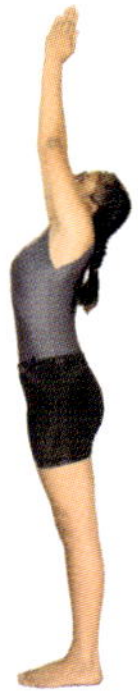

Surya Namaskara A and B

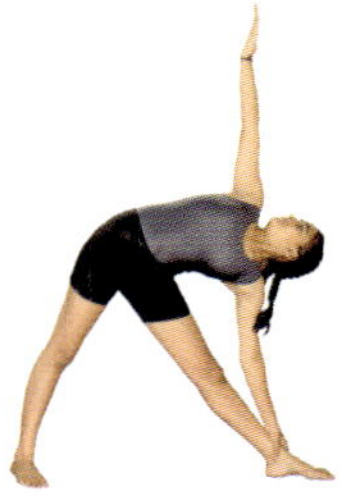

Trikonasnana – Triangle Pose

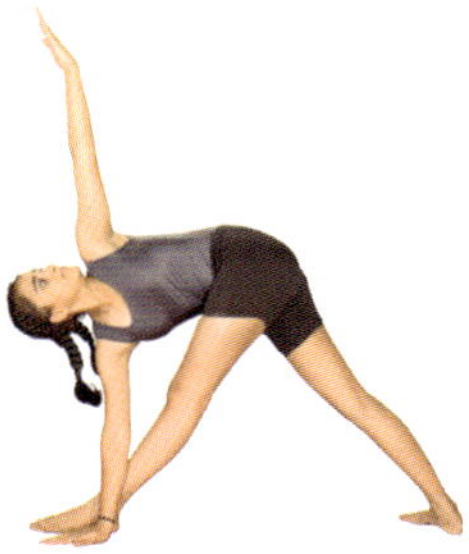

Parivritti Trikonasana – Twisted Triangle Pose

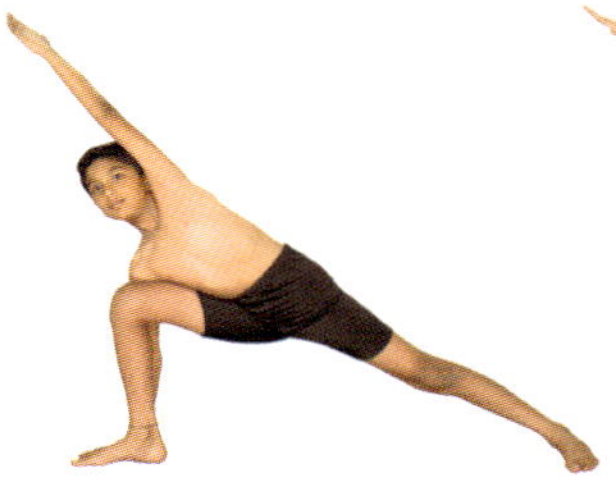

Parsvakonasana – Stretched Triangle Pose

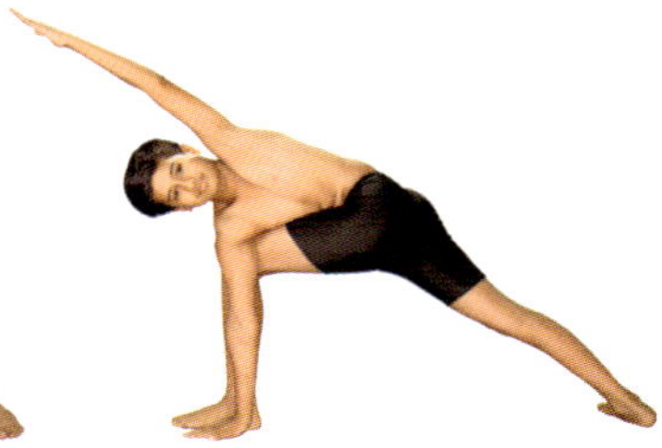

Parivritti Parsvakonasna – Twisted Stretched Pose

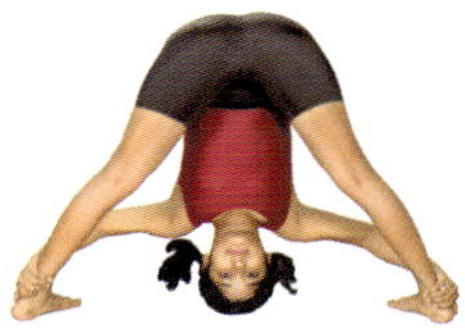

Prasaritapadottanasana – Pyramid Pose

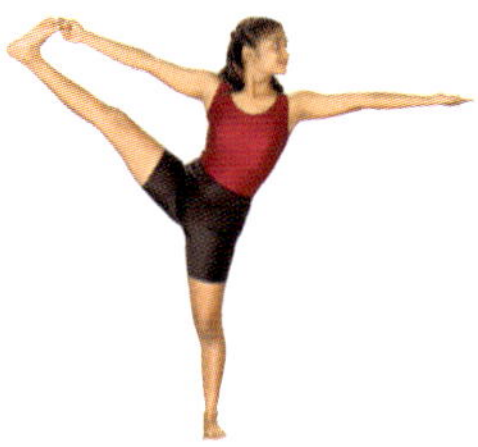

Uttita Hasta Padagustasana – Lifted Toe Hold Pose

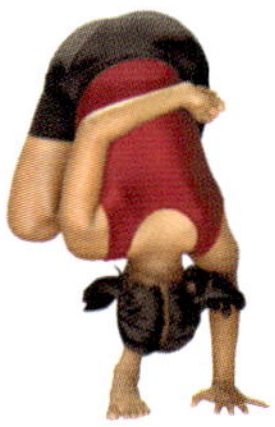

Ardha Badha Padmottanasana– Half Lotus Fold Pose

Note to parents

- There are hundreds of different viruses that can enter the body and make kids prone to coughs, colds, runny noses, headaches and stomach aches. Proper hygiene and healthy eating can reduce the symptoms of allergies and a poor immune system. Not sleeping on time is the main reason for children's low immunity, which in turn makes them susceptible to infections often. Seasonal foods help children build a strong immune system. Research has proven that yoga increases the number of natural killer cells in the body. In fact, any sports activity will help build the immune system.
- The asanas which are sequenced in this routine target to boost the immune system by reducing stress, conditioning the lungs and respiratory tract and stimulating the lymphatic system to effectively release the toxins from the body. The asanas also target blood circulation to various organs and ensure their optimal functionality.

Floor Asanas

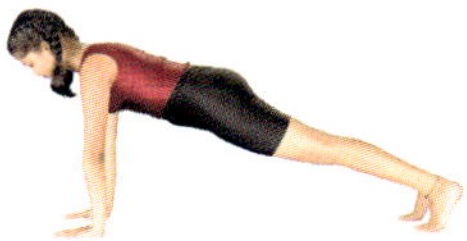

Chadurangadandasana – Plank Pose

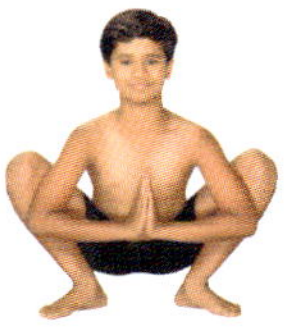

Manipurasana – Deep Squat Pose

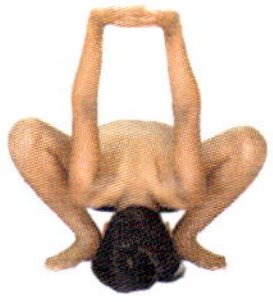

Malasana – Garland Pose

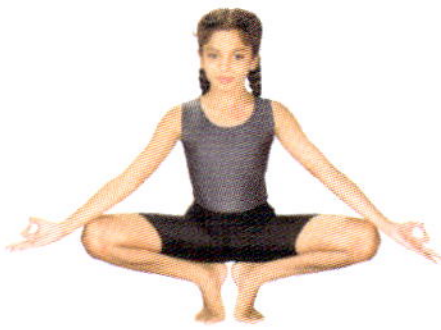

Bhadrasana – Strong Pose

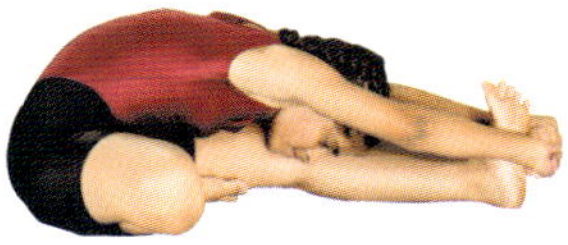

Janushirasasana – Head To Knee Pose

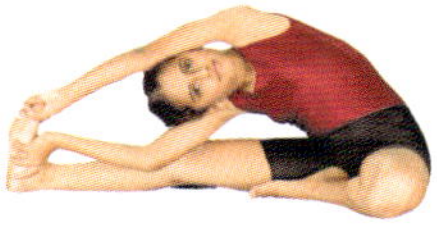

Parivritti Janushirasana – Twisted Head to Knee Pose

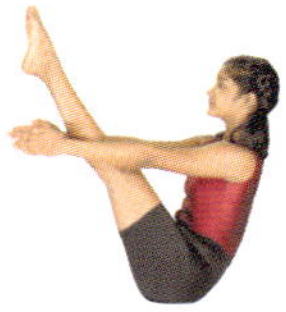

Navasana – Boat Pose

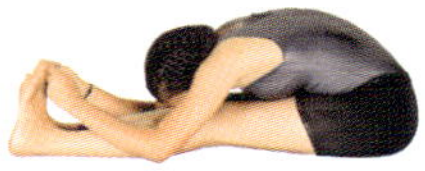

Paschimottanasana – Forward Fold

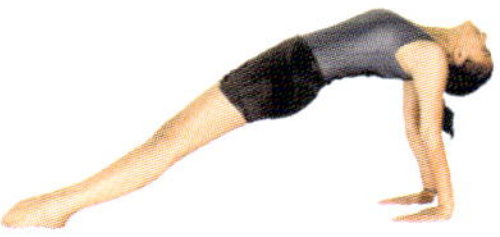

Purvottanasnana – Backward Stretch

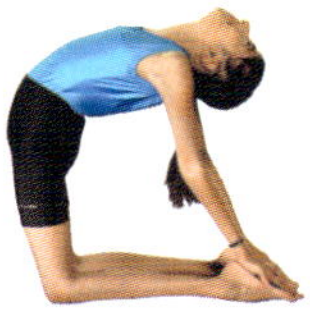

Ushtrasana – Camel Pose

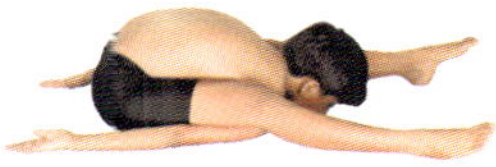

Kurmasana – Tortoise Pose

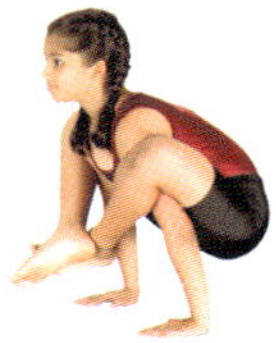

Bhujapeedasana – Shoulder Balance

Cooling Down Sequence

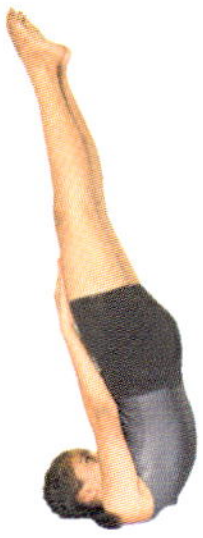

Salamba Sarvangasana – Shoulder Stand Pose

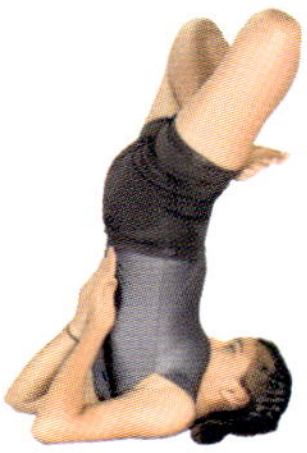

Padmasana Sarvangasana – Upturned Lotus Pose

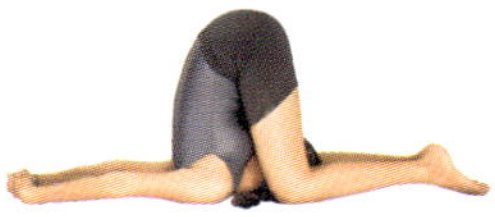

Karnapeedasana – Knee To Ear Pose

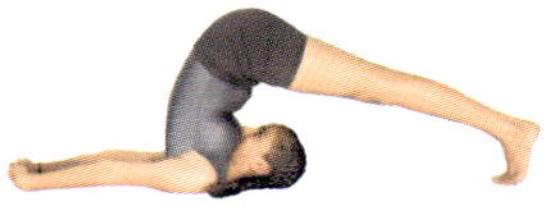

Halasana – Plough Pose

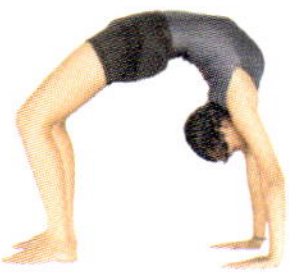

Urdwa Dhanurasana – Backward Bend

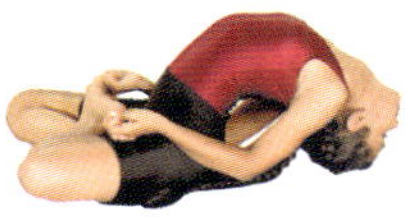

Matsyasana – Fish Pose

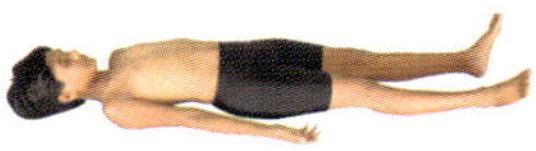

Shavasana – Total Relaxation Pose

Pranayama

As explained in **Anulom Vilom**

FRIDAY

Asanas for good posture

Standing Asanas

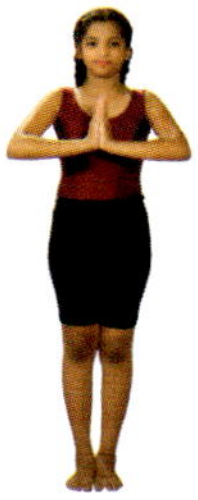

Tadasana – Pillar Pose

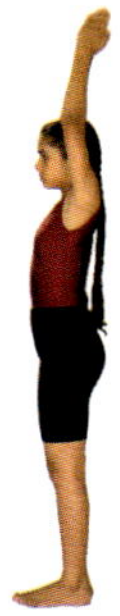

Urdwa Hasta Tadasna – Head Up Tall Pillar Pose

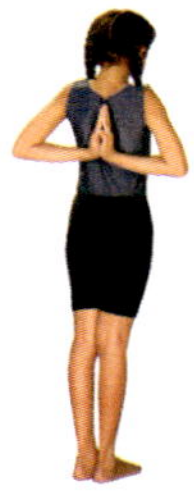

Parshwa Hasta Tadasana – Back Namaste Pillar Pose

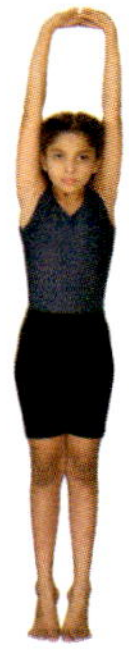

Urdwa Tadasana – Lifted Pillar Pose

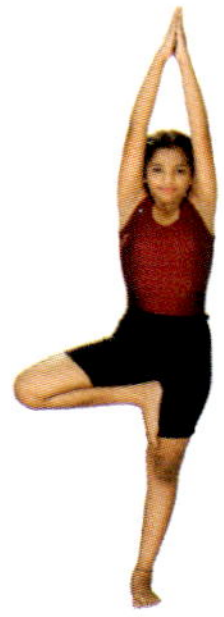

Vrikshasana – Tree Pose

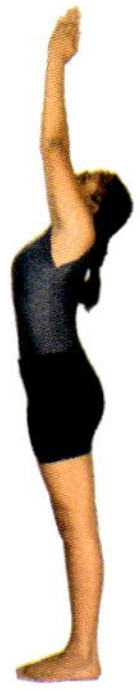

Surya Namaskara A and B

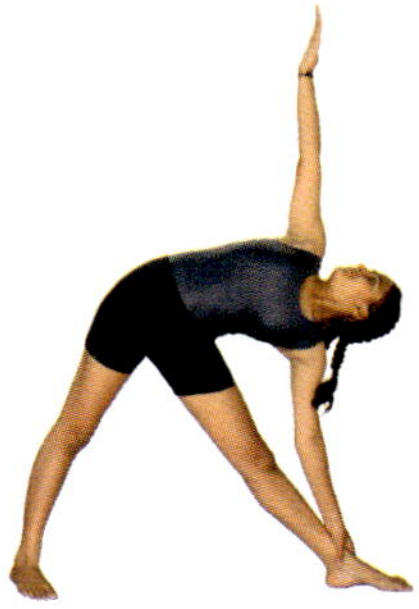

Trikonasana – Side-angle Pose

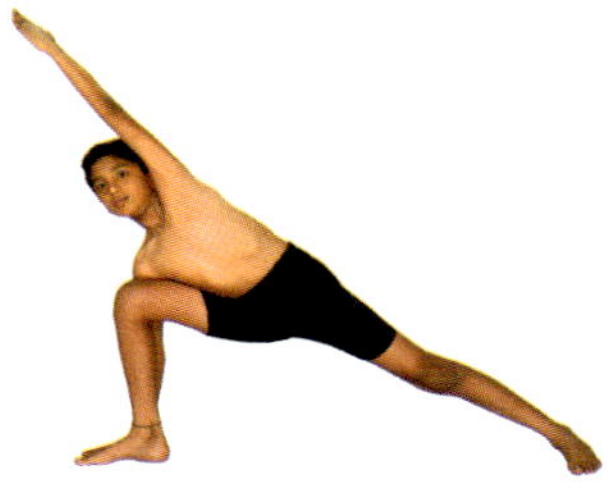

Parshwakonasana – Stretched-angle Pose

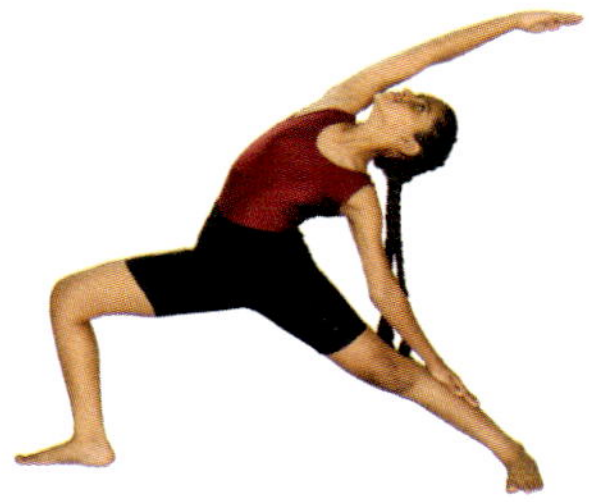

Anjaneyasana – Monkey God Pose

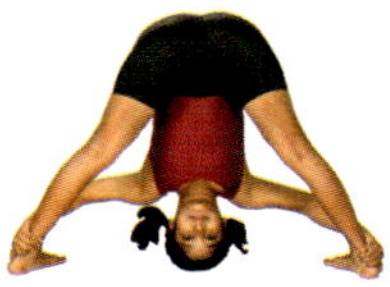

Prasaritha Padottanasana – Pyramid Pose

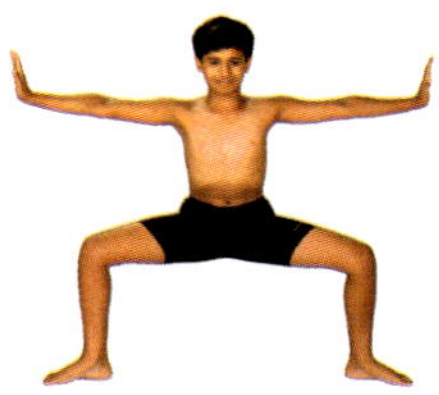

Tandavasana – Dancing Lord Pose

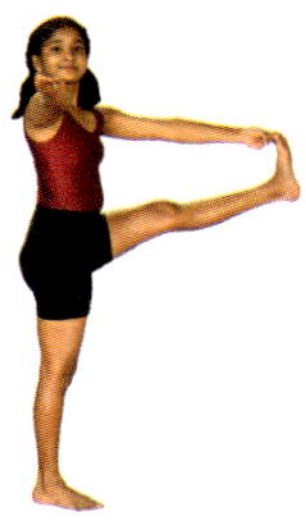

Uttita Hasta Padagustasana – Lifted Toe Hold Pose

Note to parents

- Bad posture begins early in life. If not corrected early, it will cause chronic pain and discomfort. When children develop a bad posture, it will be for life. Trying to make the child improve bad posture without strengthening the child's muscles will make it very difficult. The main areas of the body which contribute to bad posture are the head, neck, spine, arms and legs. So a good posture involves training the body to sit, stand, walk and keep the limbs in place, so that the muscles are least strained and the ligaments are performing its weight-bearing activities well. A good posture keeps the bones and muscles in place, further keeping the body comfortable.
- Sometimes when the child is emotionally stressed posture is affected. The asanas listed for practice are not only good for physical correction but also target the child's mental condition and confidence too. Consistent practice is key for progress. Yoga asanas are the best way to correct bad posture. The asanas adjust the muscular and skeletal structure and release pain and strain from the length of the body.

Floor Asanas

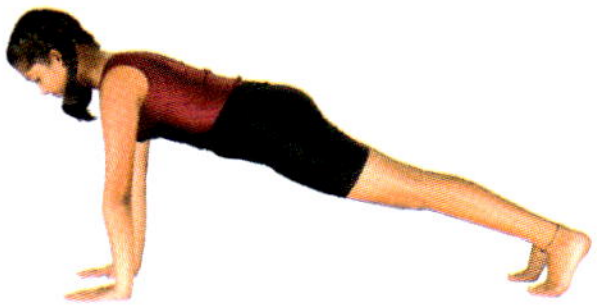
Dandasana – Staff Pose

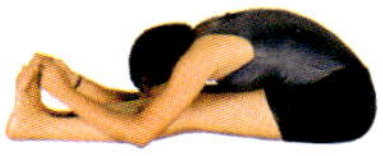
Paschimottanasana – Forward Fold Pose

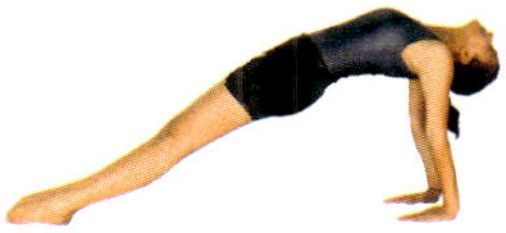
Purvottanasana – Backward Stretch Pose

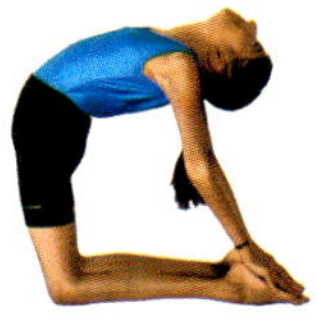
Ushtrasana – Camel Pose

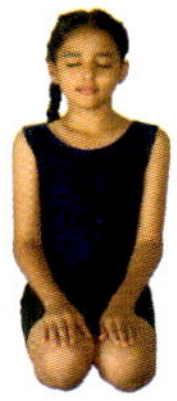
Vajrasana – Diamond Pose

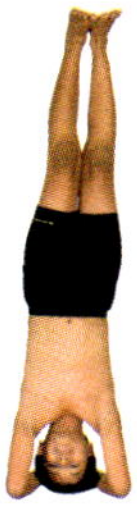
Shirasasana – Headstand Pose

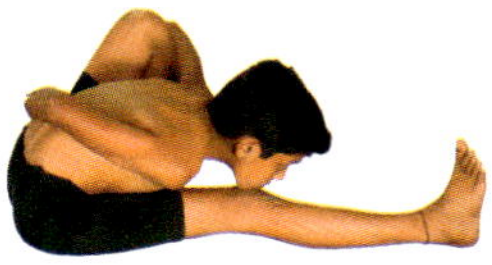
Marichasana A – Sage Pose A

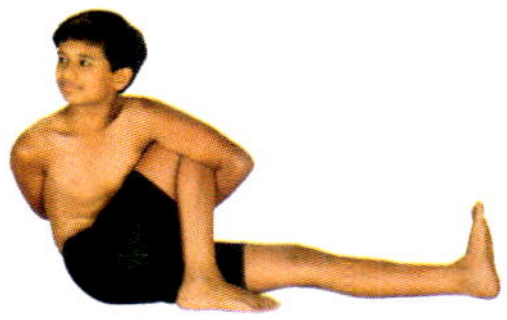
Marichasana B – Sage Pose B

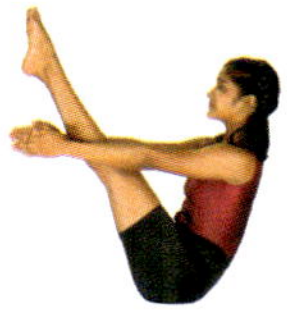
Navasana – Boat Pose

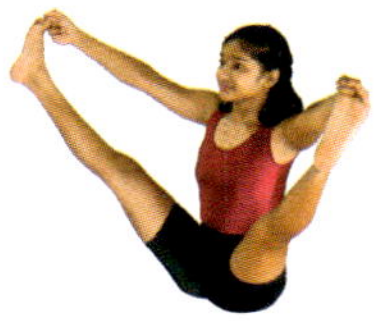
Upavistanavasana – Wide-angle Boat Pose

Cooling Down Sequence

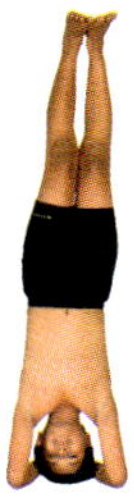
Shriasanana – Headstand Pose

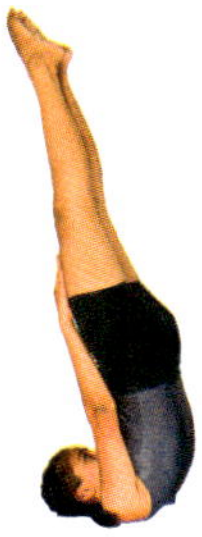
Salamba Sarvangasana – Shoulder Stand Pose

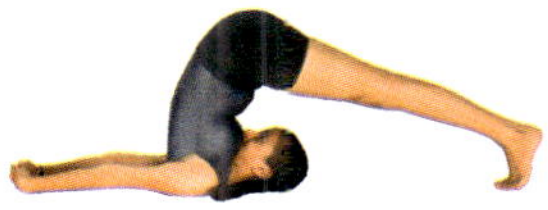
Halasana – Plough Pose

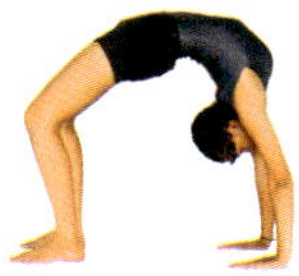
Urdwa Dhanurasana – Backward Bow Pose

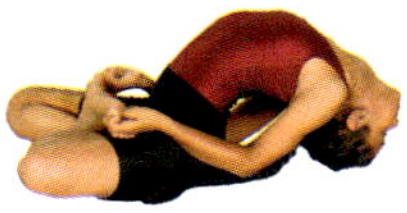
Matsyasana – Fish Pose

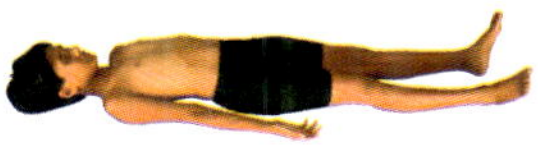
Shavasana – Total Relaxation Pose

Pranayama

As explained in **Anulom Vilom**

SATURDAY

Asanas for relaxation

Standing Asanas

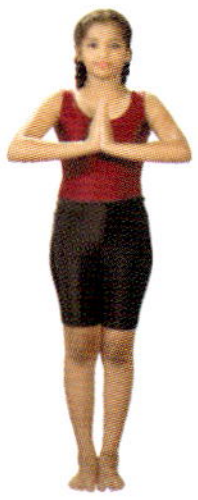

Tadasana – Pillar Pose

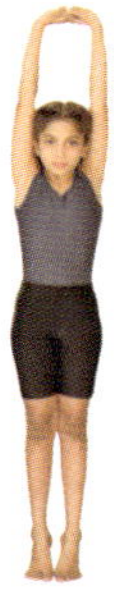

Urdwa Tadasana – Tall Pillar Pose

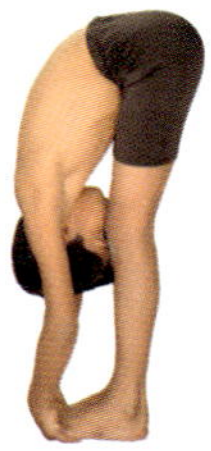

Pada Hastasana – Toe Hold Pose

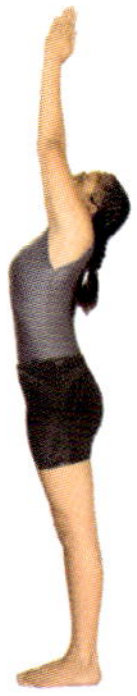

Surya Namaskara A and B

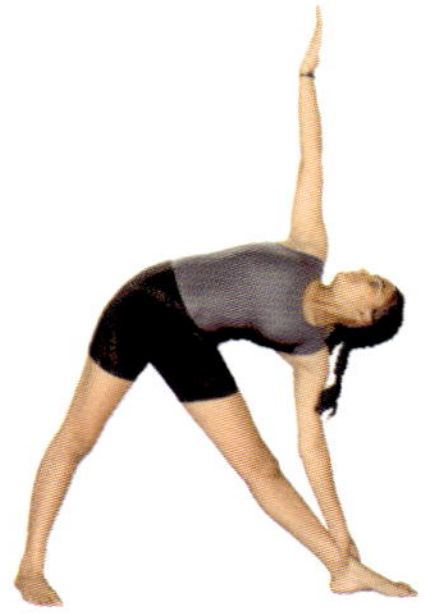

Trikonasana – Triangle Pose

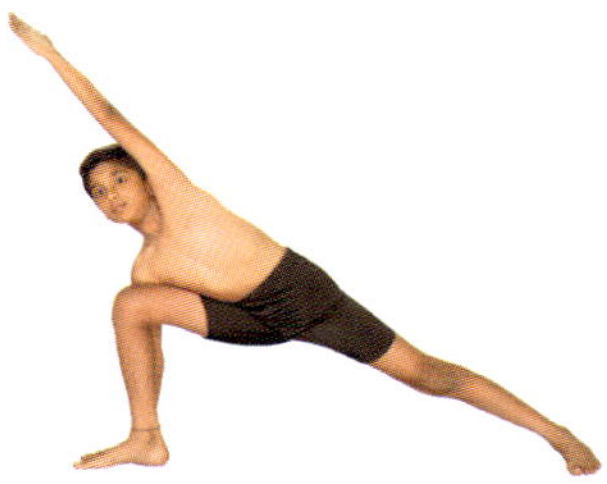

Parshwakonasana – Stretched-angle Pose

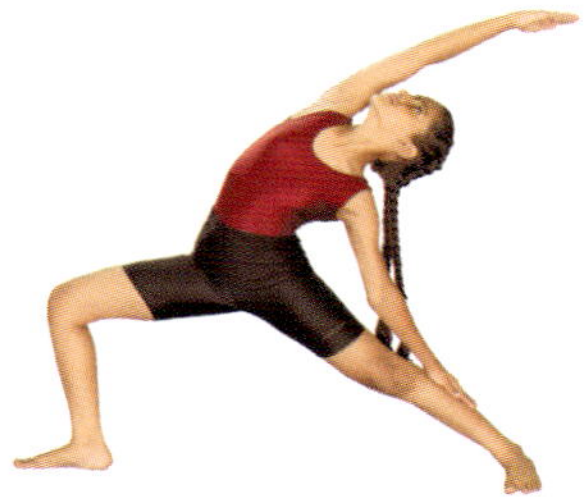

Anjaneyasana – Flying Monkey God Pose

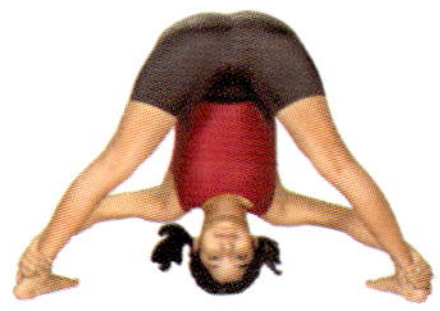

Prasarita Padottanasana – Pyramid Pose

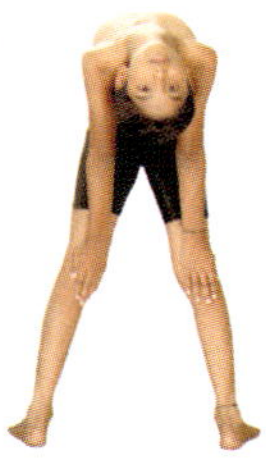

Trirangamukothanasana – Backward Stretch Pose

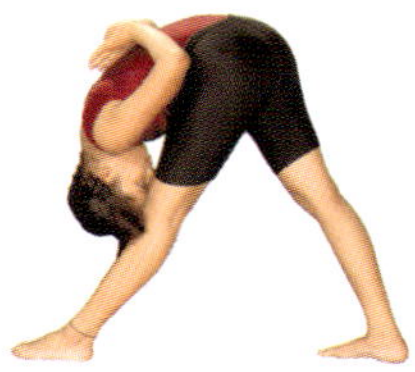

Parsvattanasna – Forward Fold Pose

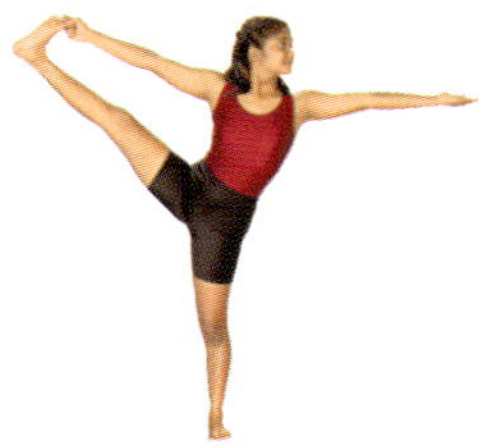

Uttitha Hasta Padangustasana – Toe Hold Pose

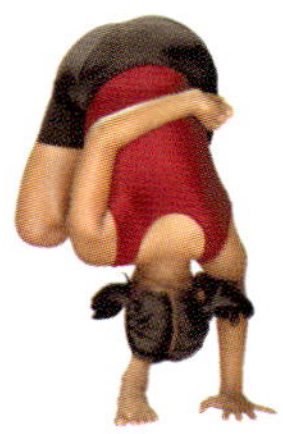

Ardhabadha Padmottanasana – Half-Lotus Toe Hold Pose

Note to parents

- Children are eager and have energetic minds, so it is natural that they are always active and engaged. To improve the quality of their energy, it would be great to relax them and change their mind fields to channelise their thought patterns. Simple asanas and relaxation techniques will go a long way to clear their thinking and bring them to be mindful.
- The asanas recommended here for practice help to slightly stress and relax the body. We will start with some standing asanas for focus and concentration and stabilise the mind by releasing tension.
- When it comes to relaxing, there are two parts of the nervous system: sympathetic and parasympathetic. These are important for understanding how to relax. I have read that the best way to understand sympathetic is to look at it like it is an accelerator, while parasympathetic is like brakes. Stress and anxiety are triggered by the sympathetic nervous system while relaxation is triggered by the parasympathetic nervous system.
- It is very important to practise breathing during this sequence. The asanas have to be done consistently to see best results. They are targetted to relax the sympathetic and activate the parasympathetic system.

Floor Asanas

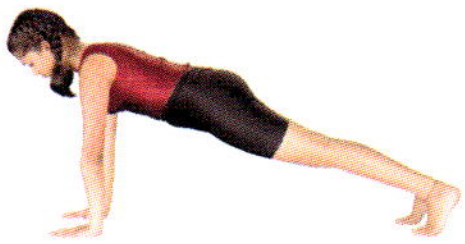

Chaduranga Dandasana – Plank Pose

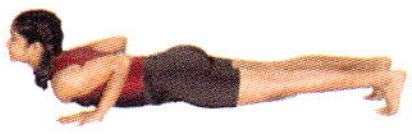

Bhujangasana – Snake Pose

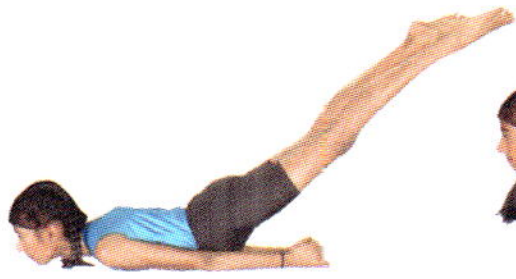

Dwipada Shalabhasana – Locust Pose

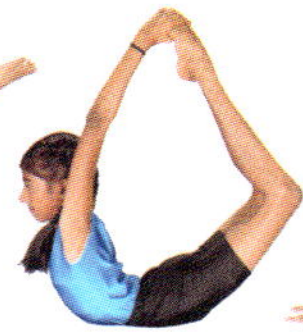

Dhanurasana – Bow Pose

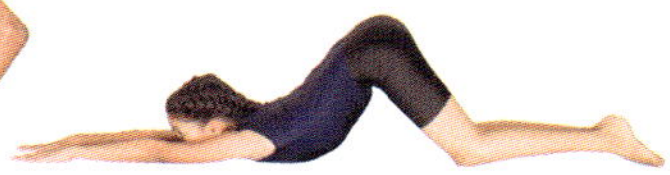

Shashankasana – Rabbit Pose

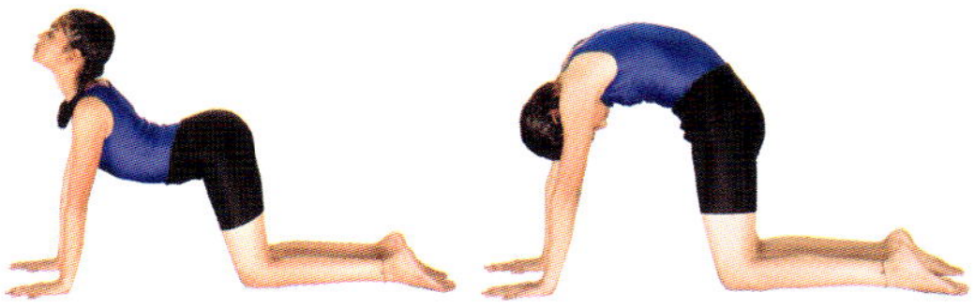

Vyagrasana A, B and C – Wild Cat Pose

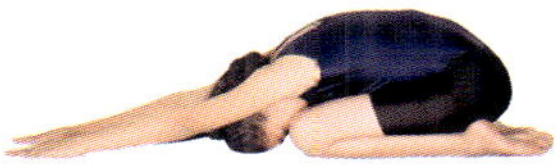

Balasana – Child Pose

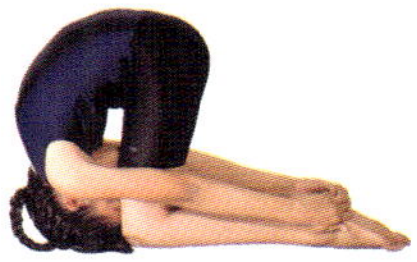

Marijariasana – Rabbit King Pose

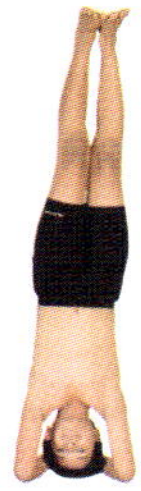

Shirasasana – Headstand Pose

Cooling Down Sequence

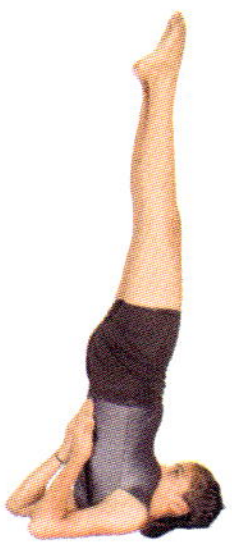

Sarvangasana – Shoulder Stand

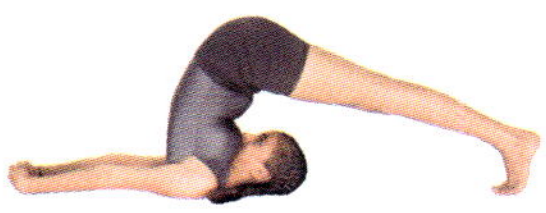

Halasana – Plough Pose

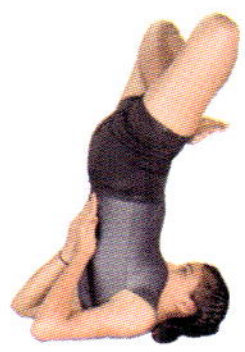

Sarvangapadmasana – Upward Lotus Pose

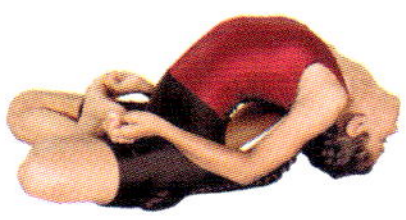

Matsyasana – Fish Pose

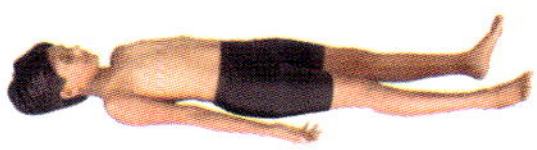

Shavasana – Total Relaxation Pose

Pranayama

As explained in **Anulom Vilom**

DIGITAL KIDS
SEQUENCE

45 Minutes to finish the sequence

Standing Asanas

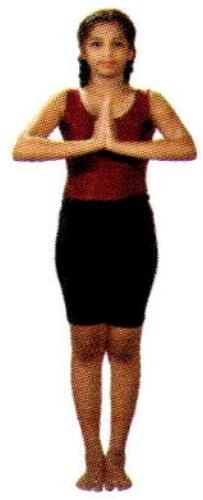

Tadasana – Pillar Pose

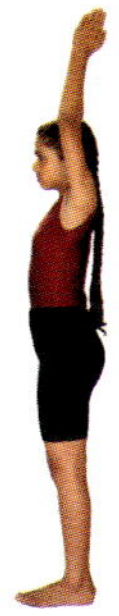

Urdwa Hasta Tadasana – Head Up Tall Pillar Pose

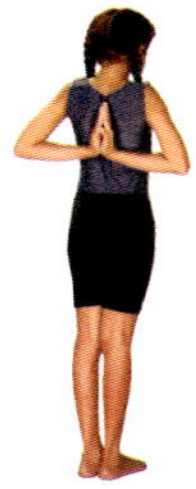

Parshwa Hasta Tadasana – Back Namaste Pillar Pose

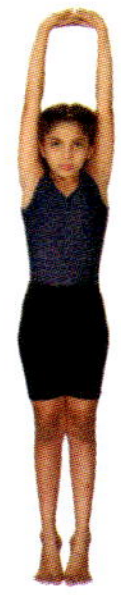

Urdwa Tadasana – Tall Pillar Pose

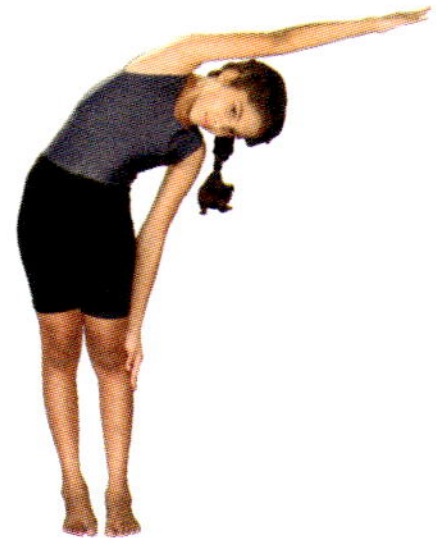

Ardha Chandra Tadasana – Half Wheel Pose

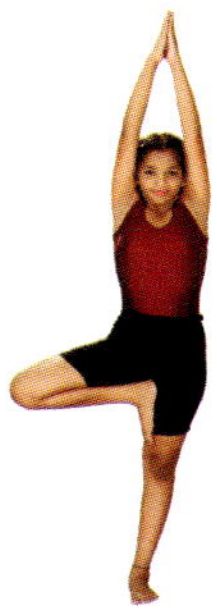

Vrikshasana – Tree Pose

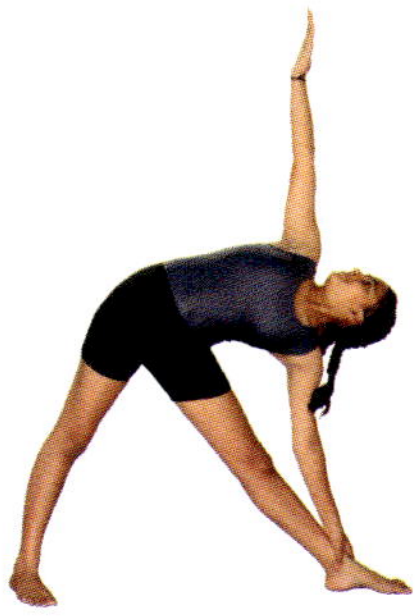

Trikonasana – Triangle Pose

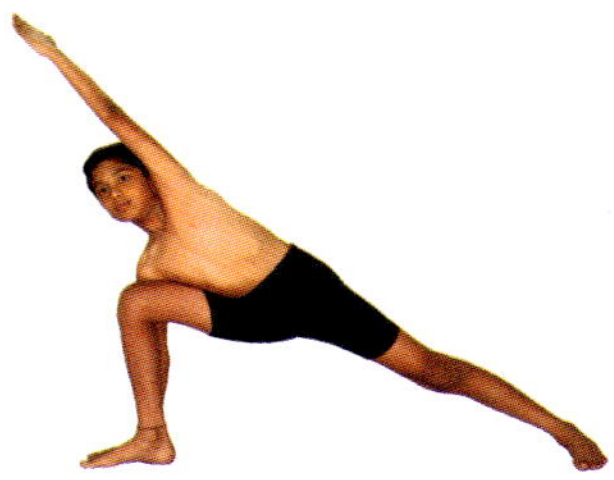

Parshwakonasana – Stretched Angle Pose

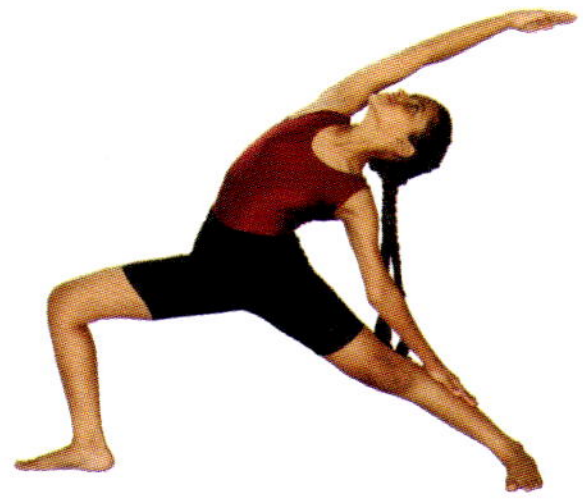

Anjaneyasana – Flying Monkey God Pose

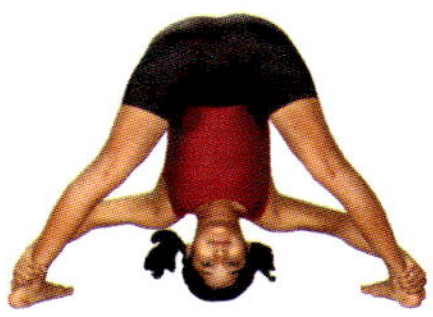

Prasarita Padottanasana – Pyramid Pose

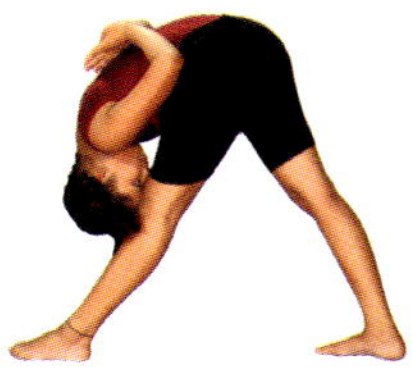

Parsvattanasna – Forward Fold Pose

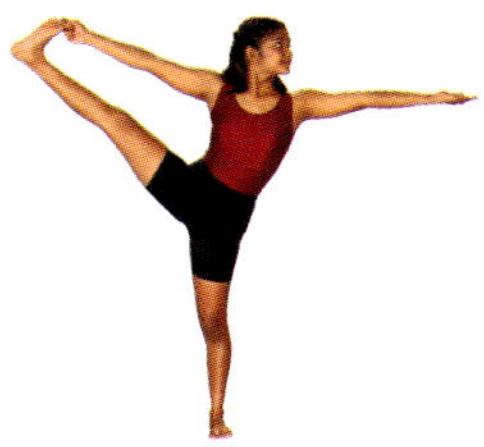

Uttita Hasta Padagustasana – Lifted Toe Hold Pose

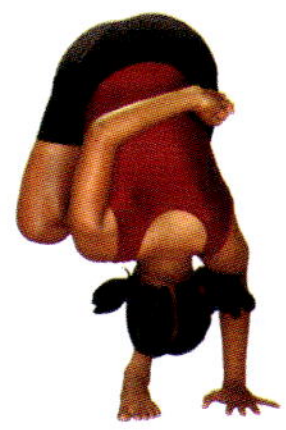

Ardhabadha Padmottanasana – Half-Lotus Toe Hold Pose

Note to parents

- While technology is good in a way, excessive use of digital devices does have a negative side to it. It does affect focus and concentration in the kids, as well as their emotional health, sleep and even empathy. It also influences growth and motor skills in children, which is a cause for concern. Though there is no scientific evidence for this however, overuse may have its impact and many school teachers have addressed this as a concern already.
- It is best to accept as early as possible that there could be a concern and help our kids to learn to adapt to change and stay ready for all those infinite possibilities ahead of them. A regular practice of yoga could help maintain children's gross motor skills, fine motor skills, sensory needs, behaviour and attention.
- Gross motor skills are larger movements made with arms, legs, feet or entire body. Fine mortar skills are coordination in small muscles, in movements. For eg. synchronisation in hands and fingers, movement of the eyes, etc. Sensory needs concern the 5 senses of sight, smell, hearing, taste and touch.
- Yoga asanas are great for strengthening and muscle coordination, particularly core and postural muscles. Developing core and postural muscles help children keep an upright posture to cope with table work such as handwriting, sitting for long hours without getting tired. Strong core and postural muscles will also keep them strong for sports activities. Yoga allows the child to explore body movements, balance, build body awareness and encourages hand and eye coordination.
- This is a sequence is a holistic solution for children of this digital age.

Floor Asanas

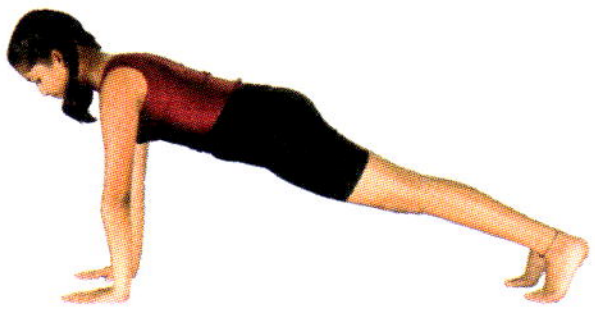

Dandasana – Staff Pose

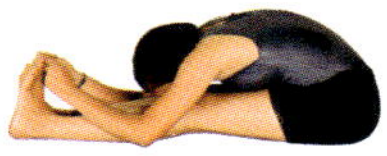

Paschimottanasana – Forward Fold Pose

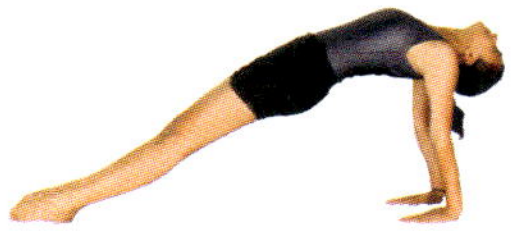

Purvottanasana – Backward Stretch Pose

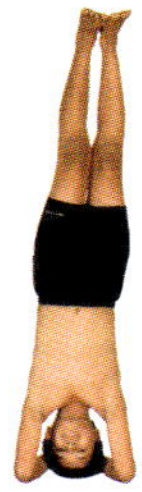

Shirasasana – Headstand Pose

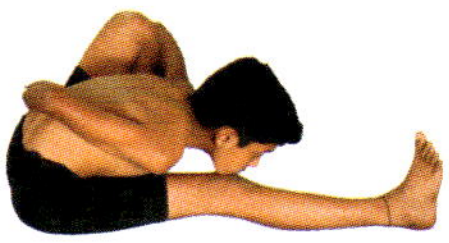

Marichasana A – Sage Pose A

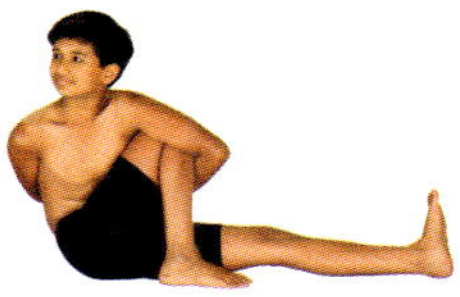

Marichasana B – Sage Pose B

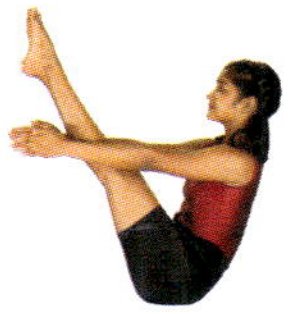

Navasana – Boat Pose

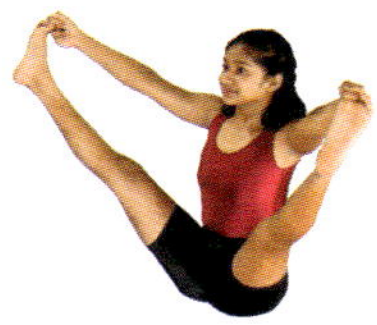

Upavistanavasana – Wide-angle Boat Pose

Cooling Down Sequence

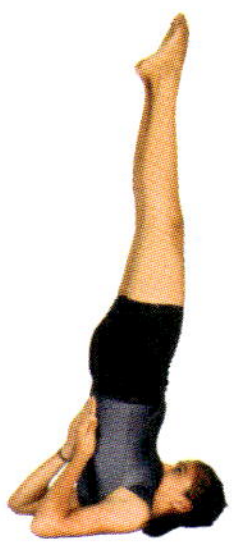

Sarvangasana – Shoulder Stand

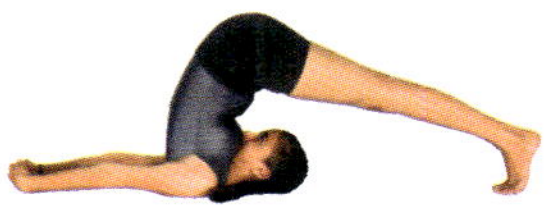

Halasana – Plough Pose

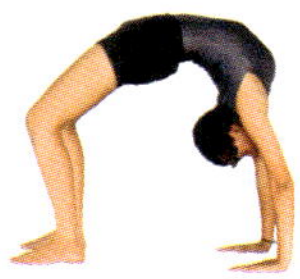

Urdwa Dhanurasana – Backward Bend

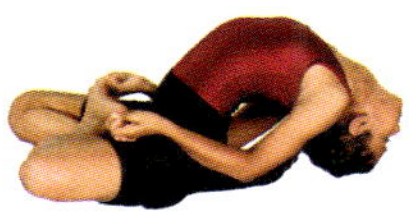

Matsyasana – Fish Pose

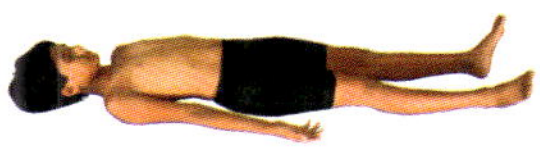

Shavasana – Total Relaxation Pose

Pranayama

As explained in **Anulom Vilom**

SPORTS STAR SEQUENCE

45 Minutes to finish the sequence

Standing Asanas

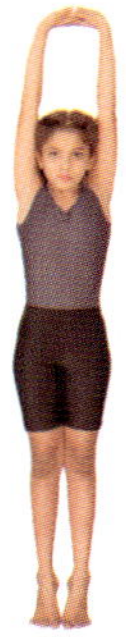

Urdwa Tadasana – Tall Pillar Pose

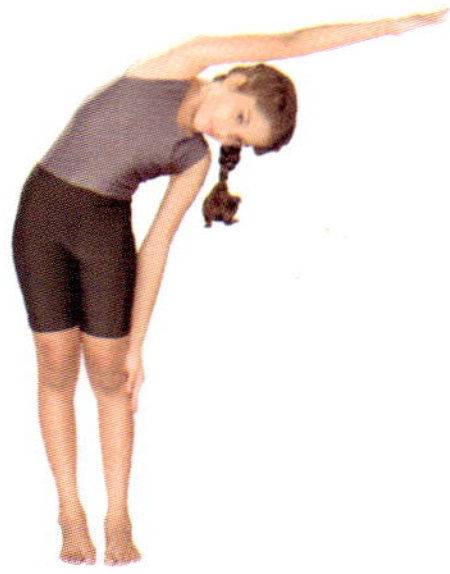

Ardha Chandra Tadasana – Half Wheel Pose

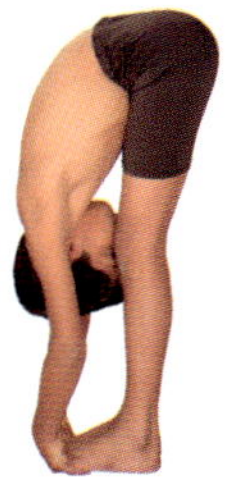

Pada Hastasana – Toe Hold Pose

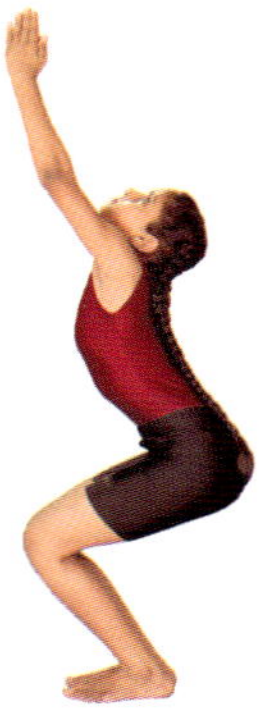

Utkattasana 2 – Chair Pose

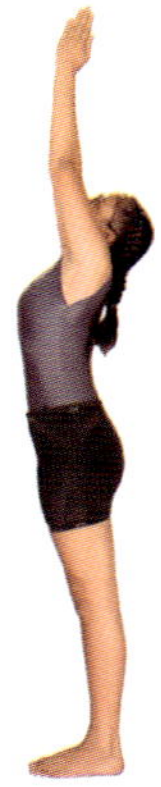

Surya Namaskara A and B

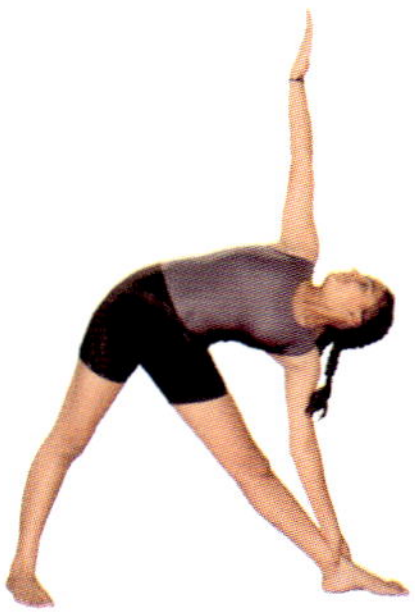

Trikonasana – Triangle Pose

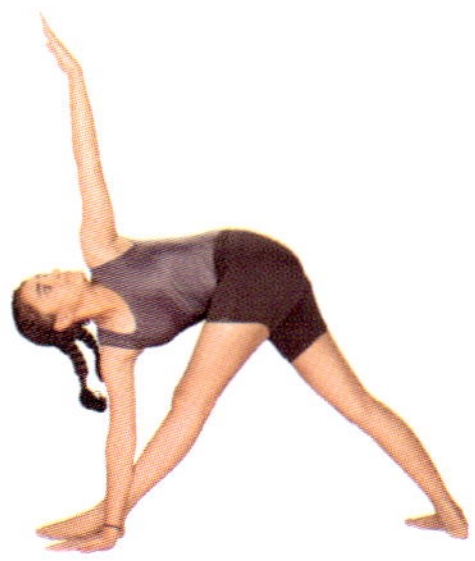

Parivritti Trikonasana – Twisted Triangle Pose

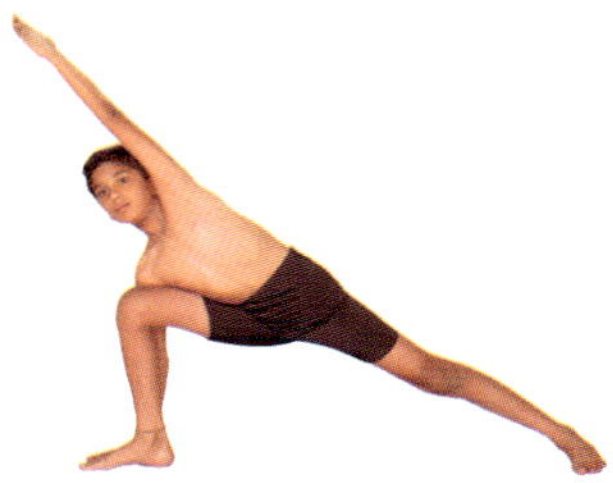

Parsvakonasana – Stretched Triangle Pose

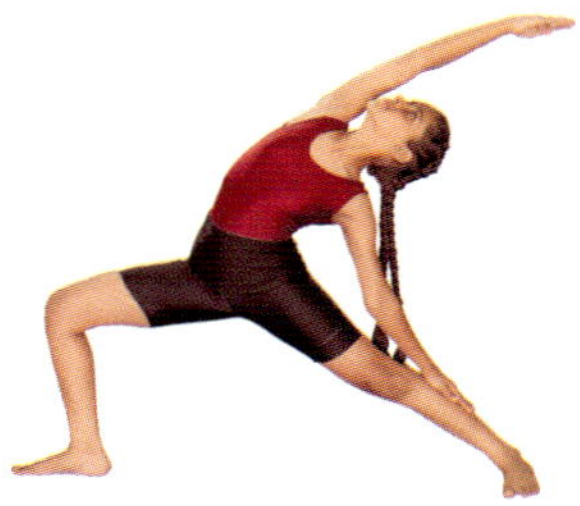

Anjaneyasana – Flying Monkey God Pose

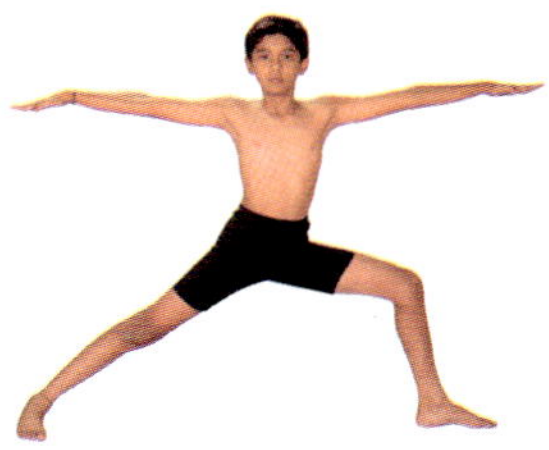

Veerabhadrasana D – Warrior Pose 4

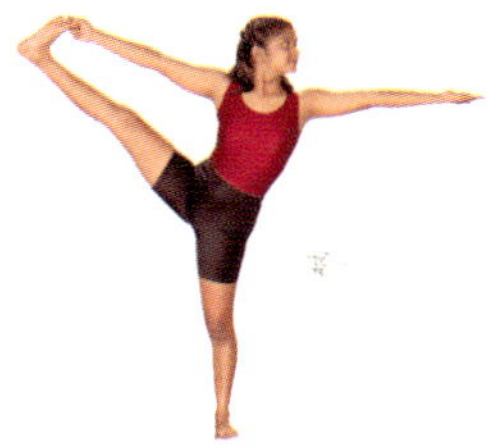

Uttita Hasta Padagustasana – Lifted Toe Hold Pose

Note to parents

- Yoga asana practice can play an important role for a child interested in sports. The practice will help the muscles, tendons and ligaments move through the full range of motions, thus cultivating balance and strength both important for sports. Yoga will also help in building up concentration and determination which are essential qualities for a sports person.
- Children who are into sports need to understand how to listen to their bodies. They should know how to take care and not get into a point of injury. The asanas listed for practice will help the child with body awareness. It will help in building up stamina, strength, alertness, concentration and courage. These asanas along with a good diet and rest will surely help the child to be successful in sports.
- The asanas sequenced here cover the chest opening asanas to encourage correct breathing and to discipline the body and regulate its functions. A regular practice with discipline is essential for best results.

Floor Asanas

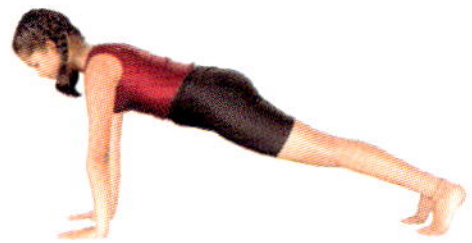

Chaduranga Dandasana – Plank Pose

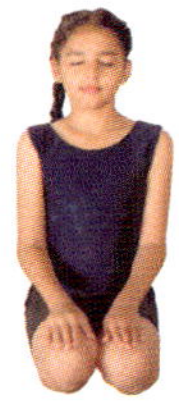

Vajrasana – Diamond Pose

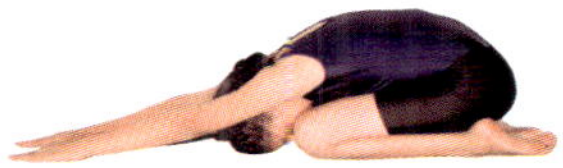

Balasana – Child Pose

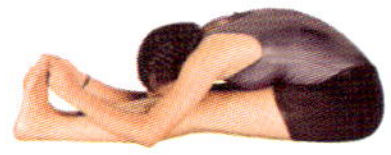

Paschimottanasana – Forward Fold Pose

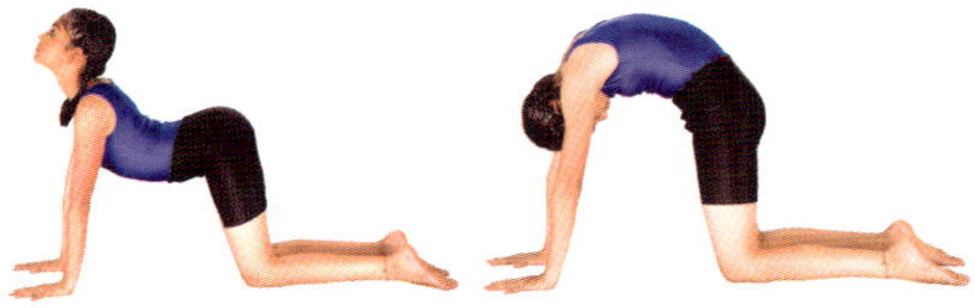

Vyagrasana A, B and C – Wild Cat Pose

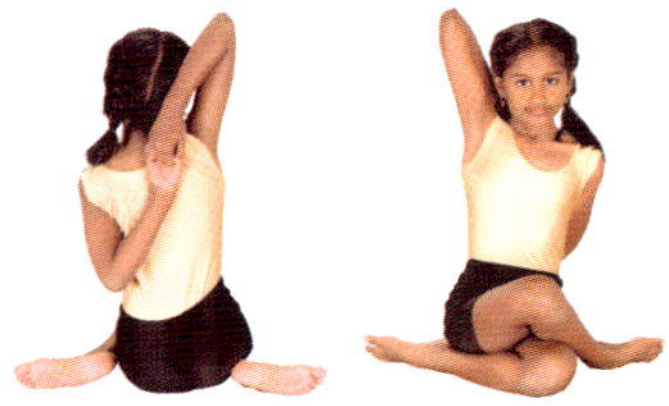

Gomukasana – Cow Face Pose

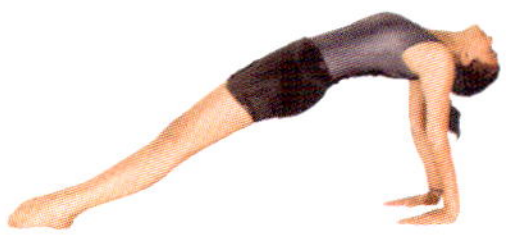

Purvottanasana – Backward Stretch Pose

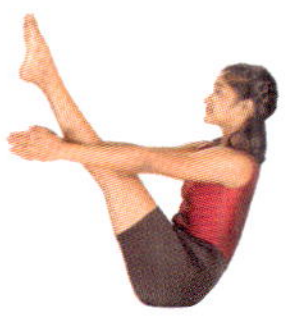

Navasana – Boat Pose

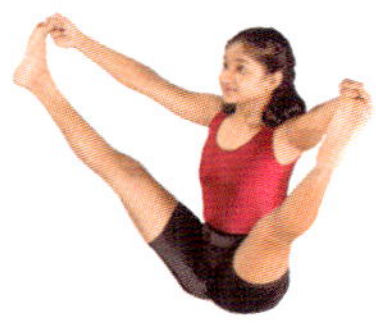

Upavistanavasana – Wide-angle Boat Pose

Cooling Down Sequence

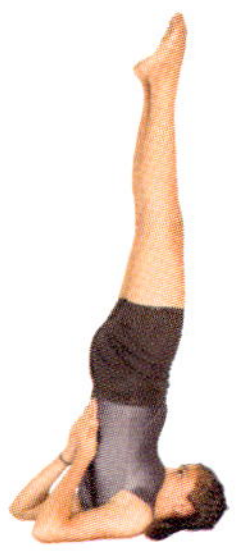

Sarvangasana – Shoulder Stand

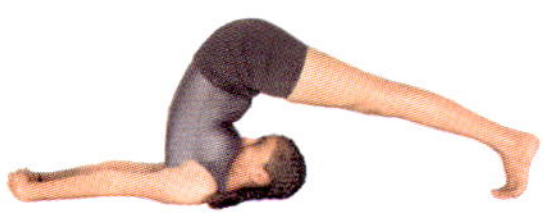

Halasana – Plough Pose

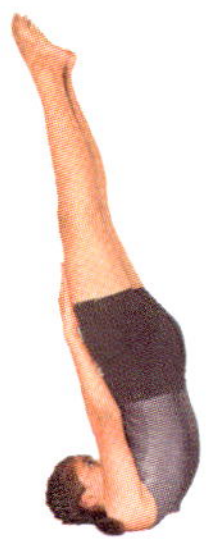

Salamba Sarvangasana – Shoulder Stand

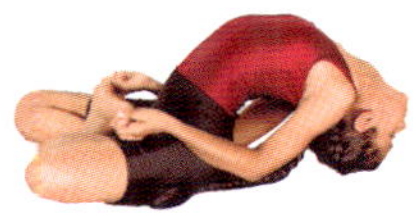

Matsyasana – Fish Pose

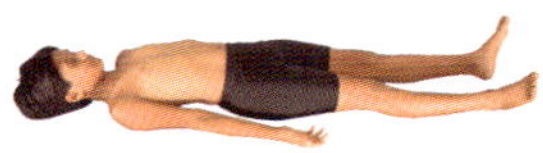

Shavasana – Total Relaxation Pose

Pranayama

As explained in **Anulom Vilom**

EXAMINATION SEQUENCE

45 Minutes practice sequence

Standing Asanas

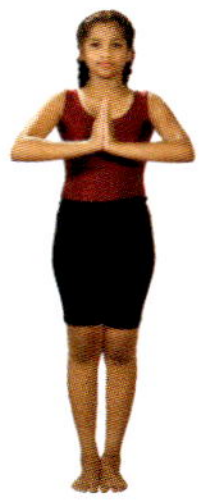

Tadasana – Pillar Pose

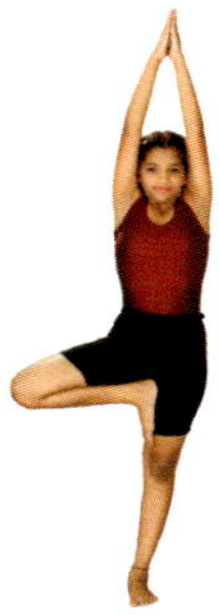

Vrikshasana – Tree Pose

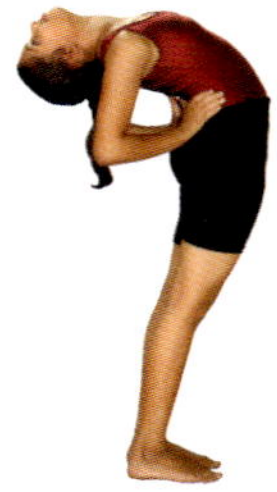

Ardha Chandra Tadasana – Half Side Wheel

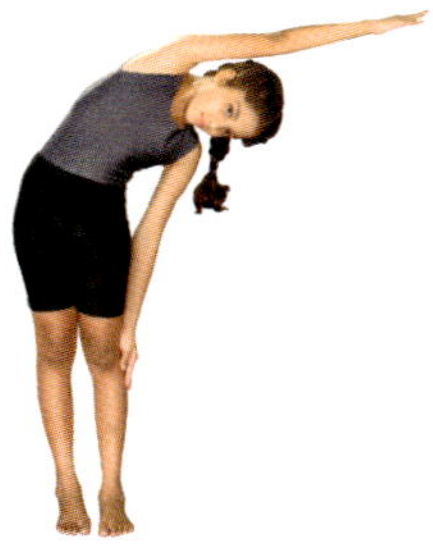

Ardha Katti Tadasana – Half Wheel Pose

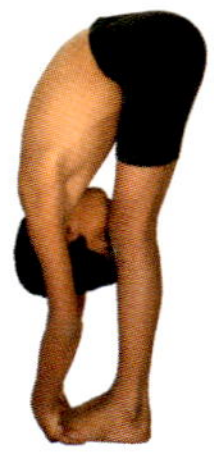

Pada Hastasana – Toe Hold Pose

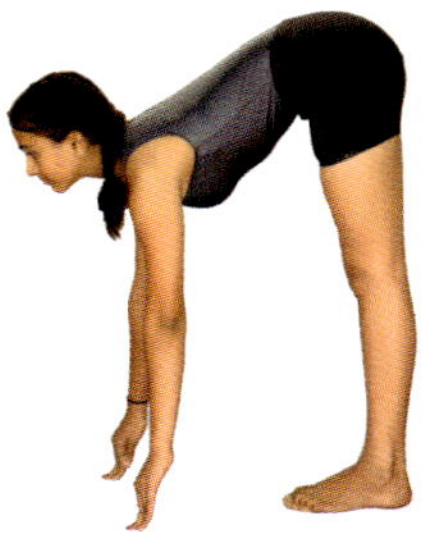

Chatushpadasana – Bear Stand

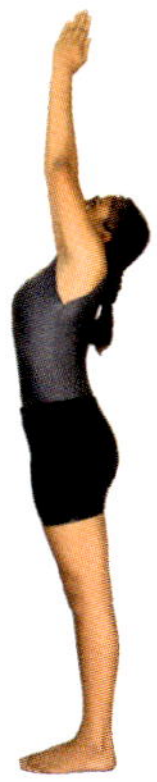

Surya Namaskara A and B

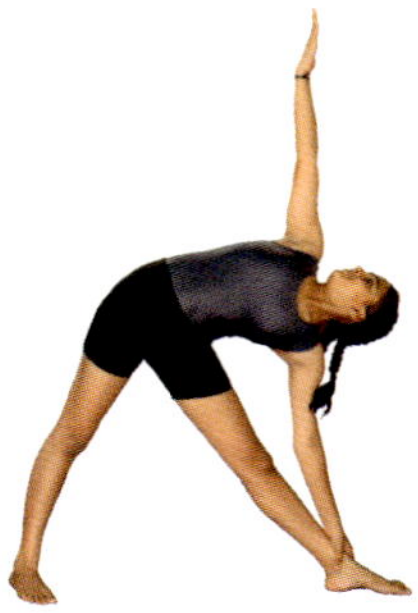

Trikonasana – Triangle Pose

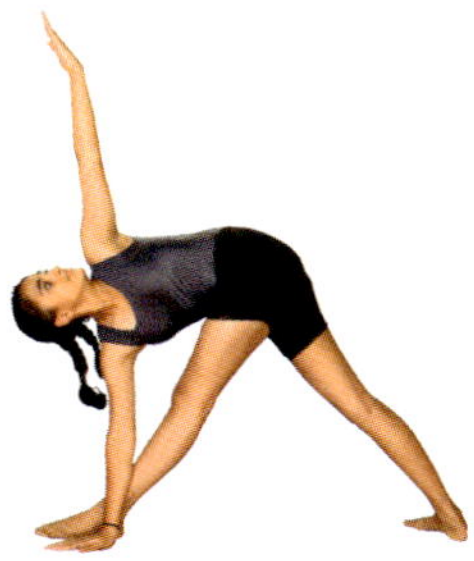

Parivritti Trikonasana – Twisted Triangle Pose

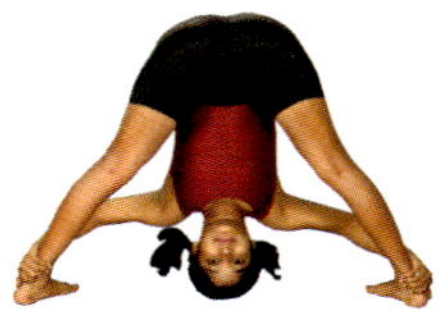

Prasarita Padottanasana – Pyramid Pose

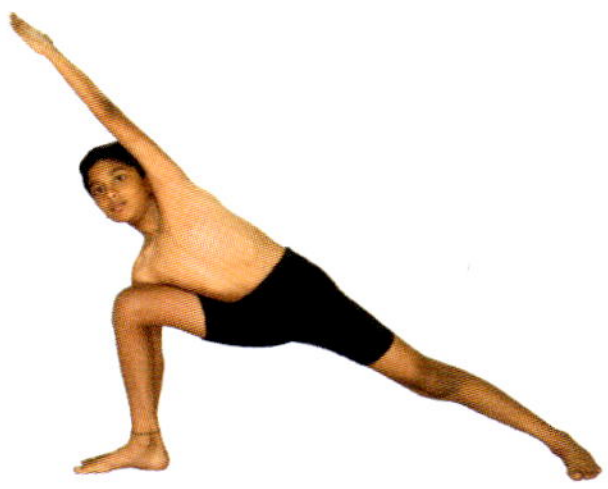

Parsvakonasana – Stretched Triangle Pose

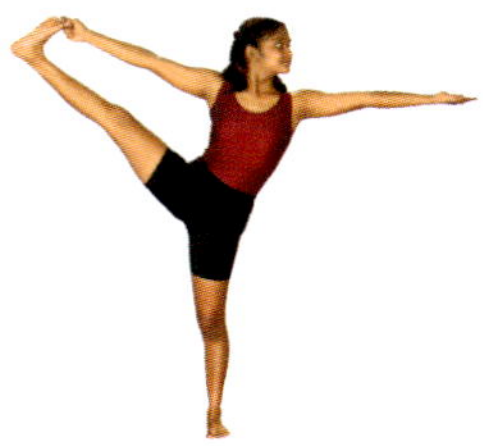

Uttita Hasta Padagustasana – Lifted Toe Hold Pose

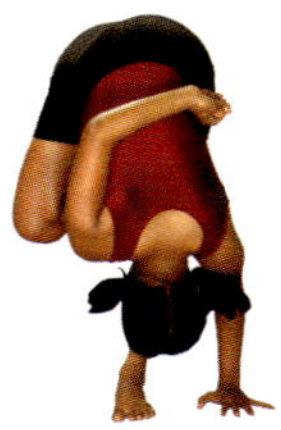

Ardhabadha Padmottanasana – Half-Lotus Toe Hold Pose

Note to parents

- The thought of exams somehow brings in panic attacks in both parents and children. The common complaint among students is not being able to remember whatthey have studied. This is when they lose a lot of energy due to stress and anxiety. Their sleep is disturbed and many have nightmares and sleeplessness too. Just telling the kids to stay calm will add to their distress. Practising yoga might help them calm down and stay alert.
- Another common problem children go through is the loss of emotional energy, the feeling of 'I don't think I will be able to do well'. Yoga practice can help the child to feel confident and calm. Yoga asanas and breathing technique has the ability to calm down an extreme and highly tense mind.
- The sequence here is for a 3`0-minute routine. This series of asanas is focused on building concentration and strength to sit for long hours of studying and academic work. These asanas when practised stretch the body and keep it comfortable to focus on studying. It will help you maintain a good appetite and take care of digestion. It will help the mind to snap out of distraction quickly. A regular practice of the above techniques will help children relax the mind and body.

Floor Asanas

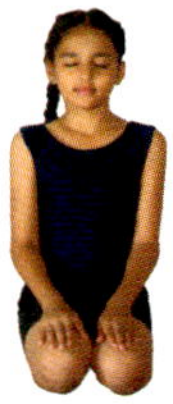
Vajrasana – Diamond Pose

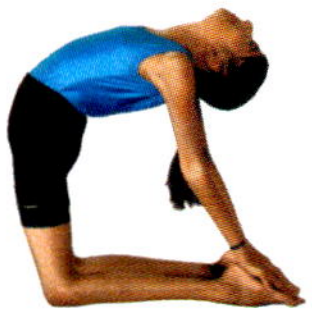
Ushtrasana – Camel Pose

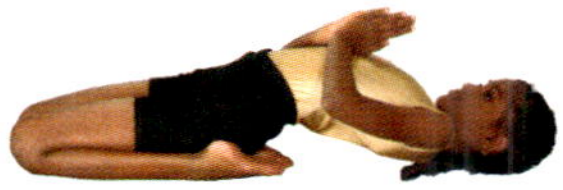
Supta Vajrasana – Backward Diamond Pose

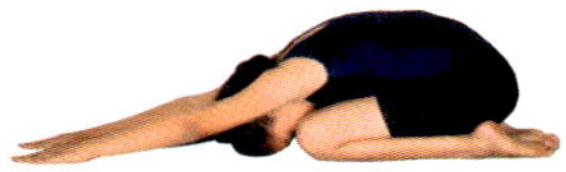
Balasana – Child Pose

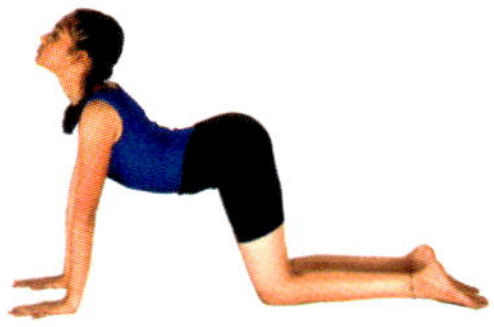
Vyagrasana A, B and C – Wild Cat Pose

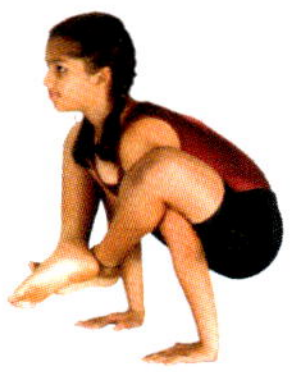
Bhujapeedasana – Shoulder Balance

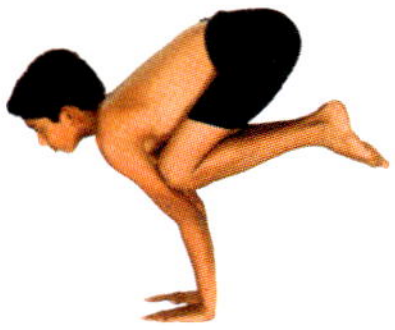
Bakasana – Bird Pose

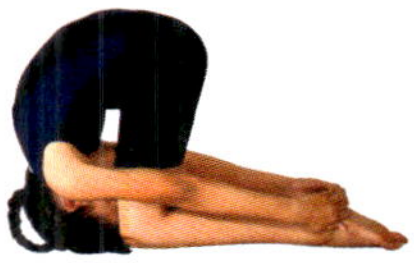
Marijariasana – Rabbit King Pose

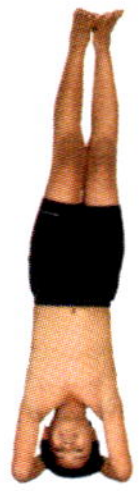
Shirasasana – Headstand Pose

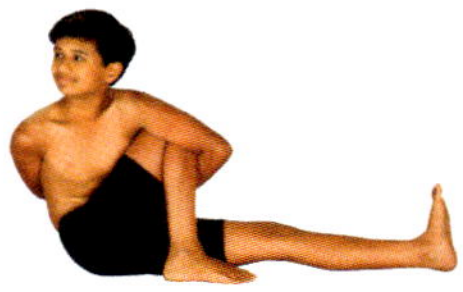
Marichasana – Sage Pose

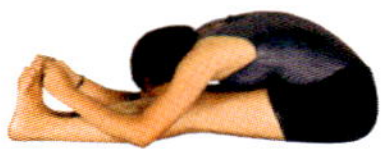
Paschimottanasana – Forward Fold Pose

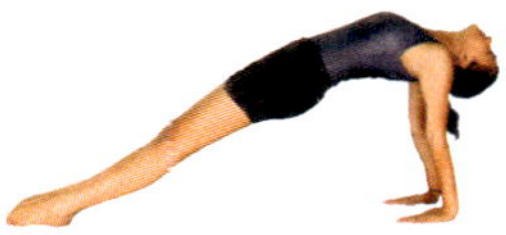
Purvottanasana – Backward Stretch Pose

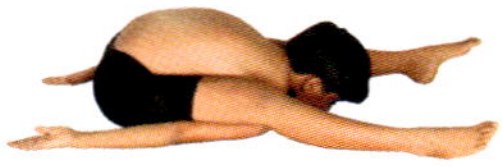
Kurmasana – Tortoise Pose

Cooling Down Sequence

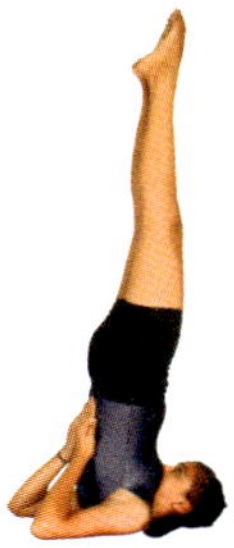
Sarvangasana – Shoulder Stand

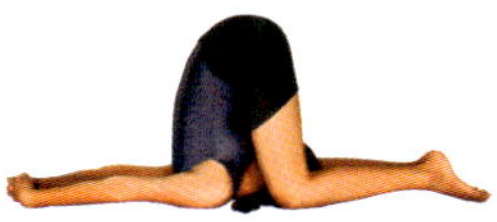
Karnapeedasana – Knee To Ear Pose

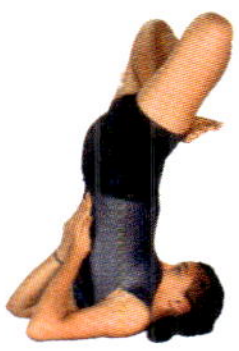
SarvangaPadmasana – Upward Lotus Pose

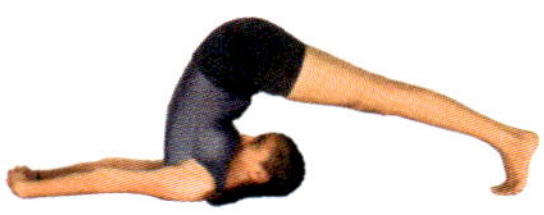
Halasana – Plough Pose

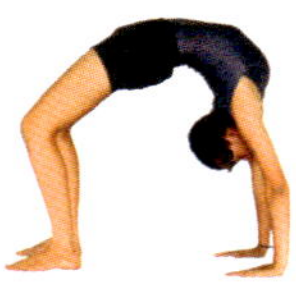
Urdwa Dhanurasana – Backward Bend

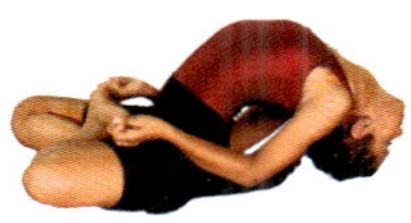
Matsyasana – Fish Pose

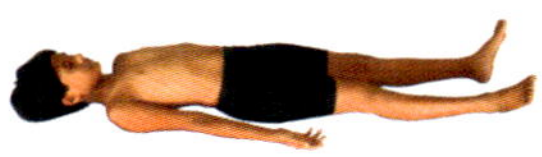
Shavasana – Total Relaxation Pose

Pranayama

As explained in **Anulom Vilom**

EXPANDABLE SEQUENCE

Standing Asanas

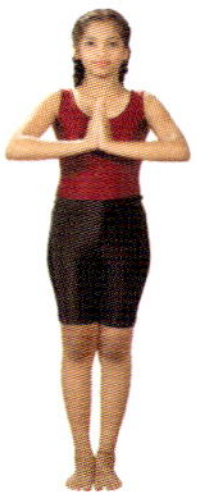

Tadasana – Pillar Pose

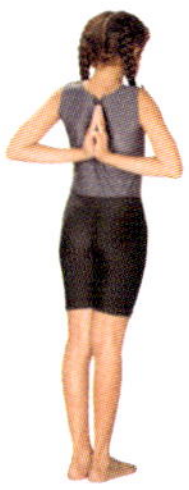

Parshwa Hasta Tadasana – Back Namaste Pillar Pose

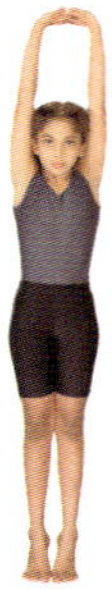

Urdwa Tadasana – Tall Pillar Pose

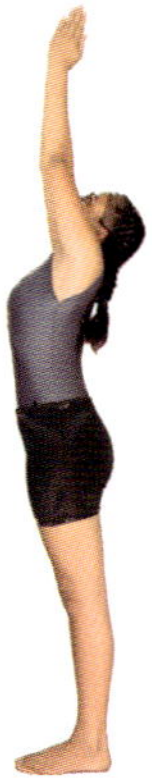

Surya Namaskara A and B

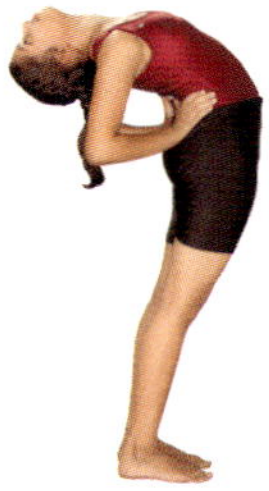

Ardha Chandra Tadasana – Half Side Wheel

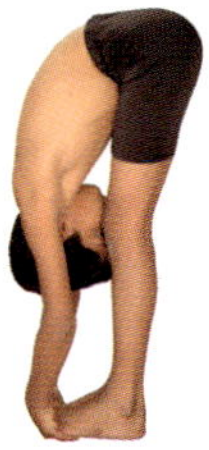

Pada Hastasana – Toe Hold Pose

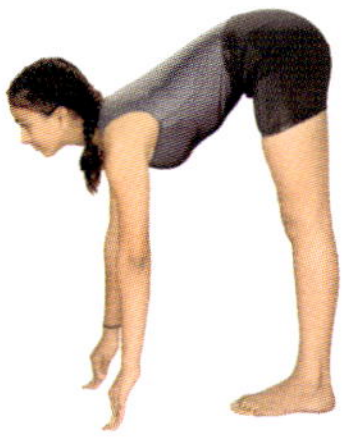

Chatushpadasana – Bear Stand

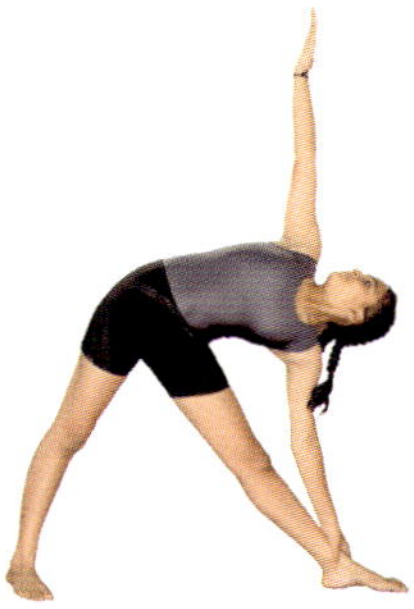

Trikonasana – Triangle Pose

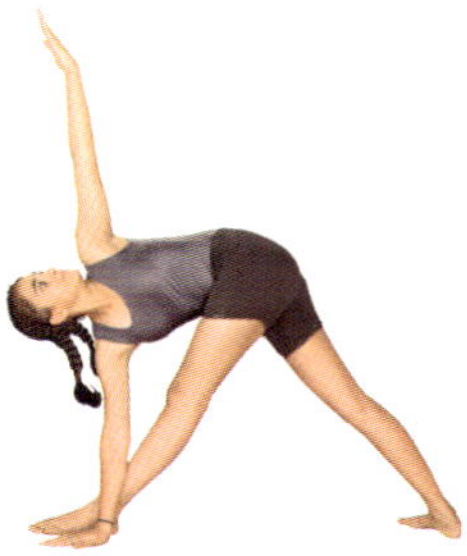

Parivritti Trikonasana – Twisted Triangle Pose

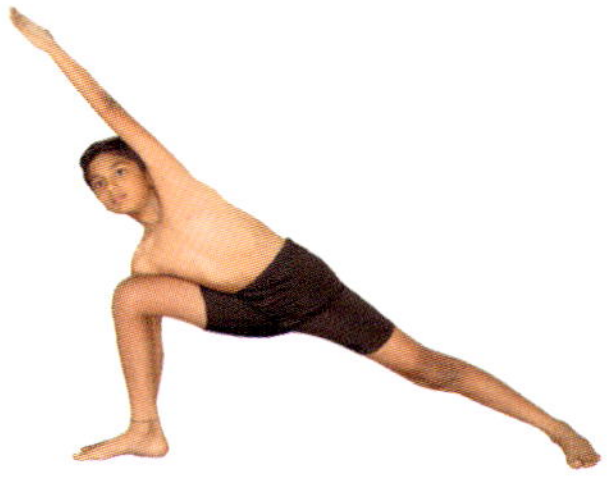

Parsvakonasana – Stretched Triangle Pose

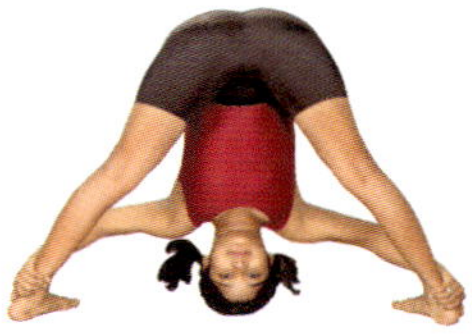

Prasarita Padottanasana – Pyramid Pose

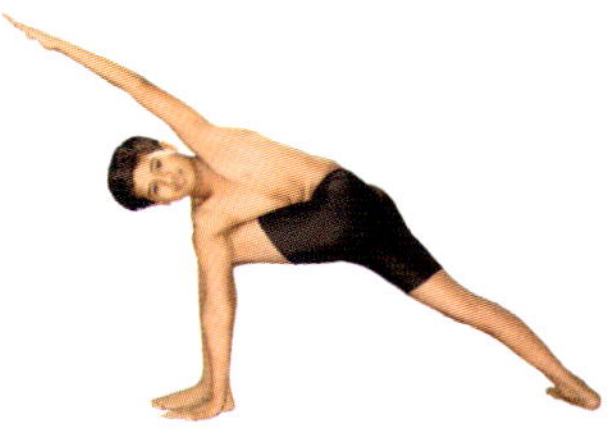

Parivritti Parsvakonasna – Twisted Stretched Pose

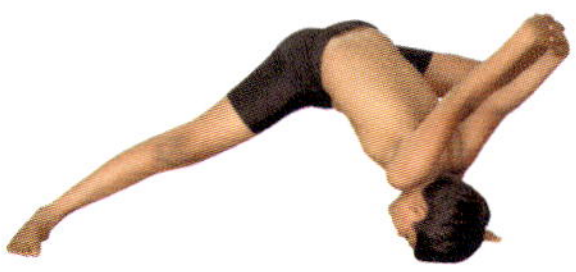

Shirasa Parsvakonasana – Forward Stretched Angle Pose

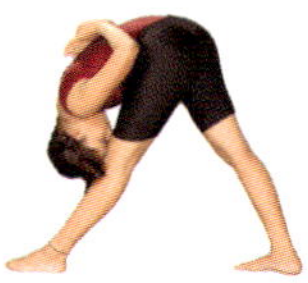

Parsvattanasna – Forward Fold Pose

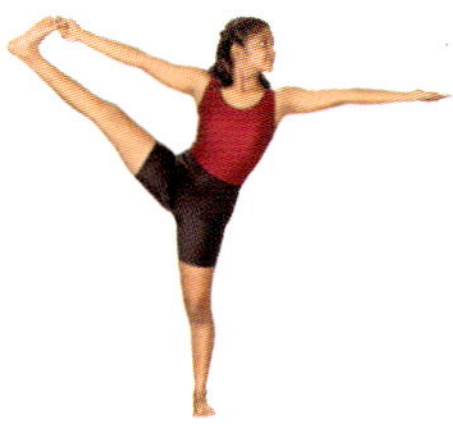

Uttita Hasta Padagustasana – Lifted Toe Hold Pose

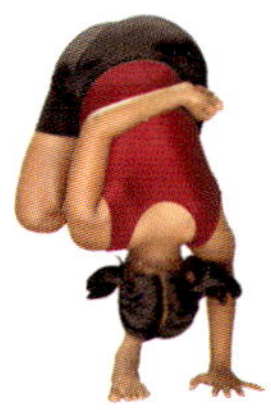

Ardhabadha Padmottanasana – Half-Lotus Toe Hold Pose

Note to parents

- Being flexible has a lot of benefits. It keeps the body supple while also building strength and stability. Yoga stretches also help the joints to get a greater range of motion, improve balance and keep the body comfortable.
- When the body is flexible children are less prone to injuries during physical activity. Muscular imbalances get corrected. The muscles are free and less stressed with fewer aches and pains due to physical activities. Posture will naturally improve. Flexibility helps to achieve a relaxed and a positive state of mind.
- The asanas should be done regularly or as often as possible. These series require proper warm up. A few favourite asanas can be picked up and done along with sports and other workout routines.

Floor Asanas

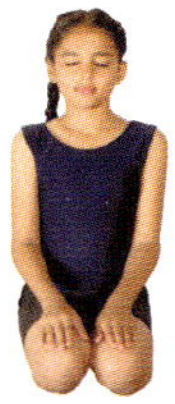
Vajrasana – Diamond Pose

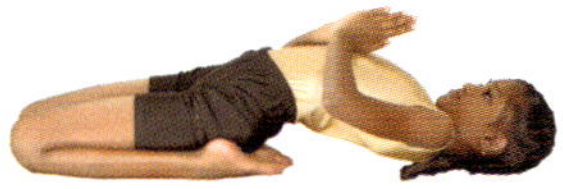
Supta Vajrasana – Backward Diamond Pose

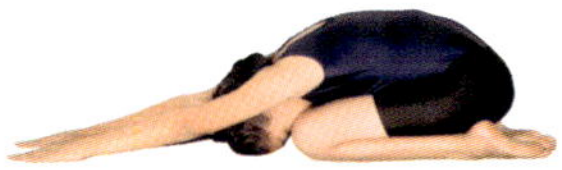
Balasana – Child Pose

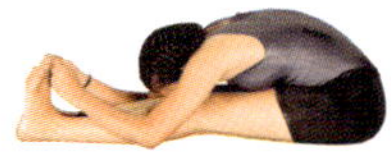
Paschimottanasana – Forward Fold Pose

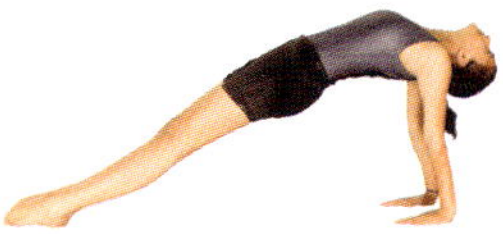
Purvottanasana – Backward Stretch Pose

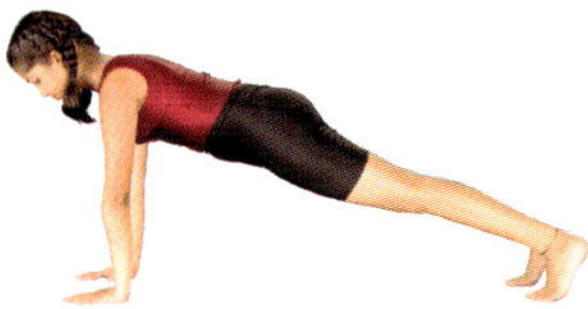
Dandasana – Staff Pose

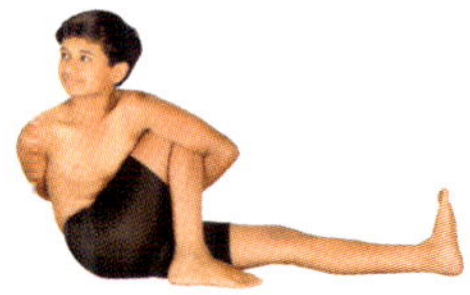
Marichasana – Sage Pose

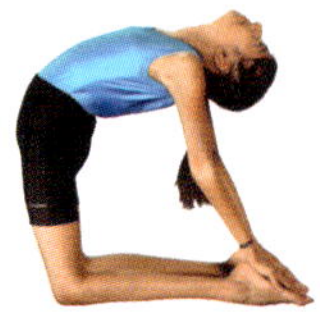
Ushtrasana – Camel Pose

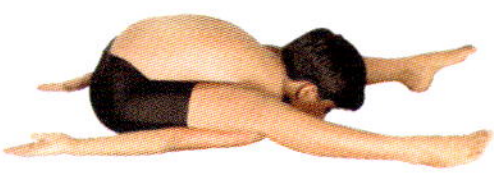
Kurmasana – Tortoise Pose

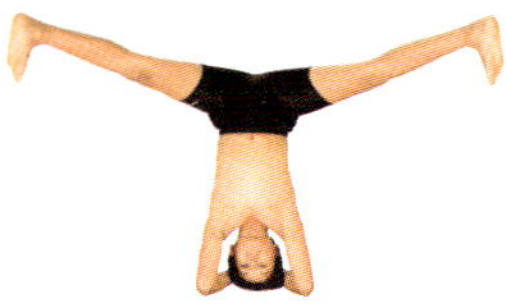
Shirasa Upavishtakonasana – Wide-angle Headstand

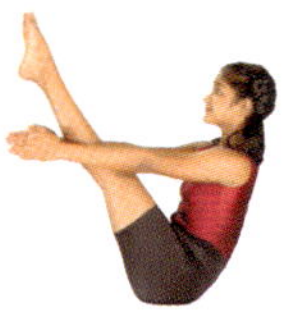
Navasana – Boat Pose

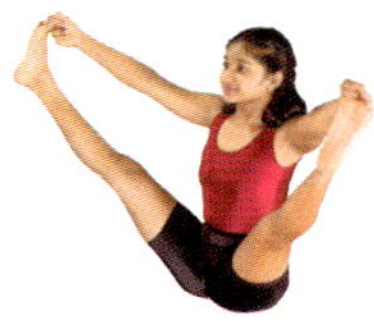
Upavistanavasana – Wide-angle Boat Pose

Cooling Down Sequence

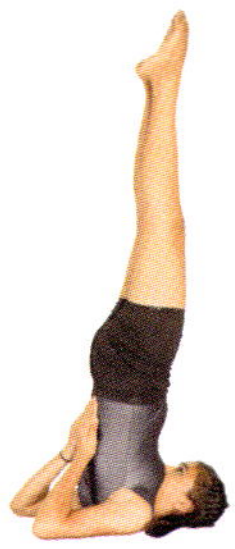
Sarvangasana – Shoulder Stand

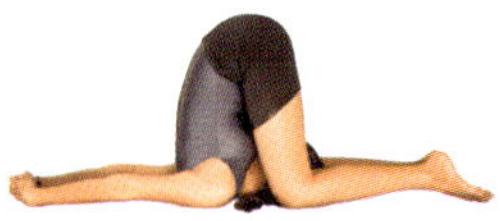
Karnapeedasana – Knee To Ear Pose

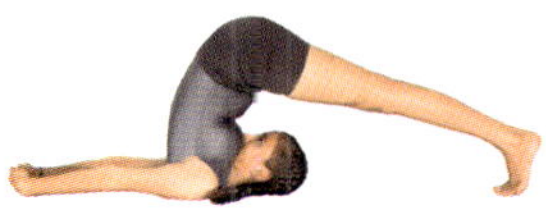
Halasana – Plough Pose

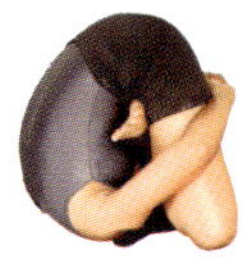
Garbha Pindasana – Baby Pose

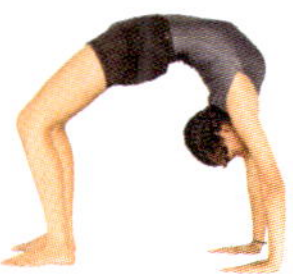
Urdwa Dhanurasana – Backward Bend

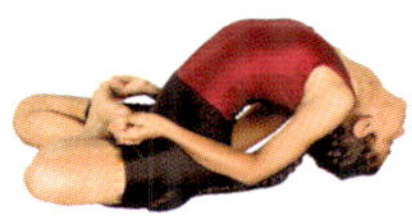
Matsyasana – Fish Pose

Pranayama

As explained in **Anulom Vilom**

TALL SEQUENCE FOR GROWTH

Standing Asanas

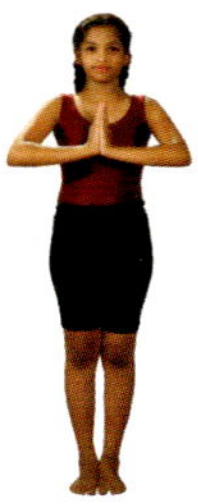
Tadasana – Pillar Pose

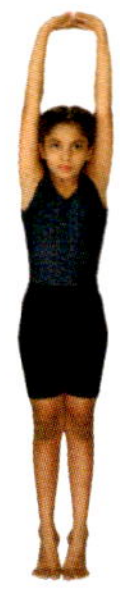
Urdwa Tadasana – Tall Pillar Pose

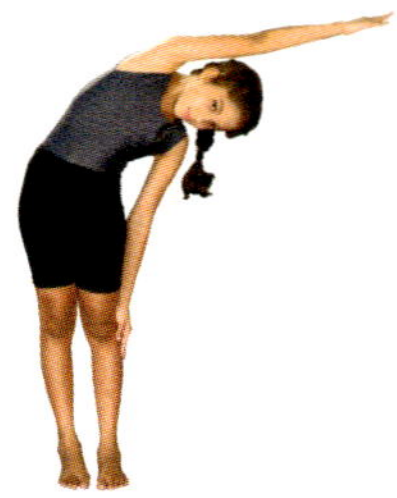
Ardha Katti Tadasana – Half Wheel Pose

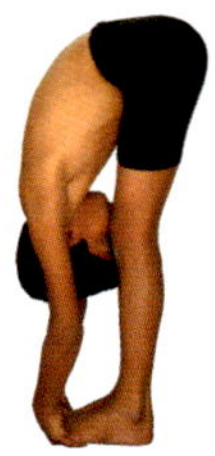
Pada Hastasana – Toe Hold Pose

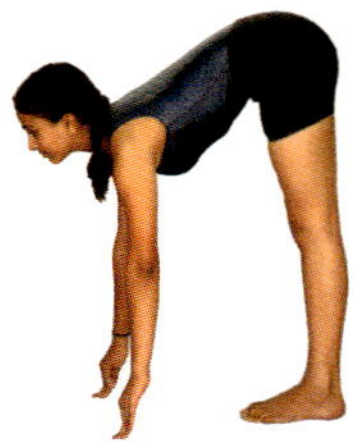
Chatushpadasana – Bear Stand

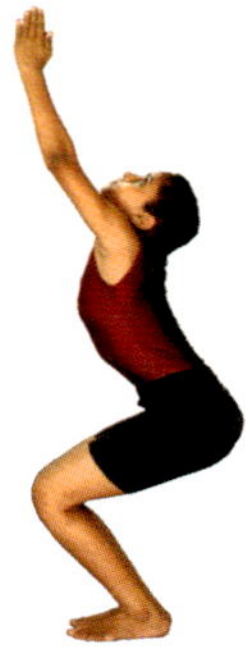
Utkattasana A B C – Chair Pose

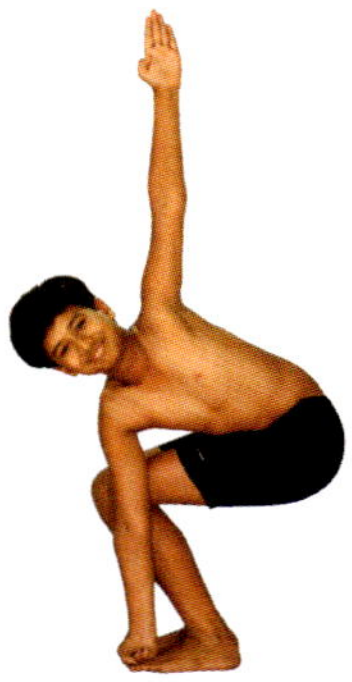
Parivritti Utkatasana – Twisted Chair Pose

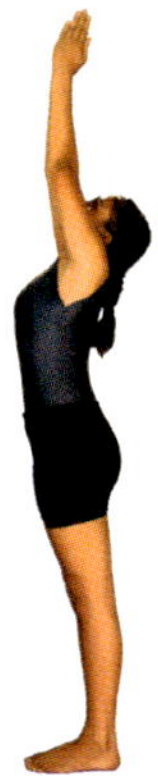
Surya Namaskara A and B

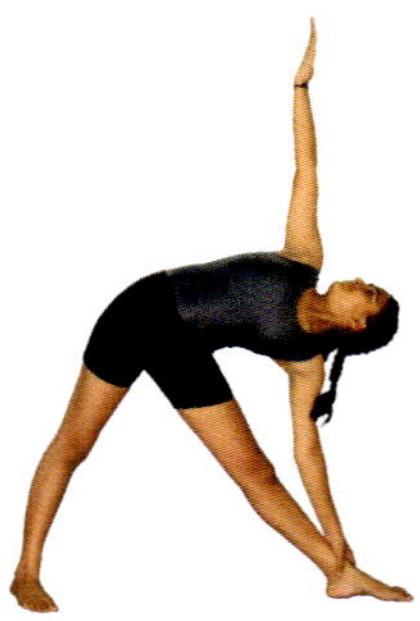
Trikonasana – Triangle Pose

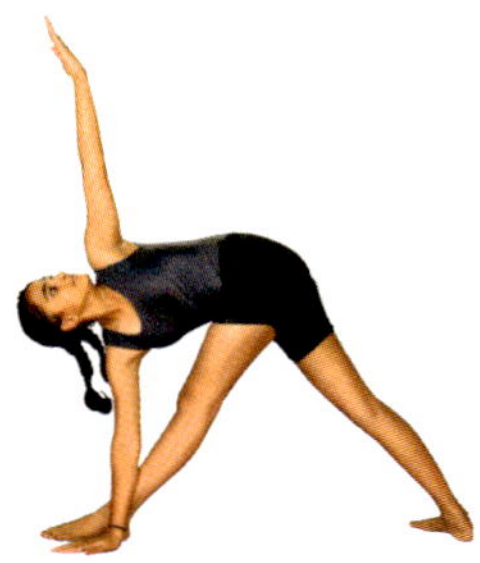
Parivritti Trikonasana – Twisted Triangle Pose

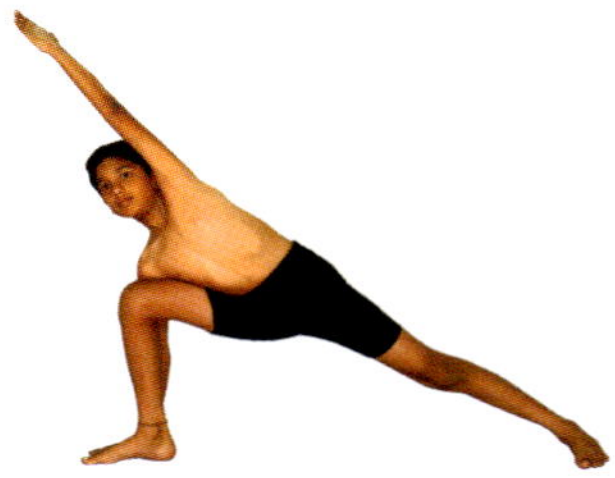
Parshwakonasana – Stretched Angle Pose

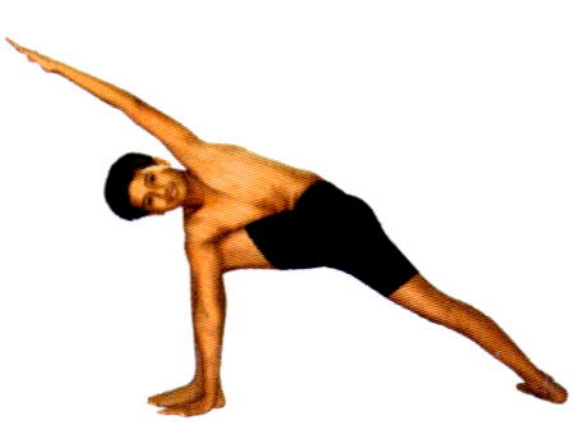
Parivritti Parsvakonasna – Twisted Stretched Pose

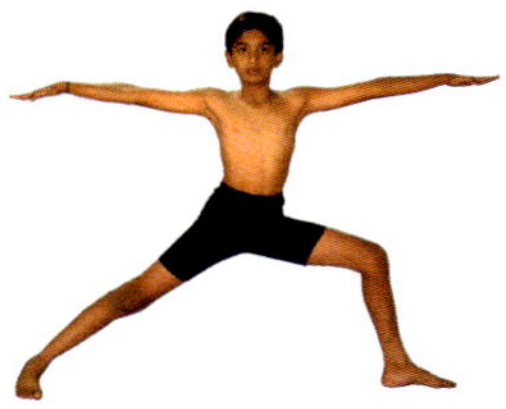
Veerabhadrasana 1, 2, 3, 4-Warrior Pose

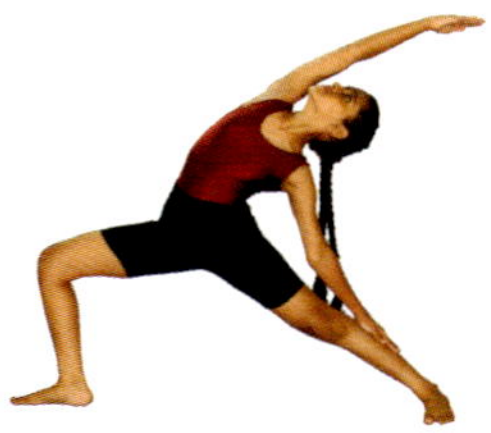
Anjaneyasana – Flying Monkey God Pose

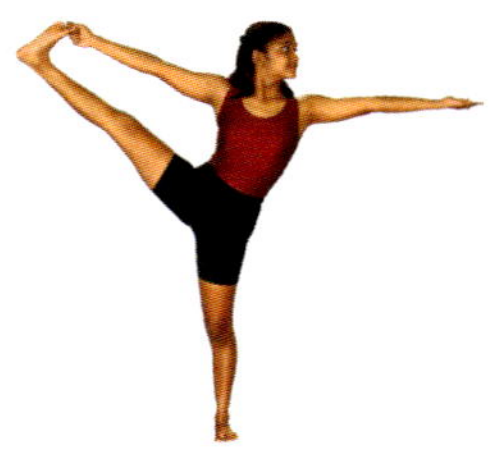
Uttita Hasta Padagustasana – Lifted Toe Hold Pose

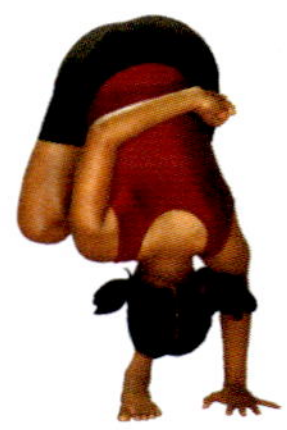
Ardhabadha Padmottanasana – Half-Lotus Toe Hold Pose

Note to parents

- The asanas listed for practice target growth hormones. Genes have the most say in determining the height of children. However, they are not the only factor. External factors like living conditions, good rest and a healthy diet also can influence the height of a child.
- Yoga stretching helps elongate the spine and improves posture. The entire body is targeted in this sequence. Stretching out the muscles of the arm, back and even the legs in a fluid motion helps. The Pranayama which follows the practices helps the child to get good and undisturbed sleep which is the most important ingredient for growth.

Floor Asanas

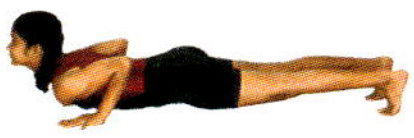

Bhujangasana – Snake Pose

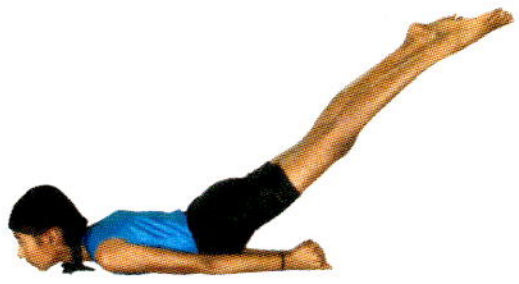

Dwipada Shalabhasana – Locust Pose

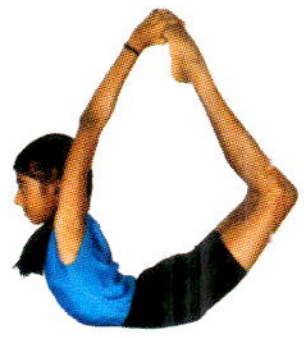

Dhanurasana – Bow Pose

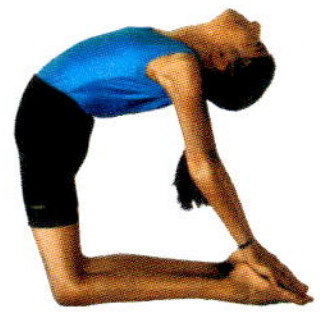

Ushtrasana – Camel Pose

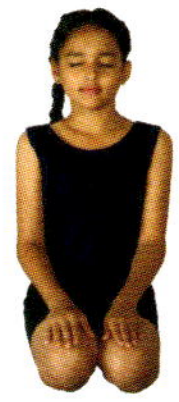

Vajrasana – Diamond Pose

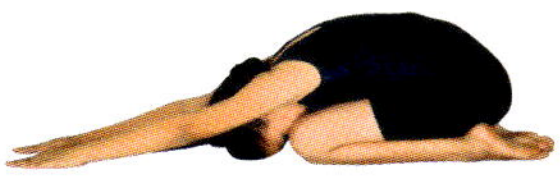

Balasana – Child Pose

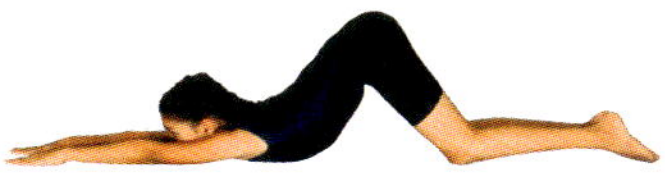

Shashankasana – Rabbit Pose

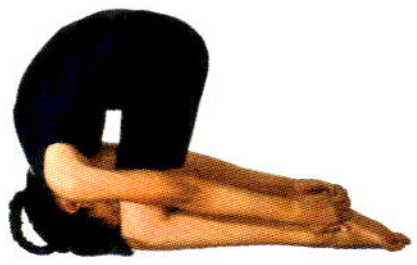

Marijariasana – Rabbit King Pose

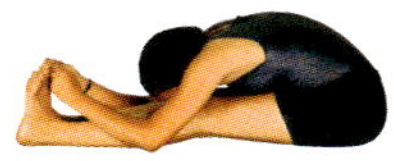

Paschimottanasana – Forward Fold Pose

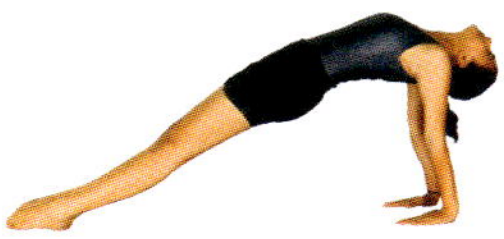

Purvottanasana – Backward Stretch Pose

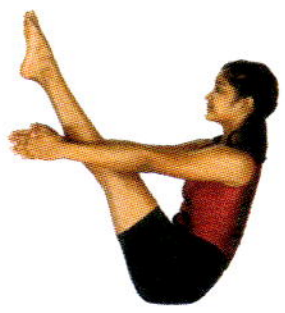

Navasana – Boat Pose

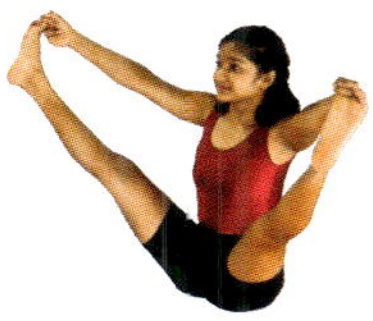

Upavistanavasana – Wide-angle Boat Pose

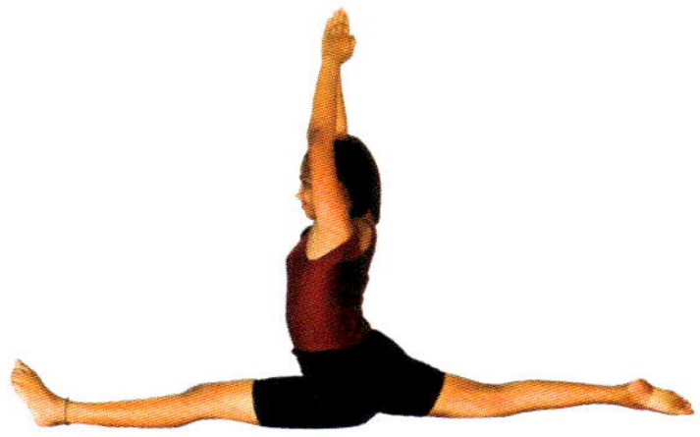

Hanumanasana – Lord Pose

Cooling Down Sequence

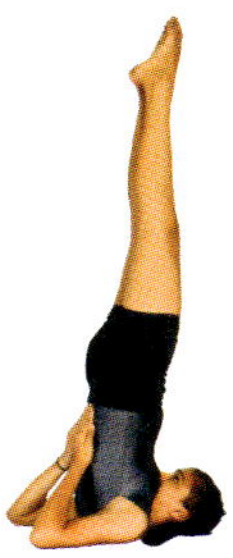

Sarvangasana – Shoulder Stand

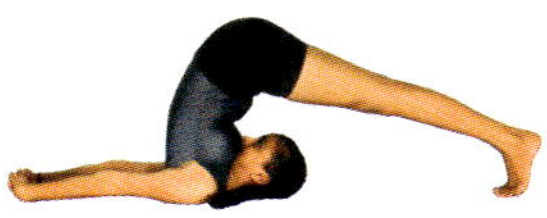

Halasana – Plough Pose

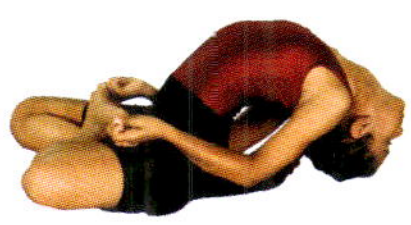

Matsyasana – Fish Pose

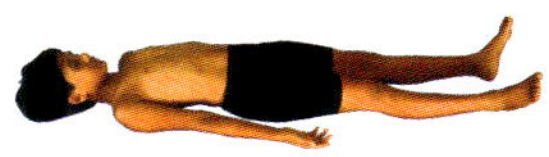

Shavasana – Total Relaxation Pose

Pranayama

As explained in **Anulom Vilom**

GIRLS' DAY SEQUENCE

DURING MENSTRUATION

Standing Asanas

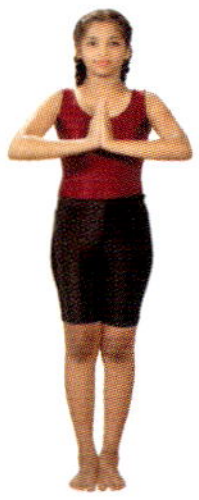

Tadasana – Pillar Pose

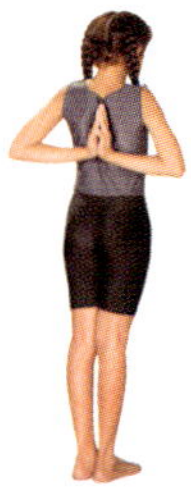

Parshwa Hasta Tadasana – Back Namaste Pillar Pose

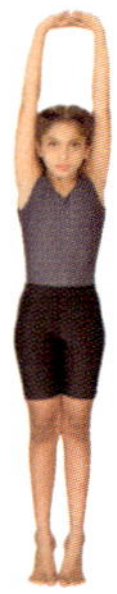

Urdwa Tadasana – Tall Pillar Pose

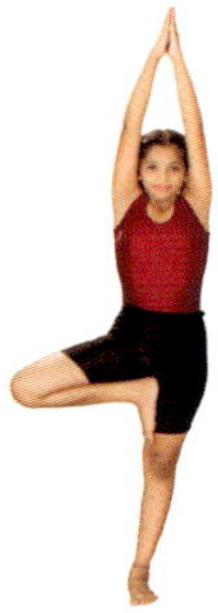

Vrikshasana – Tree Pose

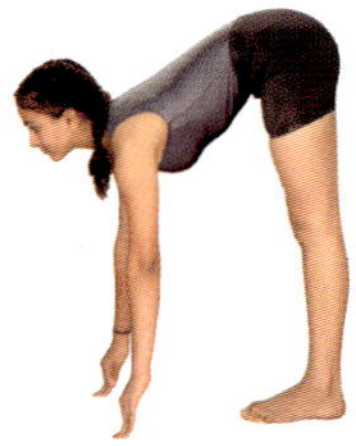

Chatushpadasana – Bear Stand

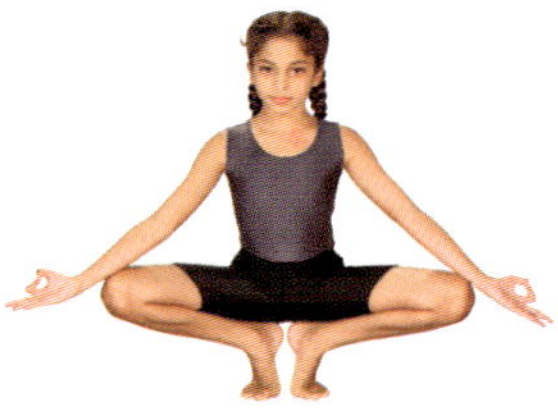

Bhadrasana – Strong Pose

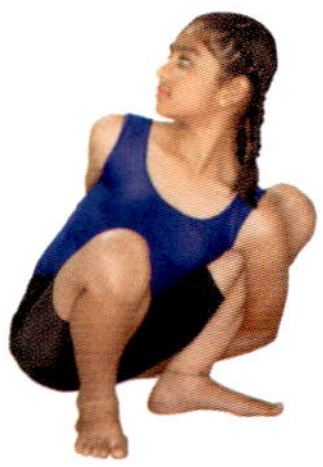

Malasana Parivritti – Garland Pose

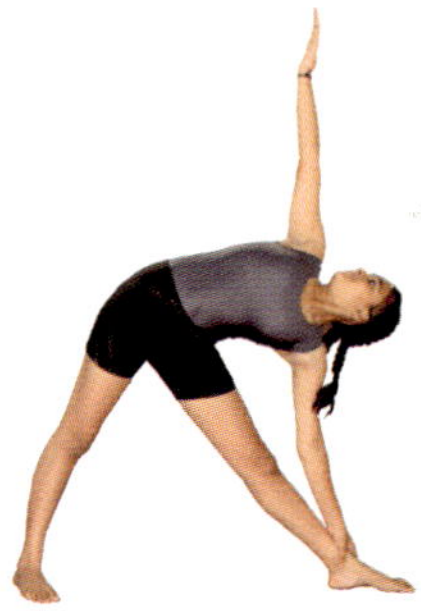

Trikonasana – Triangle Pose

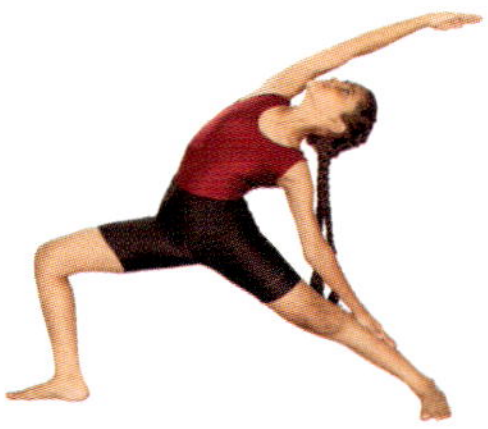

Anjaneyasana – Flying Monkey God Pose

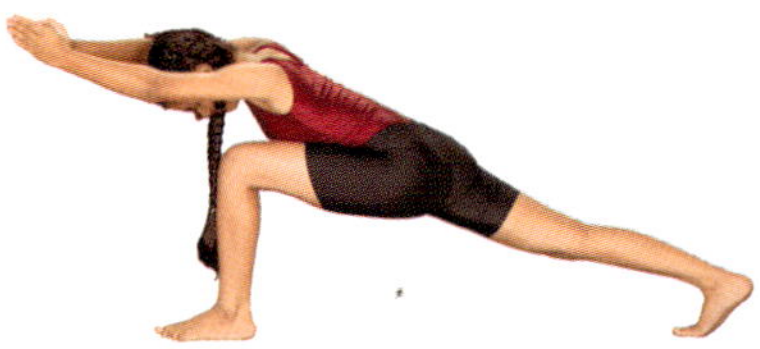

Veerabadrasana (B) – Warrior Pose B

Note to parents

Menstruation is a natural process. However, girls suffer discomfort as the date of the cycle approaches. The most common complaints include cramps, headaches, PMS, irregular periods, etc. If the problems are other than those listed above, it would be advisable to consult a doctor.

Common symptoms of PMS include:

- Mood swings • Food cravings • Backaches • Sore breasts • Bloating • Crankiness • Tiredness

Along with the yoga asanas mentioned below, it would be advisable if the following could be taken care of:

- A balanced diet will take care of food cravings and bloating abdomen
- Lots of fresh vegetables and fruits are preferable to non-vegetarian food.
- The asanas prevent mood swings and crankiness.
- Sports activities are also beneficial.

When there is irregular period, it is best to consult a doctor. Take note that the asanas listed above will not create any issues if done with care.

Floor Asanas

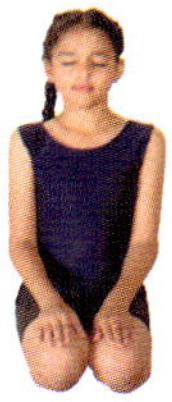

Vajrasana – Diamond Pose

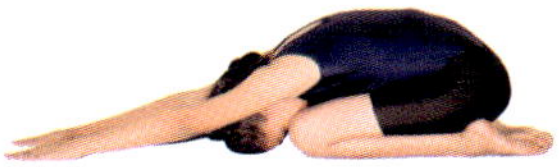

Balasana – Child Pose

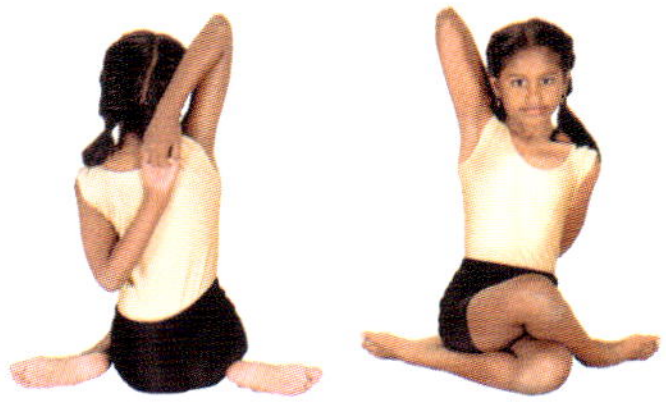

Gomukasana – Cow Face Pose

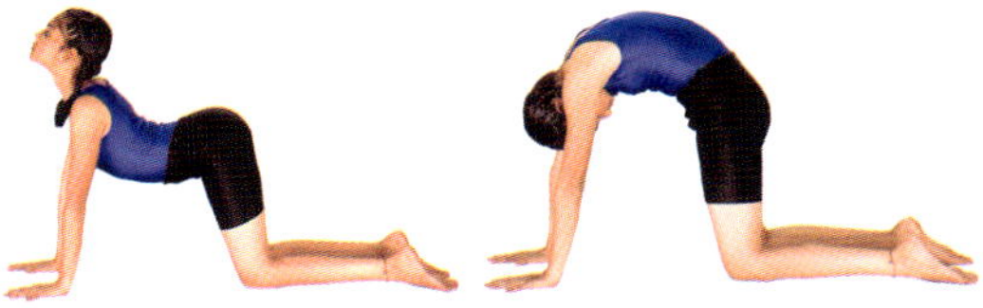

Vyagrasana A, B and C – Wild Cat Pose

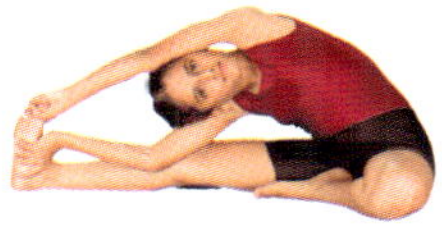

Janushirasasana – Head to Knee Pose

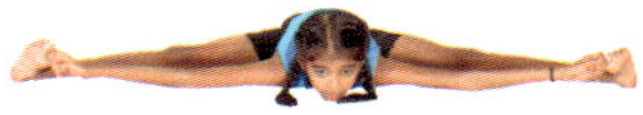

Upavistakonasana – Wide-legged Pose

Cooling Down Sequence

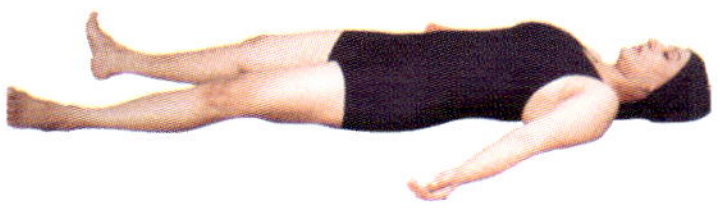

Shavasana – Total Relaxation Pose

Complete relaxation will rejuvenate the body and relax all muscular tension which is a part of the menstrual process.
Rejuvenates the body and relaxes the mind.

Pranayama

As explained in **Anulom Vilom**

Acknowledgements

This book is based on yoga and the vast knowledge of therapeutic yoga. Ancient wisdom will remain relevant in all ages and times to come. I would like to thank everyone who encouraged me to write this book on yoga for children. I thank my students for being my constant support and source of inspiration, knowledge and experience.

In Mysore, I would like to thank my childhood friend Shubha Sanjay Urs, Founder Promoter of the Mysore Literary Festival, for her support during the photoshoot in Mysore. Many thanks for always being there for me, encouraging my work and being my valuable friend.

I would like to extend my thanks to Suchita Sanjay, Proprietor, Wind Chimes, Mysore, for the beautiful venue and the freedom he gave us to move around. Thanks to my dear friend Subadra Bhattacharya for her support throughout the shoot and after it.

My gratitude to the parents of the students for their patience, encouragement and support.

I am grateful to the hardworking and dedicated Yoga Master Rudresh Yogi and his beautiful students. Thank you for training the students with the specific asanas as requested and not questioning it. Your humility and passion for your work is very impressive. Your students are indeed lucky to have found you to help train them to be Yoga Champions. The photoshoot went smoothly with your support. You are a fabulous teacher and a great human being!

Hats off to the Champions for their love and enthusiasm for the book! You kids are amazing and true champs. Thanks to Rishitha, Siyya, Shesta, Prateeksha, Priyadarshan, Kushi, Ashwarya, Hamsini, Yuktka, Amulya and Anusha for being so wonderful and posing for the book tirelessly. Thank you for all the laughs and hugs! You are fabulous examples of discipline and selflessness. Your intention to help and encourage children to adopt the practice of yoga will be cherished by all those who buy this book and learn from it. Much strength and love to you and your family members.

Thanks to Prashanth K. Nagaraja of Prashanth's Photography, Mysore for his patience and photography skills. Your cooperation and hospitality during and after the gruesome shoot is much appreciated.

I would like to acknowledge with deep gratitude the support of my husband Muthanna, son Rithwik Iyappa and daughter Manya Muthanna, for their patience and understanding of my work and passion. You keep me going!

My friends Ramki and Swarna offer me their constant support. Without their encouragement and contacts, my books would be stuck in my notepad.

Special thanks to Mr Shankar Maruwada for offering support during the photoshoots and for research expenses during the making of this book.

Thanks to my dear student and practitioner, Parmin Johar for calling the book 'futuristic' and being there during the photoshoots, for proofreading and for always being enthusiastic about helping me in my ventures. Neelima Vinod helped me with proofreading and editing. She helped me get this book into final shape.

Nikhil Korwar was a great help during the final round of proofreading and pruning. Thank you for your time and patience and for helping me to organise the contents!

Thank you, Om Books International, New Delhi, for finding value in my work and accepting my book for publication.